TotalRecall Publications, Inc.
1103 Middlecreek
Friendswood, Texas 77546
281-992-3131 281-482-5390 Fax
www.totalrecallpress.com

All rights reserved. Except as permitted under the United States Copyright Act of 1976, No part of this publication may be reproduced, stored in a retrieval system, or transmitted in any form or by any means electronic or mechanical or by photocopying, recording, or otherwise without prior permission of the publisher. Exclusive worldwide content publication / distribution by TotalRecall Publications, Inc.

Copyright © 2022 by Anton P. Sohn
Cover Photo by Anton P. Sohn

ISBN: 978-1-64883-160-7
UPC: 6-43977-41607-0

FIRST EDITION
1  2  3  4  5  6  7  8  9  10

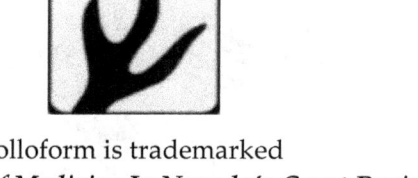

Colloform is trademarked
***1,000 Years Of Medicine In Nevada's Great Basin***
**is made possible by a grant from**
**NEVADA HISTORY OF MEDICINE FOUNDATION, INC.**

The scanning, uploading and distribution of this book via the Internet or via any other means without the permission of the publisher is illegal and punishable by law. Please purchase only authorized electronic editions, and do not participate in or encourage electronic piracy of copyrighted materials. Your support of the author's rights is appreciated.

# 1,000 Years of Medicine in Nevada's Great Basin

### Thirty-two Years of *Greasewood Tablettes*

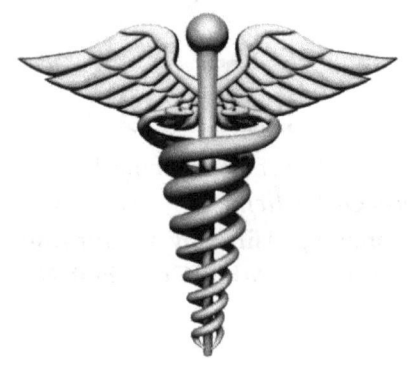

## Anton P. Sohn, MD
### Jennifer M. Grove

THIS BOOK IS DEDICATED TO THE
SOHN FAMILY
ARLENE, PHIL, LIZ, PETER
ALEX, ERIC, KERRY, BRADY, SIERRA
MAURIZA, ISABELLA, KRISTIN, MARK
AND THE
GROVE FAMILY
GROVES, ULMANS, JONES, WEBERS

## Contents

Illustrations ..................................................................................................... IX
Acknowledgements ....................................................................................... XII
Introduction .................................................................................................. XIV
History of Medicine Program University NV Reno School of Medicine ..... XVI
Greasewood Bush ......................................................................................... XVII

## I  Native American Medicine ........................................................... 1
1. Indian Remedy for Influenza, 1918 ............................................................ 2
2. Traditional Great Basin Indian Herbal Medicine ...................................... 3
3. Washoe Tribe and a Simple Herbal Remedy ........................................... 11
4. Big Mouth Charlie's Medicine Bowl, 1868 .............................................. 14
5. Nevada Indian Health Care  A Window in Time, 1958 and 1995 .......... 17
6. Healing Arts of Native Americans ........................................................... 23

## II  American Doctors ........................................................................ 36
7. Dr. Frederick Hiller, Virginia City, 1866-67 Kitchen Table Surgery and Neurosurgery ............................................................................................. 37
8. Dr. Vinton A. Muller (1892-1975)  Nevada's First Blood Transfusion ... 37
9. 1939 Carlin Canyon Train Wreck ............................................................. 38
10. Dr. Mary Fulstone's Recollections in Smith, Nevada ............................ 41
11. Dr. Mary Fulstone, Nevada's Doctor for the Ages ................................ 43
12. Dr. James W. Gerow "Call in Indian Country" ..................................... 46
13. Dr. Henry Bergstein  1874 Nevada Medical Practice Act .................... 49
14. Dr. Henry Bergstein  An Important Jewish Doctor in Early Nevada .... 51
15. Dr. Laurence D. Nelson  Adventure in the High Sierra, 1951-'52 ........ 55
16. Life History of Dr. Laurence D. Nelson ................................................ 58
17. Doctor Morris R. Walker, "Sink or Swim, 1901" ................................... 60
18. Doctor John Marsh, "Practice in the Old West" .................................... 64
19. Dr. Eliza Cook, Nevada's Fifth Female MD, 1884 ................................ 65
20. "Unverified Doctor" A.P. Lagoon, Early 1900 ...................................... 66
21. "Irregular Doctor" Simeon L. Lee .......................................................... 68
22. Doctor Harris S. Herrick  Letters to his Daughter, 1869-1891 .............. 70
23. "Colorful Doctor" Fred H. Wichmann, 1905 ......................................... 73
24. Dr. Washington L. Kistler "A Most Romantic Doctor, 1901" ............... 77
25. Dr. John A. Fuller From Las Vegas to Reno, 1910-69 .......................... 79
26. Dr. John A. Fuller, Las Vegas Years, 1910-1917 .................................. 79
27. Dr. John A. Fuller, Reno Years, 1917-1969 .......................................... 83
28. Dr. Zetus Spalding Susanville, California, 1852-1898 .......................... 87
29. Dr. T.P. Tyson, "Serious-Over-Study, 1923" ......................................... 89

30. Dr. Edwin Cantlon's Memory of Dr. T. Parry Tyson ..................... 92
31. Dr. Samuel Weaver, Paradise Valley, Nevada, 1884 ..................... 93
32. "Extraordinary Doctors" Dawson, Bergstein, Thoma, and Lewis ........ 94
33. Dr. Charles Daggett, Nevada's First Doctor, 1851 ..................... 98
34. Dr. Jack Gilbert, Twenty-six Years Of Devoted Service In Cedarville, California, 1955-'80 ..................... 99
35. "Politician Doctor" Selden McMeans, 1859-1876 ..................... 103
36. "Civil War Hero" Dr. Elias B. Harris, 1860 ..................... 105
37. Doctors Huffaker, Grisby, and Hewetson, 1800s ..................... 106
38. Dr. Anthony Huffaker's Journals, 1896-1907 ..................... 108
39. Dr. John Allen Veatch, Virginia City ..................... 109
40. Sixteen Outstanding Homegrown Doctors of Northern Nevada ..................... 111
41. Drs. Ada and Gideon Weed, Dr. A. Weed, Nevada's 1st Female MD . 112
42. "A Doctor's Doctor" Dr. Kenneth Frazer Maclean ..................... 117
43. Dr. George Thoma "Reno Street Named in his Honor" ..................... 122
44. More on Dr. George Thoma ..................... 123
45. Alfred Doten Journals, 1849-1903 "Numbing The Skin and its Contents on the Comstock" ..................... 125
46. Dr. John Edward Worden Nevada's First State Health Officer, 1936 .. 127
47. Dr. Anton Tjader, "1859 Adventures" ..................... 128
48. More on Dr. Anton Tjader, "1859 Adventures" ..................... 131
49. Acceptance of Female MDs in 19th Century Nevada ..................... 134
50. Dr. Catherine Post-Van Orden Nevada's Third Female Physician ...... 135
51. Les Moren, "Outstanding Elko MD" ..................... 136
52. Dr. Owen C. Bolstad "Stalwart" of the History of Medicine Program 139
53. Fallon Clinic ..................... 143
54. Fallon Clinic, 1949-'90, "Ding, Caffy, Si, and Len" ..................... 144
55. Dr. A. Thompson, Reno's "Blueblood" Pathologist/American Patriot 155
56. Dr. O.P. Johnstone, Nevada's First Pathologist, 1909 ..................... 156
57. Dr. Olga Kipanidze Reno's First Fulltime Anesthesiologist, 1935 ........ 157
58. Dr. Raymond St. Clair, "Saga of Missing Legs" ..................... 160
59. Nine Doctors of Washoe City, 1861-1871 ..................... 161
60. Dr. Kurt Hartoch's "Proud Dueling Scar" ..................... 166
61. Nineteenth Century Homeopathic Doctors ..................... 170
62. "Lucky" Bill Thorrington & Dr. Benjamin King, 1850s ..................... 172
63. Six Doctors Hood, "Nevada's First Family of MDs" ..................... 174
64. Doctors Hood Genealogy ..................... 175
65. DeTar Family, "Four Medical Legacies" ..................... 186
66. Dr. David "Snowshoe" Thompson, 1970 ..................... 189
67. Dr. Willian Ririe, Ely, Nevada, Leader ..................... 193
68. Dr. George "Spunky Kid" Gardner ..................... 195

69. Dr. Anton Tjader Nevada's First Autopsy, 1860................................................198
70. W.H.C. Stephenson, Virginia City Nevada's First Black Doctor, 1863....199
71. Dr. Royce W. Martin, Las Vegas' First MD ..............................................204
72. Dr. Kirk Cammack, "Frontier Desert Justice, 1960s" ...............................207
73. Dr. Jack C. Cherry, "One-of-a-Kind," 1924................................................208
74. Dr. William Patterson, "Soldier, Rancher, etc." 1899...............................213
75. Dr. John D. Campbell, "Tale of the Phantom Hand" ..............................217
76. Dr. James Barger American College of Pathologists President ............220
77. Dr. Roland Stahr Makes a House Call, 1937.............................................223
78. Reno's First Pulmonary Doctor Robert Locke, Iwo Jima and Back.....227
79. Dr. James L. Swank, "Gem of Discovery" ................................................229
80. Dr. John H. Pasek, Sixty Years Minden's Doctor ....................................231
81. "WW I Hero" Dr. Delos Ashley Turner.....................................................232
82. Dr. Louis Lombardi Nevada Board of Regents, 1950-1980 ...................234
83. Dr. Donald Pickering's "Monkey Fetus Experiment"............................235
84. Dr. Charles West, Nevada's First Licensed Black MD............................236

# III Chinese Medicine................................................................238
85. Doc Ing Hay of John Day, Oregon, 1887...................................................239
86. More on Doc Ing Hay ...................................................................................242
87. Chinese Doctors in Nevada .........................................................................243

# IV Medicine at Ninetheenth Century Great Basin Forts.....247
88. Dr. C. Kirkpatrick, Military Surgeon Fort Churchill and Fort Ruby....247
89. Dr. William P. Kendall, 1886 Forensic Examination ..............................253
90. "Saga of Nevada's Nineteenth Century Forts" ........................................259
91. Dr. George Martin Kober "Blood Ingestion to Cure Tuberculosis," ....263

# V Hospitals................................................................................267
92. Saint Mary Louise, Nevada's First Hospital The First Hospital on the Comstock, 1876................................................................................................268
93. Twenty-Nine Hospitals of West Central Nevada, 1876-1942................269
94. Las Vegas Hospital, 1932 .............................................................................272
95. Clark County Hospitals, 1904-1988 Development in a Rapidly Growing Community....................................................................................................276
96. WMC Administrator Carroll W. Ogren's "Adventures".......................282
97. First University of Nevada Hospital, 1902 ...............................................285

# VI University of Nevada Reno School of Medicine............290
98. Beginning of Medical Education in Nevada, 1969..................................291
99. Nevada School of Medicine Comes of Age, 1990 ...................................293
100. Nevada Health Service Corps, Established in 1989................................296
101. School of Medicine Psychiatry Residency ................................................297
102. Fourteenth School of Medicine's Anniversary, 1983..............................298

103. Founding Dean Dr. George Smith ..................................................300
104. Dr. Sandra Daugherty, SOM's First Female Professor .......................305
105. Dr. Fred Anderson Father of the School of Medicine .......................310
106. School of Medicine's Second Dean, Dr. Thomas J. Scully .................312
107. School of Medicine's Budget Crisis of 1981....................................313
108. School of Medicine's First Financial Officer Phillip J. Gillette.............316
109. Former Dean Dr. Ernie Mazzaferri...............................................319

## VII Dental Care .........................................................................321
110. Helen Shipley DMD, Nevada's First Female Dentist, 1905.................322
111. Harry Massoth DMD, Forensic Dentist, 1945 .................................323
112. Hermann Seyfarth DMD, 73 Years a Dentist ..................................324

## VIII Epidemics...........................................................................327
113. 1918 Nevada Flu Epidemic........................................................328
114. 1952-'53 Polio Epidemic...........................................................331
115. Dealing with Smallpox in the Old West, 1863 ...............................336
116. Steve St. Jeor PhD, and Brian Callister MD, "Hantavirus" ................337
117. Infectious Diseases in 1800s Frontier Soldiers ...............................343
118. Dr. Edward Jenner, The First Vaccination, 1796.............................347
119. "Rabies in Nevada, Muzzles and Bullets..., 1915" ...........................347
120. "Animal House" Yosemite Hantavirus Infections, 2012 ....................352

## IX Medical Events ......................................................................358
121. Washoe County Medical Society Formation, 1907............................359
122. Peter Frandsen, A Teacher to Remember, 1900-'42..........................360
123. Persia Bowers, "1874 Mystery"....................................................364
124. Professor Nathanial Wilson IV, "1899 Diabetes Guinea Pig" ...............367
125. Medical Archaeology, 1870s Virginia City Artifacts..........................372
126. West's Premier Surgical Society History of Reno Surgical Society ......374
127. History of Dermatology in Reno, 1946-2005 ..................................377
128. "The Mollie Folly," 1908 ............................................................382
129. History of Medical Malpractice in Nevada .....................................385
130. History of Grave Robbing..........................................................388
131. Prof. Walter Miller MD, PhD, Univ. Nev. 1st Prof. of Science............389
132. Robert Koch & Arthur C. Doyle, "Quest to Cure Tuberculosis" *The Remedy* (Thomas Goetz) 1890 ..................................................390
133. Public Health in Nevada, The First Fifty Years ..............................394
134. Public Health in Nevada, The Second Fifty Years...........................396
135. Galaxy 203 Crash in Reno on January 21, 1985 (30th Anniversary) Reno Led the Way in Aircraft Accident Investigations USA Today 10/28/14 Headline "Plane Crash Didn't Kill Them—Fire Did"..........................400
136. Home Remedies in Nineteenth Century Nevada..............................405

137. Ethan and Hosea Grosh, "Sad Story, 1857" ..............................................409
138. "Small-town" Veterinarian A.A. Cuthbertson .........................................413
139. Silicosis in Delmar, Nevada, 1894 ..............................................................417
140. Pharmacies in Early Nevada, 1862-1939 ..................................................423
141. More on Nevada Pharmacies .....................................................................425
142. Prison Doctor Karen Gedney, "*30 Years Behind Bars*" .........................425
143. Neonatal Intensive Care Units in Northern Nevada ..............................427
144. Southern Nevada's First Neonatal Intensive Care Unit .......................428
145. Neonatal Intensive Care Unit in Northern Nevada "Next Thing I Knew I was Hanging Upside Down" .....................................................................431
146. Reno's First Accidental NICU Death, February 1980 .............................433
147. Neonatal Intensive Care Units in Las Vegas ............................................434
148. Another Dr. Christensen, "To the Rescue" ..............................................437
149. Nevada's Medical Heritage Great Basin History of Medicine Museum and Library ....................................................................................................439
150. Dr. Christian B. Zabriske, "1868 Disinfectant" .......................................443

# X  Nursing ...........................................................................................................**446**
151. Midwives in Nevada, 1878-1908 .................................................................447
152. Dorothy George RN, "Content to Help People" .....................................452
153. Ellen House DNSc, History of Nursing in Nevada ................................454

    Books By Nevada History of Medicine Foundation, Inc. .................. 456
    Abbreviations .............................................................................................. 458
    Chronology of Medical Events ................................................................. 460
    Postscript Photos ........................................................................................ 463
    Index ............................................................................................................. 468

# Illustrations

| | |
|---|---|
| Greasewood Bush ................ XVIII, XIX | Dr. Zetus Spalding ............................ 89 |
| Granite Medicine Bowl and Pestle: . 17 | Dr. Martin Robinson, 1918 ................ 89 |
| Big Mouth Charlie, 1902 ..................... 17 | Dr. T. Perry Tyson, 1920s .................. 92 |
| Shaman Johnny Shoshone ................ 27 | Dr. Samuel and Mrs. Weaver ............ 94 |
| Shaman Tayoni ..................................... 31 | Dr. John Lewis, 1909 .......................... 97 |
| Shaman Dick Mawee ......................... 34 | Dr. A. Parker Lewis, 1913 .................. 97 |
| ca. 400 BC Asclepius ......................... 36 | Dr. Henry Bergstein, 1890s ............... 97 |
| Dr. Mary Fulstone MD, 1987 ............ 44 | Dr. Jack C. Gilbert, 1980s ................ 102 |
| Fred & Dr. Mary Fulstone, 1973 ....... 45 | Dr. Selden McMeans ........................ 104 |
| 1939 Carlin Canyon Train Wreck ..... 45 | Dr. E.B. Harris, late 1800s ............... 106 |
| Nevada Mental Health Hospital ...... 48 | Dr. John Allen Veatch ...................... 110 |
| Dr. Henry Bergstein ........................... 48 | Dr. Anthony Huffaker ...................... 110 |
| Dr. Laurence Nelson, 1949 ................ 59 | Dr. Gideon and Ada Weed, 1860s .. 117 |
| Dr. James Wiggins Gerow ................ 62 | Dr. Ken Maclean, 1950 ..................... 120 |
| Dr. Laurence Nelson, 1953 ................ 63 | Dr. George Thoma, 1900s ................ 123 |
| Dr. Morris R. Walker, 1900 ................ 63 | Dr. Anton Tjader, 1860s ................... 132 |
| 1951 Snowbound Train near Donner Summit ........................................... 63 | Dr. Frederick Hiller, 1860s .............. 133 |
| | Dr. Leslie Moren, mid-1900s .......... 138 |
| Dr. Simeon L. Lee ............................... 73 | Dr. John Worden .............................. 138 |
| Alfred Doten, 1866 ............................. 76 | Dr. Catherine Post-Van Orden ....... 139 |
| Dr. V.A. Muller, 1920s ........................ 76 | Dr. Owen Bolstad, 1980s ................ 143 |
| Dr. Eliza Cook, 1900s ......................... 76 | Dr. Leonard Miller, 1979 ................ 150 |
| Dr. John Marsh, 1900s ........................ 77 | Fallon Clinic, 1979 ........................... 152 |
| Dr. Frederick H. Wichmann, 1900s .. 77 | Dr. Darius Caffaratti ........................ 153 |
| Dr. E. Cook in Front of her Home .... 77 | Dr. Conrad Frydenlund ................... 153 |
| Dr. Washington Kistler, 1910 ............ 79 | Drs. Michael Dingacci ..................... 154 |
| Dr. John A. Fuller .............................. 86 | Dr. A.J. Dingacci .............................. 154 |
| Dr. John Pickard ................................ 86 | Dr. F. Anderson, 1985 ...................... 154 |
| Dr. Fuller's ENT Instruments .......... 86 | Nev. State Med. Assoc. Rep. Dr. Si Elliott ............................... 154 |
| 1958 St. Mary's Staff .......................... 87 | |
| Dr. John Detar ..................................... 87 | Nevada Governor Mike O'Callaghan ..................... 154 |
| Dr. John Fuller .................................... 87 | |
| Dr. Henry Valenta ............................... 87 | Nev. State Senator Norm Glazer, 1971 ..................... 154 |
| Dr. John Scott, Sr. ............................... 87 | |
| Dr. Walter Quinn ................................ 87 | Dr. Alice Thompson, 1920s ............. 156 |
| Dr. Leslie Gould ................................. 87 | Dr. Kurt Hartoch .............................. 159 |

Dr. Sidney Morrison, 1910 ............... 159
Dr. Olga Kipanidze .......................... 159
Washoe City, Nevada, 1865 ............ 165
1860 Map of Nevada Territory ....... 165
Dr. William. H. Hood ...................... 176
Dr. Charles John Hood .................... 178
Dr. Arthur James Hood I ................ 180
Dr. A.J. Hood II ............................... 182
Dr. Dwight L. 'Dutch' Hood ........... 183
Dr. Tom Hood .................................. 185
Dr. David "Snowshoe" Thompson 193
Dr. George Gardner, 1915 ............... 197
Dr. George Gardner, 1975 ............... 197
Dr. Stephenson Ad., 1864 ................ 204
Dr. Royce W. Martin, 1930s ............ 206
Dr. Jack C. Cherry, 1960s ................ 213
Dr. William H. Patterson, ca. .......... 217
Dr. John D. Campbell, ca. 1910 ...... 219
Dr. James Barger, 1940s ................... 223
Dr. John Pasek, 1980s ...................... 232
Dr. Delos Ashley Turner ................. 233
Dr. Louis Lombardi, ca. 1970 ......... 235
Artificial Monkey Womb ................ 236
Dr. Charles I. West, ca. 1970 ........... 237
Chinese Herbs .................................. 238
Wm. Thompson, Guide Carolyn
   Mienhimer, L.E. Toole, and
   Wm. Payne ................................ 242
Kam Wah Chung Store, 1999 ......... 242
Herbalist Wai Tong, Carson City ... 246
Fort Churchill Hospital Ruins ........ 247
Civil War Amputation Kit .............. 256
Ft. McDermitt Officers' Quarters ... 257
Guide James Prida ........................... 257
Dr. Owen Bolstad ............................ 257
Roy Hogan ....................................... 257
Colonel William P. Kendall MD .... 258
Fort Ruby Sutler's Cabin, 1993 ....... 258
Ft. Ruby Officers' Quarters, 1993 ... 264

Fort Scott Enlisted Men's Quarters 265
Measuring Tape on Fort Scott
   Hospital Foundation, 1993 ...... 265
Dr. George M. Kober, 1873 ............. 266
Surgeon E.P. Vollum, 1874 .............. 266
Saint Mary Louise Hospital, 1867 .. 267
Dr. Gerald Sylvain, 1972 ................. 274
Las Vegas Hospital, 1976 ................ 275
Washoe General Hospital, 1903 ..... 275
Bolder Hospital, 1931 ...................... 276
Carroll W. Ogren, 1997 .................... 284
University of Nevada Hospital ...... 288
Dr. Gerorge R. Magee ...................... 289
UNRSOM Entrance, 1990 ................ 290
Dr. George Smith ............................. 304
Dr. Bill Tappan, 1976 ....................... 304
Dr. Sandra & Robert Daugherty .... 307
DR. R. Daugherty Reading Room .. 309
Dr. Thomas J. Scully ........................ 312
Dr. Frederick Anderson .................. 313
Philip John Gillette ......................... 320
Dr. Ernie Mazzaferri ........................ 320
Dr. Helen Shipley DDS ................... 321
Dr. Harry Massoth DDS .................. 324
Dr. Hermann Seyfarth DMD .......... 326
Nurse Lawson, Iron Lung, 1950 ..... 327
Dr. William E. Simpson ................... 335
Seven-week-old baby with Polio ... 335
Reno Flu Masks, 1918 ...................... 336
1878 NSMA Medallion .................... 358
Persia Bowers ................................... 369
Dr. Ben Cunningham ...................... 369
Prof. Wilson IV & son Nathanial ... 370
Prof. Peter Frandsen ........................ 370
Dr. Raymond St. Clair & Family .... 370
Reno Public School, 1874 ................ 371
"Hamilton Main Street"
   in Harper's Weekly, 1869 ........ 371
Virginia City Needle & Syringe ..... 374

Reno Surgical Society, early 1960... 376
Dr. John Cline (President AMA).... 376
Dr. Michael DeBakey....................... 376
Dr. Wesley Hall, Sr. .......................... 376
Dr. William O'Brien, Jr. ................... 376
Professor Walter McNab Miller .... 393
Dr. Reine Hartzell ............................ 393
Mollie Harrison, 1908 ...................... 393
Dr. George McKenzie ...................... 394
Dr. Donald Maclean, Jr.................... 394
Dr. Donald Kwalik........................... 400
Reno Galaxy 203, 1985..................... 405
Grosh Brothers, 1857 ....................... 413
Dr. Arlynn Cuthbertson DVM ....... 416
Delmar Building Ruins, 1990s........ 421
Delmar Map...................................... 422
Pharmacy Exhibit............................. 424
Dr. Bill Stephan, 1974 ...................... 435
NICU Transport Crash, Mt. Rose .. 436
Erin Madsen RN................................ 436
Brian Walsh RT, Renown NICU .... 436
Dr. Feldman, Sunrise NICU, 1976 . 437
Dr. Pickering, 1973........................... 437
Dr. G. Norman Christensen............ 438
Byblos Column With Snake............ 443
Wooden Stethoscope, 1863 ............. 443
Dr. Lee's Microscope, 1900 ............. 443
1747 Book on Medicine ................... 443
Dorothy George RN, 1943............... 446
Midwife Dr. Bethenia Owens, MD 451
Dr. Ralph Bowdie, 1920................... 463
Dr. John L. Robinson, 1922 ............. 463
Dr. Horace Brown, 1923 .................. 463
Dr. R.P. Roantree, 1930..................... 463
Dr. Charles E. Secor, 1936 ............... 464
Dr. Daniel J. Hurley, 1942 ............... 464
Dr. Edwin Cantlon, 1956.................. 464
Dr. Stanley L. Hardy, 1957.............. 464
Dr. Roland Stahr, 1958..................... 465
Dr. Ernest Mack, 1959...................... 465
Dr. Joe George, 1965 ........................ 465
Dr. V.A. Salvadorini, 1969 ............... 465
Capt. Treat Cafferata, 1987 ............. 466
Capt. Tom Brady, VN 1968.............. 466
Lt. Richard Ganchan, VN 1969....... 466
Capt. Anton Sohn, VN 1968............ 466

# Acknowledgements

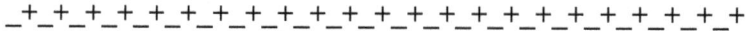

A book of this scope cannot be accomplished without the help of numerous individuals. First and foremost are Drs. Owen Bolstad and my daughter, Dr. Kristin Sohn Fermoile, who share my love for history of medicine. Kristin has written articles on the history of medicine but also has edited *Greasewood Tablettes* and *1,000 Years of Medicine in Nevada's Great Basin*. Owen helped with naming *Greasewood Tablettes* and contributed to its success.

Reno colleague, Dr. S.N. "Nick" Landis, told me about an Indian patient who had metastatic cancer. He told the patient, there was no treatment, return to Fallon, and contact the Indian medicine man. When he returned to see Dr. Landis, the cancer was gone. He said the shaman prescribed tea from Greasewood leaves. As a result of Indian use of the Greasewood plant, I suggested the name Greasewood for the bulletin. Owen added *Tablettes*, French for tablet, to give the bulletin's name sophistication.

Guy Rocha was a great source of information and suggested people who were important in our medical history. John Marschall PhD was a frequent speaker at our history of medicine meetings and brought Dr. Henry Bergstein to our attention. For years, Gussie Burgoyne organized and formatted *Greasewood Tablettes*. Jennifer Grove followed in her footsteps and helped by copying articles for *1,000 Years of Medicine in Nevada's Great Basin*. For this reason, she deserves to be co-author of *this book*. Lynda McLellan has been involved in promoting our program and helped organize the history of medicine museum and library. Eileen Barker was a great help in 1985 when our program started. Peter Aylworth started as an intern and later was an employee in the pathology department. Dr. Bob Daugherty was instrumental in providing space for the Great Basin Museum and Library.

Phyllis Cudek deserves credit for writing articles on the history of medicine. Her husband, Dr. Ron Cudek alerted me to the opening of a pathology position in Reno in 1967, which led to the birth of Nevada's history of medicine program. Dr. Don Kwalik added the history of the Nevada State Health Department.

Numerous others provided information for this book, including Annie Blachley, Dr. Tom Brady, Dr. Curtis Brown, Dr. Norm Christensen, Dr. John Dooley, Phil Earl, Dr. Fred Elliott, Mike Ezell, Dr. Bernard Feldman, Teresa Garrison, Dr. Tom Hall, Martha Hildreth PhD, Dr. Tom Hood, Ellen House DNSc, Dr. John Iliescu, Tom King PhD, Dr. Trudy Larson, Dr. Bob Locke, Dr. Colleen Lyons, Blair McGirk, Anne McMillian, Dr. Ali Monibi, Bruce Moran PhD, Dr. Dick Newbold, Carroll Ogren, Cynthia Pinto, Lisa Puleo, Rick Pugh, Dr. Gary Ridenour, Elmer Rusco PhD, Dr. Rod Sage, Dr. Elwood Schmidt, Dr. Bill Stephan, Louis E. Toole, Linda Valle, Lynne Williams, and Joan Zenan.

# Introduction

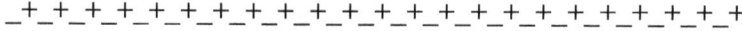

This is the story of medicine in the Great Basin and adjacent areas from the beginning of known life in the Great Basin to the twentieth century. The title of this book emphasizes that Shoshone and Paiute Indians lived in the Great Basin for thousands of years. They practiced medicine using all parts of the Greasewood plant and other native plants to treat aliments.

We tell the story of Indian herbal medicine that developed over thousands of years. In more recent times, Native Americans successfully treated the flu epidemic of 1918.

In the nineteenth century, American doctors came west in wagon trains to settle the West. Later, Chinese labor was brought across the Pacific Ocean to build the railroad over the Sierra and work in mines. They brought their medicine men and medical traditions with them.

Newly arrived American doctors expanded healthcare to towns along the railroad, to mining camps, and to settlements throughout the Great Basin. The following chapters also tell the story of the establishment and development of the first medical school in Nevada. Its development led to a history of medicine section in the department of pathology and the following record of Nevada's history.

I am writing this book so Nevada's medical history will not be forgotten. I tried to record the history of nursing in Nevada but was informed by the Nevada Nursing Association they would do it. They came through, and I have added Nevada's nursing history by Ellen House DNSc.

In 1989, we initiated a program to give pathology students a perspective on history of medicine by requiring them to do a research paper on history of medicine. Student history of medicine research was a carry-over from my education requirement at Indiana University School of Medicine. At University of Nevada School of Medicine a winning essay is selected; some are included. Others are about medicine outside the scope of this book and are not included.

Before I came on the scene at UNSOM in 1985, there was little organized effort to record and preserve the medical history of our state. I developed a centralized source for publishing and preserving items of historical significance. Dr. Fred Anderson deserves recognition because he had an interest in Nevada's history of medicine and gave priceless articles of historical significance to the School of Medicine, which were added to the Great Basin History of Medicine Museum/Library.

# History of Medicine Program
## University Nevada Reno School of Medicine
### By Dr. Anton Sohn

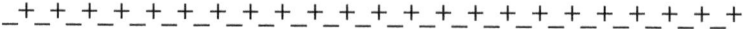

After I was appointed chairman of pathology, I approached Dean Robert Daugherty for the Department of Pathology to create a medical history of medicine division. He agreed and the division was formed with the help of Martha Hildreth PhD, Bruce Moran PhD, and Tom King PhD. Numerous individuals, who are named on page 277, donated information, time, and money to create the new division and the museum/library.

The division publishes a quarterly bulletin, *Greasewood Tablettes,* on a quarterly basis with historical information relating to medicine in our state. Most of the articles and information in this book are from previous issues of *Greasewood Tablettes*. We also developed a facility for collection of photographs, artifacts, manuscripts, documents, records, oral histories, and other memorabilia. This material provides a valuable resource for future authors and researchers.

We realize there have been previous efforts by individuals and historical societies to record parts of Nevada's medical history. We used these resources to supplement our information on Nevada's history of medicine.

# Greasewood Bush
## By Blair McGirk

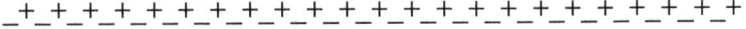

Greasewood, alias Creosote Bush, specifically the genus *Larrea,* is the dominant desert plant from California to Texas and south to Argentina. It boasts among its members the oldest know living plant—at 12,000 years it makes the Sequoias and Bristlecone pines look like youngsters. *Larrea* is remarkably resistant to bacterial, fungal, and insect attack, is generally unpalatable to animals, and deters most plants from growing nearby. It copes with extremely arid conditions and is currently expanding its range in overgrazed and disturbed areas.

The creosote bush (*Larrea tridentata*) has a long history in folk medicine and Indian lore. It was used to treat complaints including cancer, wounds, infections, ulcers, and dental caries. It has antineoplastic, antibiotic, and antifeedant properties (adversely affects insects). One of its major constituents, nordihydroguaiaretic acid (NDGA) inhibits the mitochondrial respiratory chain, glycolysis, prostaglandin synthesis, and was used as an antioxidant in fats and oils for many years before being replaced by less toxic antioxidants. NDGA is currently undergoing clinical trials for the treatment of basal and squamous cell carcinoma and shows promise towards mammary carcinoma as well.

The antineoplastic clinical trials of NDGA represent one of the success stories at the University of Nevada, Reno. The antineoplastic and mitochondrial inhibitory properties of NDGA were identified in the laboratory of Ron Pardini PhD, a member of the Department of Biochemistry. His work, in collaboration with Chemex, a private pharmaceutical corporation, laid the groundwork for the development of a potentially marketable drug. Proceeds from the collaboration established the Chemex

Natural Products Laboratory at the University of Nevada, Reno, but Greasewood plant is no longer is being studied. The bush was grown in tissue culture, and its natural production, metabolism and antioxidant enzyme activities were studied.

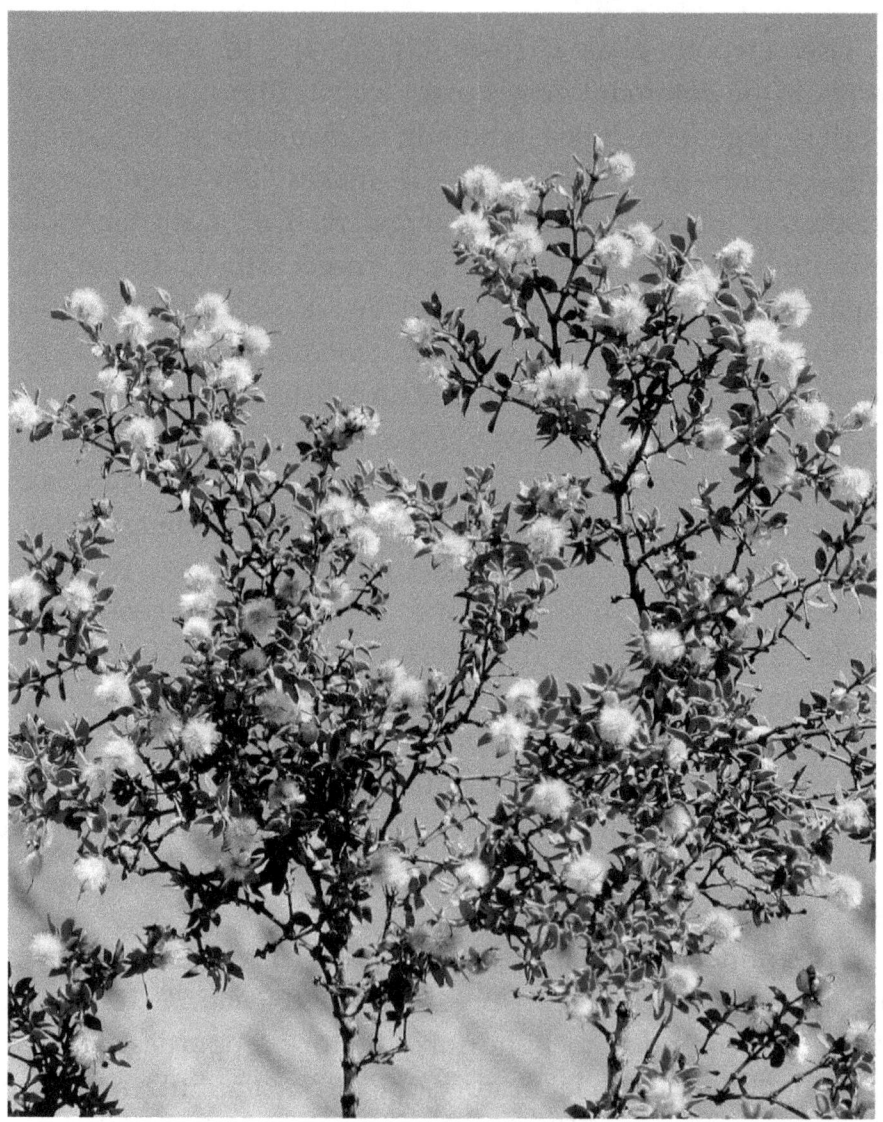

Greasewood Bush

# More on Greasewood Bush
## By Dr. Anton Sohn

_+_+_+_+_+_+_+_+_+_+_+_+_+_+_+_+_+_+_+_+_+

After we adopted the greasewood bush as the banner for our newsletter, I had to admit a certain amount of chagrin about my lack of knowledge about the plant. After living in Nevada, much time spent enjoying the out-of-doors, I was not confident I could identify the greasewood plant.

Although Blair McGirk's article contained much information about the pharmacological properties of the greasewood plant, it didn't say much about what the plant looked like.

To learn more I referred to a copy of Shrubs of the Great Basin by Hugh Mozingo, University of Nevada Press, 1987. This book is a splendid resource devoted to the natural history of the Great Basin vegetation. Greasewood, also called creosote bush grows in very alkaline soil where few other plants can survive. Its ability to grow in dry desert conditions may be due in part to its very long taproot, which is able to penetrate twenty to fifty feet deep to reach groundwater. Native Americans used the creosote bush in a variety of ways. The Northern Paiute name for the greasewood plant is TONOBI. Greasewood bush smells like creosote, making identification easy.

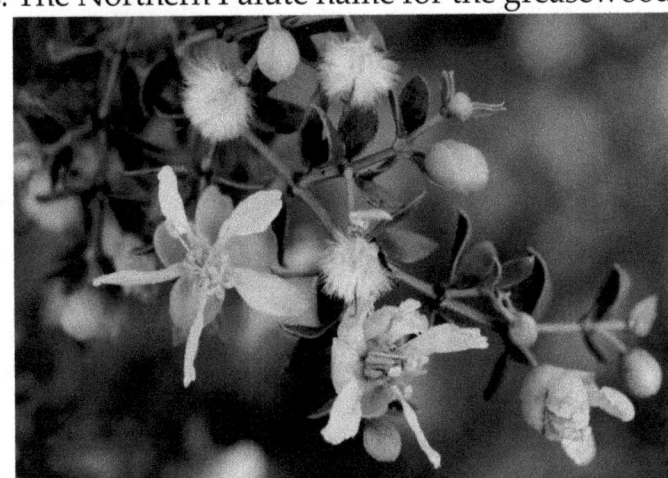

Greasewood Bush Flower

# I

+_+_+_+_+_+_+_+_+_+_+_+_+_+_+_+_+_+_+_+_+_+_+_+

# NATIVE AMERICAN MEDICINE
### "WALKING IN BEAUTY, LIVING IN BALANCE"
### NAVAJO PHILOSOPHY OF HEALING

**Native Voices:**
**Native Peoples' Concepts of Health and Illness**

Traveling Exhibition Host Guide
(rev 11/30/15)

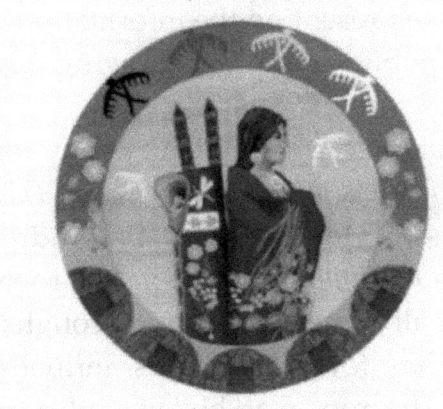

 NIH  U.S. National Library of Medicine

+_+_+_+_+_+_+_+_+_+_+_+_+_+_+_+_+_+_+_+_+_+_+_+

## Indian Remedy for Influenza, 1918

While doing some research on sources of medical interest, graduate student Mike Ezell came across an article in the *Bulletin of the Nevada State Board of Health,* No. 1, January 1920, compiled and edited by Gustav F. Ruediger MD. This article, entitled *"An Indian Remedy for Influenza"* described the use by the Washoe Indians of a root, *Leptotaemia dissecta,* in the treatment of influenza.

There was not a single death from influenza or its complications in the Washoe tribe during the 1918 epidemic, although Indians living in other parts of the state, where the root did not grow, died in high numbers. According to this report, it was also used among white settlers to treat mild to virulent types of influenza and proved to be the nearest approach to a specific therapy in epidemic influenza and the accompanying pneumonia.

The Nevada Board of Health, in presenting these facts did make the disclaimer that they did not give their endorsement to the remedy but were presenting the information with the idea of giving the matter publicity and encouraging others to give it a trial.

The use of *Leptotaemia* as an Indian remedy for influenza was described in *Medicinal Uses of Plants by Indian Tribes of Nevada* by Percy Train, James R. Heinrichs and W. Andrew Archer. The plant is *Leptotaemia multifidi.* In his book, the root is described as a panacea for most all ailments, including coughs and colds, and disorders such as hay fever, bronchitis, influenza, pneumonia, and tuberculosis. The root was boiled and decocted as a tea, pulverized, and smoked (sometimes mixed with tobacco), inhaled by burning the root on live coals, and mixed with various other plant remedies. Often raw pieces of the root were chewed for sore throat. Treatment of gonorrhea was suggested using the root in combination with plants of *Achillea lanulosa,* when boiled together to be drank as tea.

Oily sap collected from the freshly cut root was applied to skin cuts and sores, and the same oil was dropped into the eye as a treatment of trachoma or gonorrheal infection of the eye. Decoction of the root was used as a wash in treatment of smallpox, as well as for various skin rashes and sores. The raw root was pulped and applied to cuts and sores.

Pulped root was applied to the umbilical cord of newborn babies by Washoe Indians. In some of the Indian settlements, the root was even used to treat distemper in horses! Many other uses have been described.

Both the Paiute and Shoshone name for the root is *toh-aw save* or *toh-sa*, while the Washoe name was *dosa* or *dozaz*. There is much confusion regarding names of the various roots and herbs used medicinally by the Indians. Common names for *Leptotaenia multifidi* are wild carrot, Queen Anne's Lace, cough root, and Indian balsam.

## Traditional Great Basin Indian Herbal Medicine
## By Janet K. Holmes

The following article does not advocate the use of these traditional Native American remedies. These plants may be toxic and require special preparation to be made safe for medicinal purposes. In addition, many of these plants were harvested on a seasonal basis, which may affect the medicinal or toxic properties. The Food and Drug Administration (FDA) may even ban some substances listed in this article. There also could be side effects that occur when taken with other medications. For these reasons, one should not use any of the following plants unless under a physician's supervision.

Over the past few decades, a growing segment of modern American society has embraced health food stores, which offer holistic and traditional herbal medicines, as well as traditional home remedies. This can easily be demonstrated through article titles on the covers of popular magazines, television infocommercials, telephone directory yellow pages, and the popularity of homeopathic physicians. Regular American medical practitioners realize the importance of cultural medical traditions and therefore include some of these traditional medicinal alternatives as part of their treatments. The acceptance of integrating modern medicine and traditional cultural medicine has even reached the University of Nevada, Reno campus. On February 11, 2002, Dr. Lori Alvord gave a lecture at the University of Nevada, Reno School of Medicine entitled, "Walking in Beauty, Living in Balance" (Navajo Philosophy of Healing).

This was based on Dr. Lori Alvord's book, *The Scalpel, and the Silver Bear: The First Navajo Woman Surgeon Combines Western Medicine and Traditional Healing*. We will examine Great Basin Indian ethno-botanical medicine in the hopes that modern Great Basin inhabitants may appreciate Navajo traditional healing.

One may ask the question: "How knowledgeable were the Great Basin Indian groups about the medicinal plants in their respective areas?" To answer this question, first, we must understand that extensive numbers of common plants were used. In addition, many were used for thousands of years and were shown to be effective through trial and error. Over two hundred varieties of roots and plants were used to treat ailments. In *Handbook of the North American Indians Vol. 11*, the authors state in their article entitled *Western Shoshone*: Fifty-two plants are said to constitute medicine for colds, 57 for venereal diseases (with occasional distinctions between gonorrhea and syphilis), 44 for swelling, 34 for diarrhea, 37 for rheumatism and 48 for various stomach indispositions including stomachache.

Because of the hundreds of varieties of plants used within their ethnobotanical medicine, it is not possible, within this venue, to cover every plant the Great Basin people used for herbal cure or to cover the traditional preparation of each remedy. Therefore, we will briefly examine only approximately fifty species of plants and their uses. The list is alphabetically listed by common English plant names.

**NOTE:**

Common names of all plants differ from locality to locality, and a specific named plant may mean something quite different to different individuals. Native American Indians used many plants that were pharmacologically active, such as Ephedra, and were used appropriately. Great Basin Native Americans did not suffer from scurvy because many of the plants were dried and used during periods when fresh plants were not available. Consequently, Vitamin C was ingested from these dried leafy plants.

*Alumroot* was used to make a tonic for use in general debility, as well as for heart trouble, venereal disease, high fevers, eyewash, liver problems, and diarrhea. In addition, it was used as an astringent and as a treatment for colic.

*Arrow weed* was used for bloody diarrhea, indigestion, or a "sour" stomach.

*Balsamroot* was used for severe stomach problems as well as bladder troubles.

*Biscuit root, Toza, cough root, fern leaf or carrot leaf* was employed to treat trachoma, swellings, sprains, sore throat, gonorrhea, hay fever, colds, coughs, bronchitis, fevers, chest congestion, influenza, pneumonia, and as an antiseptic for smallpox, rashes, sores, and cuts. Biscuit root was also considered a curative for tuberculosis. It is still commonly used to treat arthritis, colds, and influenza.

*Black cottonwood* was used for headaches, venereal diseases, tuberculosis, stomach disorders, and general disability (blood tonic).

*Brass buttons* was used for constipation, stomachaches, and cramps. It also acted as an emetic and physic, as well as was used as eyewash.

*Bristlecone pine* was used to draw out boils and administer to sores.

*Butterball* was used as a cold medicine, eye medicine, a remedy for stomachaches, and venereal diseases.

*Button snakewood* was used for diarrhea.

*California incense cedar* was considered to protect against contagious diseases.

*Cow parsnip* was used for toothaches, sore throats, coughs, colds, diarrhea, tuberculosis, rheumatism, and to benefit healing of wounds.

*Creosote bush* or *Greasewood bush* was a general cure-all. It had analgesic and antiseptic properties. It was used to stimulate urination, to cure venereal diseases, colds, rheumatism, chicken pox, burns, and bowel cramps, and to aid in new skin formation. It worked as a styptic and, in recent years, it has been useful for treating cancer It was also called Greasewood and because of its extensive medicinal use by native Americans, our quarterly bulletin is named after it.

*Dodder* was believed to induce sterility.

*Ephedra, Mormon tea, Indian tea, or squaw tea* was used as a treatment for venereal diseases like syphilis and gonorrhea. It was also used for ailments of the kidneys and cramps. It was also used for bladder disorders, colds, blood purifier, circulation, delayed or difficult menstruation, and stomach disorders. When combined with other plants, it treated diarrhea, cure for sores, and burns. Some considered it to be a curative for backaches and anemia.

*False hellebore or skunk cabbage* was used as a contraceptive. Guess why!! In addition, it was used for venereal diseases, sore throats, heavy colds, inflamed tonsils, swellings, rheumatism, sore nipples, infections, sores, cuts, boils, blood poisoning, and as a liniment. It was also applied to snake bites. Other uses include burns, bruises, toothaches, and fevers.

*Gourd* was used for venereal diseases (gonorrhea and syphilis) as well as an emetic and physic. It was a remedy for bloating and for worms. Gourd plants were also considered to be a cure-all by some indigenous people.

*Horehound* was believed to stimulate blood circulation. It also acted as a cough, cold, and respiratory aid.

*Horsetail rush* was taken for kidney problems. It was used as a diuretic, eyewash, and for urinary tract infections.

*Jimson weed* was not known to have been used for medicinal purposes. However, it was known for its narcotic properties. It was used on occasion to render a person unconscious.

*Juniper* was used by Great Basin Indians as a blood tonic or treating venereal disease. It was also used for headaches, colds, disinfectant, fever, measles, burns, and wounds.

*Lovage* was made into a cough treatment.

*Manzanita* was used for venereal disease. In addition, manzanita was used for poison oak rash and wounds.

*Mint, spearmint, or peppermint* was used in a large variety of afflictions like colic, stomachaches, indigestion, diarrhea, headaches, colds, fevers, sore throats, and to reduce swelling. It was also used for heart problems. Spearmint leaves cured an upset stomach; and was used as a cough syrup. Peppermint was used for gas pains.

*Milkweed* was employed for headaches and ringworm. It also could draw out snakebite poison.

*Pink sand* was applied to burns.

*Prince's plume, desert plume, or Indian cabbage* was used to treat sore gums and teeth, earaches, rheumatic pains, and general weakness after an illness. It was also used during a diphtheria epidemic to relieve pain and congestion of the throat.

*Puffball* was considered beneficial for swellings and sores.

*Quaking aspen* was used for venereal diseases. Some indigenous people insisted this had no medicinal value, but rather the *black cottonwood* should be used instead.

*Rabbitbrush* was made into remedies for colds, stomach disorders, and bloody diarrhea. It was also rubbed into the scalp to stimulate freer breathing. A general tonic was also made from Rabbitbrush. A liniment came from rabbitbrush as well.

<u>Sagebrush</u> was used as a headache remedy and used for rheumatism. Sagebrush was also used in healing ceremonies. Old black leaves were used on baby rashes.

<u>Sand wort</u> was used as an eyewash.

<u>Serviceberry</u> was used for snow blindness.

<u>Single-leaf pinyon</u> was frequently mixed with other plants and used for colds, venereal diseases, rheumatism, tuberculosis, fevers, nausea, chronic indigestion, influenza, pneumonia, bowel trouble, diarrhea, kidney problems, smallpox, ruptures, sciatic pains, chest congestion, and as a post-childbirth tonic. It was also used as a treatment for insect bites, swellings, sores, rashes, and cuts, or for drawing out boils and slivers. In addition, it was a sore throat remedy. Intestinal parasites, worms, and muscular soreness were also symptoms this was used to treat.

<u>Smokebush</u> was used as a cough and cold remedy, as well as used to treat pneumonia, tuberculosis, influenza, whooping cough, stomachaches, toothaches, smallpox, measles, venereal diseases, muscular pains, diarrhea, sores, rheumatism, face neuralgia, incontinence, kidney trouble, or to induce urination.

<u>Snowberry or waxberry</u> was used for stomach pains and indigestion. These plants also helped to relieve the pains of childbirth.

<u>St. John's wort</u> was used for bullet wounds, cuts, swellings, aching feet, toothaches, and venereal diseases.

<u>Sulphur flower</u> was for rheumatism, lameness, stomachaches, & colds.

<u>Tobacco</u> was employed to expel worms, as well as treat athlete's foot, asthma, tuberculosis, swellings, rheumatism, cuts, sores, snakebites, hives, eczema, skin infections or irritations. Tobacco was also used for decayed tooth pain. It also functioned as a cold remedy. It functioned as a physic and an emetic. The tobacco plant that is found in the Great Basin has much less

nicotine than its relative from eastern U.S. that is used in cigarettes, etc. Great Basin tobacco plant was also used in healing rituals.

<u>Violet</u> was a sweat inducer. Canadian violets were used for lung trouble.

<u>White fir</u> was believed to cure tuberculosis, venereal diseases, sores, boils, cuts, and lung troubles.

<u>White-sage or winterfat</u> was used as an anti-lice treatment, as well as a general scalp and hair tonic. It was believed to hold anti-graying and anti-baldness properties, as well as a potential hair-restorer. It was also used to relieve eye soreness. This helped to alleviate intermittent fevers and it aided in relieving respiratory ailments.

<u>White sand</u> was employed for swellings.

<u>Wild buckwheat</u> was used for tuberculosis, lameness, rheumatism, cough, and bladder trouble.

<u>Wild geraniums</u> were used for upset-stomach, swollen feet, venereal diseases, sore eyes, colds, and as a contraceptive. They were also used for ulcers.

<u>Wild mustard</u> was used as treatment for burns.

<u>Wild rose or Woods' rose</u> was used for cuts, sores, wounds, intestinal influenza, bloody diarrhea, burns, swellings, boils, as a general tonic, or physic. It also was a cold remedy.

<u>Yellow dock, Indian rhubarb, curly dock</u> is a common weed across the Great Basin. Depending on the preparation, it was used to treat rheumatic swellings, bruises, burns, liver disorder, and venereal diseases.

<u>Yellow dock</u> was also used as a pain reliever, a blood purifier, cure for diarrhea, and as a general tonic. In addition, it was used for a variety of ailments (e.g. scurvy, scales, running sores, skin eruptions, and itch reliever). It was used to treat stomachaches. It was also smoked.

<u>Yucca, Spanish bayonet, Lord's candle</u> was used to treat blindness and skin irritation.

**NOTE:**
Many of these herbs were also used for veterinary purposes. Beyond botanical remedies, there were many non-plant remedies used by the Great Basin people as well. These included such treatments as using breast milk for a nursing baby's sore eyes, skunk grease on chapped skin, and horse urine for broken and itching pustules. In addition, fat from animal hearts was thought to be a cure for tuberculosis. We have only begun to "glimpse" the extensive medicinal knowledge used by Great Basin's indigenous people.

It is clear to see that these Great Basin natives were creative in their cures. One can tell by the wide variety of plants for certain diseases (venereal diseases and rheumatism) that they had difficulty in finding reliable remedies. This seemed to be especially true for ailments that were brought in by European contact. It was also well known that various cures were adapted from their immigrant neighbors, and they, in turn, borrowed from the Native Americans. By looking at these curatives, one can also gain perspective about the kinds of maladies that were most common. The indigenous Great Basin people found a wealth of medicinal riches amongst what would be a wasteland of worthless desert by modern Americans.

These herbs and plants played an important role in healing. Data indicates the Paiute were highly sophisticated botanists. Beyond the Paiute, the Shoshone were probably the most advanced tribe in terms of medicinal plant lore. For the Goshute, it appears all members of the tribe had some working knowledge of the medicinal herbs. The Washoe were considered to have the least plant lore and borrowed from neighboring tribes. The Shoshone and Paiute were known to have traded medicinal plants with Indians outside of the Great Basin. They also traveled across the Great Basin seeking medicinal plants.

# Washoe Tribe and a Simple Herbal Remedy
## Fifty Million Deaths May Have Been Avoided

By David Prosser
Winner History of History of a
Disease Essay for Second-year Students in Pathology

The 1918 flu pandemic has gone down in history as one of the most devastating diseases to sweep the world (before COVID-19). Commonly known as the Spanish Flu due to its misperceived severity and beginning in Spain where it was uncensored and more widely publicized.

However, the first documented cases occurred in the United States at Camp Funston, Kansas. In two years, roughly one third of the world's population and 28% of Americans had contracted the virus. It is estimated that 675,000 Americans died due to contracting the virus, a number ten times greater than the number of Americans who died in World War I. Though these numbers paint the picture of a disease that left no stone unturned, a small native American tribe in northern Nevada may in fact have been the most successful population in combating the disease by employing a simple herbal remedy extracted from the root of *Lomatium dissectum*, a plant indigenous to the Great Basin.

As the state with the smallest population in 1918, Nevada was lacking the infrastructure manpower to reach the sparsely located rural populations comprising most of the population and was thus slow to report cases of disease. Once able to assess the spread of influenza, it was found that thousands of the state's residents had died from the virus.

Though many of those thousands who died had been inhabitants of Indian reservations, Dr. Ernst Krebs, a physician working near Carson City, Nevada, discovered two striking facts concerning the local Washoe Indians. The first was the fact that, though members of the tribe had become ill with the virus, not one member of the tribe died from influenza or its complications.

The second was the fact the tribe had been using the root of the *Lomatium dissectum* plant to treat those who contracted the illness.

*Lomatium dissectum*, colloquially known as biscuitroot, is a rare species of plant in the parsley family that grows in semi-arid climates in the northwest region of the United States and parts of Canada. Up to the time of the flu outbreak, it had been used by the Washoe tribe to treat all fever causing ailments. The method used by the Washoe tribe to extract the active product used for treatment was peeling the root of the plant, then boiling this root and skimming the oil off the top. A large dose of broth containing this extract was then given to the patient. One pound of the root was used to produce the medicinal product and it was given over a three-day period to tribal members who had contracted the Spanish Flu. Within one week's time of initiation of treatment, all patients reportedly had a full recovery.

Dr. Krebs conceded to the fact that the use of the plant and the survival of all Washoe tribesmen were given it as treatment for influenza may have been coincidental. Further supporting the utility of this plant extract in treating influenza, however, was Krebs's report that another physician used it in his practice to treat those infected with influenza that were described as hopeless cases. It was found that treatment of these patients using the extract alone led to a full recover. Other physicians began catching on started using preparations of *Lomatium dissectum* to treat many Caucasians who had contracted the Spanish Flu, which they found a great success. Krebs even went so far as to describe it as the most effective treatment of that time in treating influenza and any accompanying pneumonia. He praised the plant extract for its versatility, recording that it was more efficacious at treating a cough and longer lasting than the opiate expectorants of the day. He also noted it was a bronchial, intestinal, and urinary antiseptic, and it also was able to slow the heart rate and lower the blood pressure.

Supporting Krebs's assertion that this treatment had great

versatility, in addition to treating the flu, native tribes used biscuitroot for ailments such as the common cold, arthritis, tuberculosis, and rheumatism. The constituents of *Lomatium dissectum* have since been determined. It contained furanocoumarins and pyranocoumarins.

Both have been shown to have significant antimicrobial activity. The furanocoumarins, for example, have been shown to be effective in inactivation of both DNA and RNA viruses, and they also have antibacterial and antifungal activity. Also present are saponins, which are present in herbs used historically for medicinal purposes. For example, these herbs have been used as tranquilizers, expectorants, and antitussive agents. Ascorbic acid is also found in the plant and is thought to have immune stimulating activity. Coumarins, which have been shown to be vasodilating agents and thus capable of lowering blood pressure, are found to be present in the plant as well.

*Lomatium dissectum* has further been shown to have both bactericidal effects to varying degrees against some of the most common infectious organisms, including Streptococcus pyogenes, Escherichia coli, Pseudo-monas aeruginosa, Corynebacterium diptherium, and Mycobacterium tuberculosis. When adjusted for concentration, these effects were on par with penicillin. In addition, another study testing the plant's bacteriostatic and bactericidal activity against 62 strains of bacteria and fungi found at least partial inhibition of growth in all these organisms.

As a result of the successful healing effects of *Lomatium dissectum* in treating influenza found both in the Washoe tribe and the subsequent trials performed by physicians, the plant enjoyed a short period of popularity with four manufacturing plants producing extracts. However, this period proved to be short lived, as its utility was somehow unable to catch the attention of medical professionals outside of its region of distribution. Interest in the extract waned soon after the end of the influenza pandemic and production on a commercial scale ceased.

The legend of the Spanish Flu and the devastating toll it took on the world is well known. Though modern-day technology, in conjunction with the breadth of information concerning disease, allow, for the most effective methods of treatment to be employed, it can only be described as amazing that the seemingly simple remedy used by the Washoe tribe was so effective as to not lose a single tribal member to one of the most infamous viral infections the world has seen to date.

A disease that took the lives of so many of the world's population was no match for *Lomatium dissectum*. In the perspective of modern day, whether *Lomatium dissectum* could have had a greater impact by reducing the death toll of the flu of 1918 throughout the American population under the right circumstances is a moot point considering the theoretical basis of the question. However, there is no denying the impact this one plant had on a little tribe in Northern Nevada that defied the odds and cheated imminent death. Was it due to the plant, or did they have natural immunity?

## BIG MOUTH CHARLIE'S MEDICINE BOWL, 1868

Judge Ernest Chappel Bonner, who lived in Alturas, California, was an avid collector of Native American artifacts. Over his lifetime he collected an extensive collection of Indian beadwork, baskets, historic relics, and artifacts. This collection has been carefully preserved by his descendants and is still largely intact. Much of this famous collection has been exhibited at the Nevada Historical Society's Museum in Reno in past years. Big Mouth Charlie's Medicine Bowl was passed down through the family and has come into the possession of Judge Bonner's great grandson, Dr. Curtis Brown. Curtis, graduate of the University of Nevada School of Medicine, was kind to loan Charlie's Medicine Bowl to the Great Basin History of Medicine Museum.

The stone 12-inch mortar and pestle was used by the last

Modoc Indian Medicine Man, Big Mouth Charlie, to mix medicines. The story of Medicine Man Charlie told by Judge Bonner and others makes this ancient artifact interesting. As the story goes, a group of renegade Modoc Indians had plotted to trap General George Crook and his party near Likely, California, in 1868. The soldiers were saved by the intervention of a "friend" of the white men, an Indian named Tom Dickens. As a result of his treachery, families of the renegades held great resentment for the traitor, Tom. Sometime later, one of the "friendly" Indians fell sick and Charlie was called to mix a potion for him, using this same ancient mortar passed down through generations of medicine men. When the patient died, civil authorities stepped into the picture and arrested Charlie for murder. He was convicted and served a term in California's prison.

After serving his time, Charlie returned to the tribe and assumed his old position of authority. Many of the tribesmen avoided contact with Charlie, fearing the curse of the medicine man they believed to be as deadly as any weapon. One night, one of the renegades crept into Tom Dicken's camp and beat him savagely. Tom refused to be treated by Charlie and while they were talking together the conversation became heated, and Charlie invoked a curse upon Tom. He stated, "one year from today, you will die!' The creeping paralysis of fear preyed upon Tom's mind, and each time they met Charlie would remind Tom of the number of "suns" he had left. It was said, on the very day Charlie specified, Dickens died.

There was an old tribal law that if a medicine man lost three patients in a row, he must be executed, and now Charlie had lost two. The threatening countenance that Charlie presented was exaggerated by his large, deformed mouth-which was, supposedly, the result of a gunshot wound to his face, hence the name Big Mouth Charlie. In the summer of 1902, Charlie had traveled on a royal Indian pilgrimage to a camp about 50 miles from Alturas. During that encampment an enraged Indian had attacked Charlie, emptying his revolver into Charlie's mouth. Every one of the witnesses affirmed Charlie spat out the bullets as fast as they came!

During an argument with the Steele brothers, Charlie turned to Wes Steele and raising his powerful right arm, invoked the curse, "One year from today, you die, like Tom Dickens." Like Tom Dickens, Wes began to weaken month by month and on the appointed day he died quietly. That was Charlie's third death. Friends of Steele decided to take no chances and repeatedly laid plots to kill the medicine man. Time-after-time, Charlie managed to escape. Finally, one dark night a lone Indian stalked Charlie's camp. Taking him by surprise, he shot the old medicine man in the back of the neck, then emptied his rifle into Charlie's body before he could utter another curse.

The tribe was greatly relieved by Charlie's death, since no one seemed to know who killed him, and no one signed a complaint, District Attorney Ernest Bonner refused to prosecute anyone. Not long after that incident, Mr. Bonner was called before the tribal council.

By acclamation the judge was made an official member of the tribe. On that same day, Charlie's widow, together with Wes Steele's brother, Sam, came to the Bonner home. Since the squaw could speak no English, Sam spoke for her: "Charlie told her if anything happens to him, he wants Ernest Bonner to have his medicine bowl and pestle." With that passed the last of the Modoc Indian doctors, for without this bowl no other medicine man can serve the tribe. Since that time, the Modoc Indians go to the doctors provided by the Bureau of Indian Affairs.

**NOTE:**

Some of the material in this article was taken from *The Nevada State Journal,* March 23, 1952. Dr. Curtis Brown and his father, John Webster Brown, brought Big Mouth Charlie to our attention and loaned Charlie's bowl from their vast collection of Indian artifacts to the HOM Museum.

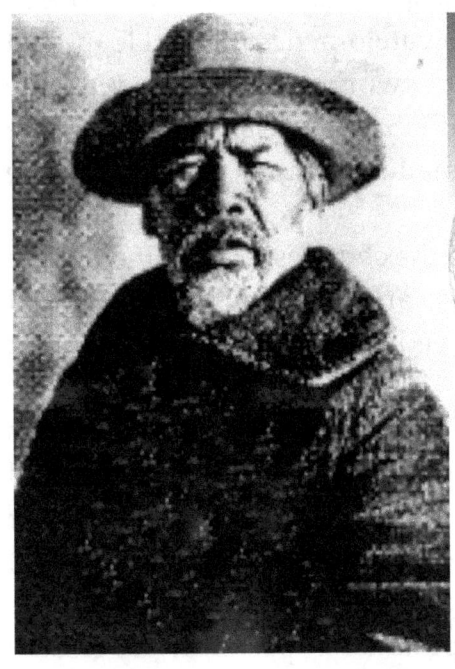

Big Mouth Charlie, 1902

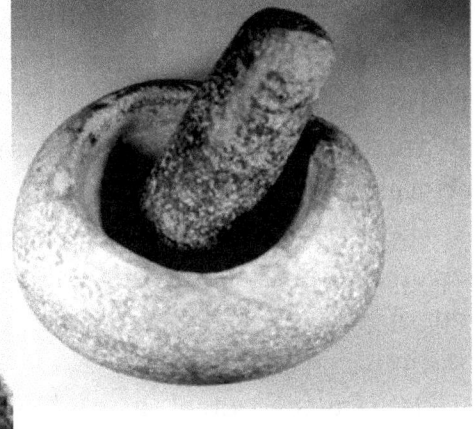

Granite Medicine Bowl
and Pestle:
ca. 12 in. diameter
(History of Medicine Museum
Exhibit)

## Nevada Indian Health Care
## A Window in Time, 1958 and 1995
### By Dr. Elwood L. Schmidt

This essay shows snapshots of windows in time of U.S. Government healthcare to the Indians of Nevada. The people we served were called Indians, a name they did not recognize as insulting, and by no means meant to be insulting.

The Bureau of Indian Affairs provided Indian healthcare until 1954-55 when Congress mandated the U.S. Public Health Service (USPHS) establish a Division of Indian Health Service (DIHS) and assume direction and staffing of the various hospitals and clinics in the continental U.S. and Alaska. The new division treated Indians and Alaska natives using primarily commissioned USPHS medical officers and some contract physicians. The total budget in 1957 was about $40,000,000.

Doctors B.A. Winne and Verlyn "Si" Elliott ably staffed the

Schurz Indian Health Service Hospital and Clinic until about 1956 when Dr. Elliott went into private practice in Ely. He moved to Fallon in 1958. Dr. Winne went to work with the Nevada State Health Department. Two USPHS physician-officers were assigned to Schurz, and they made multiple changes to the services.

The tribes, severely upset with the changes, complained to the Nevada congressional delegation, and the USPHS discharged one of the physicians and moved his colleague to another location.

Dr. James Stoetzel, a graduate of the University of Illinois Medical School, had recently completed his rotating general internship and joined the USPHS. They assigned him to Schurz to help restore service. I had served one year in Keams Canyon, Arizona, on the Hopi reservation that also provided care to the many Navajos who lived on Hopi lands in proximity to Keams Canyon. My commanding officer recommended me to the area headquarters as being congenial and able to work well with the Indian people.

As a result I was sent to Schurz to reestablish the tribes' trust in the USPHS and Schurz personnel. I reported to duty July 1, 1958, as Medical Officer-in-Charge.

Dr. Stoetzel and I established a fine working relationship at the office and hospital and resumed hours and services much as Dr. B.A. Winne and Dr. Si Elliott had provided.

Walter Voorhees of Schurz was the inter-tribal council chairman at the time. He helped by connecting me to most of the groups served by Schurz. We traveled to Nixon, Yerington, Fallon, and the Reno-Sparks colony to reassure them of our renewed services and commitment to their needs. Retrospectively, we were limited in our services because patients had to travel to Schurz to be seen by a physician for most non-emergency services. The clinics in Fallon, Yerington, and Nixon were either non-existent or only occasionally staffed. Tribal medical services in Winnemucca were provided in Owyhee by the other USPHS facility in the state.

In Schurz, we delivered pregnant women and cared for them 1-5 days postpartum. We did 4-6 tonsillectomies on the day set aside for procedures. We brought patients to Schurz Indian Health Service Hospital from Hawthorne, Yerington, Fallon, Carson City, Lovelock, and Reno hospitals if their stay was expected to be more than a day or two. These patients were usually post op from an appendectomy, cholecystectomy, or C-section. Also a significant number were post trauma victims from fights, auto accidents or other mishaps. Our ambulance and crew transported the patients to Schurz.

Stewart Indian School in Carson City was fully functioning at the time. One day a week Dr. Stoetzel or I would go to Carson City and do physical exams on the Indian Health Service (IHS) students.

Frequently, we discovered unexpected pregnancies and other situations in need of treatment. We also admitted students who needed tonsillectomies according to the standards of the time. The day-to-day needs of the students were served by Miss Hershey RN, a seasoned and well-respected nurse who helped guide neophyte physicians who were her putative supervisors.

A contract physician in Carson City saw students in need of more care than Miss Hershey or our weekly visits could offer.

He, name unremembered, was cordial and helpful to our service, even inviting us to the Carson Medical Society meetings several times. This attitude of cooperation was not universal. Many of the physicians in the area were dismissive of physicians who would work for the government. They also resented Indian patients who had little sense of time for office hours, for proper use of hospital facilities, and for whom they had to fill out a small form for reimbursement. In 1958-59, and for several years afterward, patients were responsible for paying their own bills. If they had insurance, they were expected to file the claim, but they were still responsible for payment.

How quaint that seems now that every medical office provides staff to submit third party claims and arrange referrals, etc.

A problem that vexed all Indian stations was determination of eligibility for service. Who was an Indian? Who certified his/her eligibility? This problem lingers to some extent to this day.

We were responsible for services to Indians living at Moapa and Reese River. My trip to Moapa was depressing because of the general lack of sanitation used by the people and their general sense of hopelessness and unwillingness to work with the Clark County Health Department. I visited the Reese River Reservation accompanied by a dedicated state public health nurse in the spring of 1959.

Miss Hershey administered immunizations and tuberculin skin testing on students at the school. A married couple taught at the school. New western style houses had been erected 2-3 years previously and looked fine at first, but a closer look showed most interior walls had been breached as the inhabitants wanted different passageways.

Our patient mix included a small but significant number of people with tuberculosis, several people with grand mal seizures, very few patients with diabetes, and a scattering of the other maladies that a general medical practioneer of the time would see, e.g. rashes, upper respiratory infections (URI), seasonal allergies, hypertension, gonorrhea, digestive problems, and significant seasonal diarrhea.

Alcoholism was our biggest problem, as many of the trauma cases, infants with malnutrition, and patients with cirrhosis were alcohol related.

We had no effective means to address this problem, except in a limited, case-by-case basis and some use of Antabuse to help maintain sobriety for the short term.

Medicines we had available included Dilantin and

phenobarbital for seizures; penicillin, streptomycin, tetracycline, erythromycin, and sulfonamides (I recall triple sulfa) were our antimicrobials. Chloramphenicol was available but not used because of the fear of its side effects. Isoniazid for tuberculosis, Reserpine and Apresoline for hypertension, whole leaf digitalis and I think digitoxin for heart failure were in our pharmacy. Priscoline for peripheral vasodilation, Demerol and morphine for pain, Nembutal, Seconal, and chloral hydrate for sedation, Thorazine for psychosis and as an antiemetic, Dramamine for nausea, Benadryl for allergy, adrenalin for anaphylaxis, and insulin for diabetes completed our drugs. We used ether, by drip and then intubation with ventilation for anesthesia for tonsillectomies.

Mr. Christensen, a Washoe Indian, was our X-ray and laboratory technician. Lab tests were limited as was true of lab tests in civilian practice at the time. Complete blood counts (CBCs) performed by hand and electrolytes were sent off but were out of date by the time results were available. A blood urea nitrogen (BUN) a kidney function test was available. I don't recall but protein bound iodine (PBI), a chemical test for thyroid function, might have been in general use. Mr. Chris, as he was fondly and respectfully known, continued in Schurz until 1974 or 1975 when he retired.

I am sure many of our patients used traditional medicines, herbs, ceremonies, for treatment of their ailments, but unfortunately, I did not know of their practices.

In 1995, I returned to Nevada and had the good fortune to be *locum tenens* for the PHS in northern Nevada by treating patients in Fallon, Yerington, and Gardnerville clinics. Schurz by this time was only an outpatient facility.

The convenience to the population served, the testing, and medications available at that time was truly amazing.

In this limited group, I saw much less alcoholism and its effects. I saw much, much more diabetes and hypertension. It appears the tribes have recognized and addressed the problem of alcohol and spousal abuse, and the need for much more mental health services.

## "Never use your Gun for a Baseball Bat"

A most memorable patient was a Reno-Sparks Colony member who, with a fellow tribesman, went rabbit hunting at Stead AFB. He shot a rabbit but found it still alive.

He held his double barrel shotgun like a baseball bat and swung the butt at the rabbit. The other barrel of his gun discharged with the muzzle against his left upper abdomen. His great good fortune occurred when the MPs from Stead AFB, already on the way to evict the trespassers, arrived on the scene almost immediately and raced him to Reno.

Dr. Gil Lenz was standing by and immediately set to work to repair and/or remove his spleen, left kidney, large bowel, and part of his stomach, plus repair a large skin defect in the abdominal wall. He was transferred to the Schurz Hospital for care, most particularly of his skin graft, and we confiscated the alcohol and various other psychoactive drugs his hunting buddy smuggled to him on weekly visits.

## "A Rock and Roll Delivery"

One night I was in the delivery room with a patient ready to deliver. I had my left hand on the perineum and my right hand on the baby's head. Suddenly the patient was several inches away from me and to the side, my stool was moving, and the patient was moving. There was a rumbling sound, and I was disoriented for a second. One of the nurses said, "Earthquake!"

I finally managed to stabilize myself in contact with the patient and deliver the baby with no "drops" involved. Several days later I went to Yerington to assist on a hydrocele repair in their newly built operating room (OR), proudly billed as earthquake proof. When we left the OR at completion of the procedure, we found an excited group of staff asking, "Did you feel it? Wasn't that a big one?" We had been totally unaware of the earthquake in the OR.

## HEALING ARTS OF NATIVE AMERICANS
## By Dr. Anton Sohn

The health of North American natives was probably better off before their country was invaded by Europeans. Life was harsh in the Great Basin and starvation a threat during the harsh, cold winters, but the inhabitants were free of the many diseases that killed thousands in Europe, Africa, and Asia. This article and future ones will deal with how the American Indians treated native diseases as well as diseases brought to this country.

Nine tribal groups roamed the Great Basin, and each had its unique practices when dealing with illness. The nine groups, anthropologists recognize in the Intermountain West. Are Western Shoshone, Northern Shoshone/Bannock, Eastern Shoshone, Ute, Southern Paiute, Kawaiisu, Owens Valley Paiute, Northern Paiute, and Washoe. Although these nine groups had distinct and separate practices, they dealt with disease in a similar fashion. They not only respected each other's practices, they borrowed from each other.

The Native Indian's health system dealt with health, disease, mental illness, and rites of passage—birth, naming, puberty, and old age. Various individuals in the tribe had their place in this coordinated and coherent system that had a rich, strongly conservative tradition.

The women of the tribe oversaw menstrual rites and the birth process. On occasion a shaman might be called during a difficult birth. The men were concerned with hunting and the passage of young men into the warrior class. On a more profound level, medicine men accompanied the war parties for religious and medical needs. The cause and treatment of diseases of the American Indian were a complex combination of medicine and religion. A healthy individual had a harmonious relationship with the supernatural, while disease was a disturbance of this balance. Healing brought about in one of several manners, reestablished the balance. In the Great Basin there were three classes of health providers: the herbalist, the medicine man, and the shaman.

The herbalist treated minor ailments such as broken bones, minor trauma, indigestion, etc. He or she mixed concoctions and had knowledge of plants and herbs. In some tribes they practiced bloodletting.

On another level was the medicine man who had some power in his curing activities, but his powers were considerably less than the shaman who healed in deep trances and went on soul journeys to rescue the soul of his patient. Modern medicine would recognize the shaman as a psychotherapist. All Great Basin tribal groups used these healers in a similar manner, but there were subtle differences.

## WESTERN SHOSHONE MEDICINE

The Western Shoshone occupied the largest territory extending from the depths of arid Death Valley and adjacent Panamint Mountains to the north to the Idaho border and east to include the Great Salt Lake. Most of this area was sparely inhabited and, in fact, was the last area in the United States where settlers and the U.S. Army displaced the resident native Americans. Forts Halleck and Ruby were in the western half of the Western Shoshone land.

The Western Shoshone practiced medicine on two levels—curing supernatural disease by the shaman and treating other diseases by the herbalist. Most injury and common minor illness were not considered to be caused by a supernatural phenomenon and were treated with herbs and home remedies like folk medicine as it was practiced by non-native settlers. To accomplish this task, various members of the tribe gathered the plants during the appropriate seasons, dried them and pulverized them for later use.

Several plants used in modern pharmacology, for example ephedra, were used by Great Basin Indians. Of all the native American groups in the Great Basin, the Western Shoshone had the greatest knowledge of plants and their medicinal uses. Furthermore, they carefully guarded their identification.

In contrast, the Washoe Indians had little knowledge of herbs and traded for them with neighboring Indian tribes. To illustrate the extent of the Western Shoshone's knowledge of herbal medicine: 52 plants were used for upper-respiratory disease, 57 for venereal disease, 44 for swelling, 34 for diarrhea, 37 for rheumatism, and 48 for stomach disorders.

Most serious illnesses among the Western Shoshone required treatment by a medicine man. Some medicine men healed in a light trance while others became more deeply entranced. Only in a deep trance could the shaman leave his body, become ecstatic, and rescue the soul of the sick person who was usually suffering from a disease with altered consciousness such as a coma or delirium.

The shaman was either a generalist with general curing ability or a specialist who was known to cure a specific disease such as a rattlesnake bite. This power was usually acquired in a dream in which the shaman saw himself curing a patient with a specific problem.

Central to medical practice of the shaman was the concept that disease was caused by the intrusion of an object within the body. The Shoshone believed an arrow-shooting dwarf caused disease. Therefore, the shaman healed by sucking out a foreign object such as stick or blood and displaying the object for all to see.

Each shaman in the Western Shoshone tribe practiced the sucking or healing ritual in his distinct and unique manner. In one healing ritual the shaman piled sagebrush around a fire pit and placed the sick person on a pile of sage. The shaman sang and meditated, and then placed his mouth on the diseased area and sucked out the pain. If the illness was more serious the shaman gave a longer treatment with chanting and singing, fasting, making sacrifices, and more important, he used sacred eagle feathers.

In another healing ceremony, the native American shaman drew lines with a sacred diatomaceous rock on his patient and instructed the patient to go to the river early the next day to sprinkle water, pray, and make a sacrifice.

In addition, disease could be due to a transgression or the soul leaving the body. Laying on hands was also an important part of the ritual. This practice is like the Christian practice of healing by laying-on-of-hands, an important psychological factor in healing.

The Western Shoshone also believed evil medicine doctors or sorcerers practiced witchcraft and caused disease. A shaman who refused to treat a patient or who failed to invoke a cure was considered evil.

If a healing ceremony did not produce a cure, the fee was returned. On a much more serious level there was an unwritten law that if a shaman lost three patients he should die—malpractice punishment at its extreme.

At Fort Ruby near Elko, Nevada, a shaman lost his third patient, and members of the Shoshone Tribe decided to kill him. Mr. Wines, a pioneer 19th century rancher who was trusted, called them together and informed them he would send for the soldiers if they murdered the shaman. A compromise was reached, the Shoshones returned to their wikiups with a guarantee from the shaman that he would give up the practice of medicine.

In addition to shamanism and herbs, the Western Shoshone believed in hydrotherapy. Since ancient times, they used water from medicine springs in eastern Ruby Valley to cure various ailments. On occasion, family groups camped near the springs to use its curative water. If necessary, they carried the spring water to distant camps for use.

Hydrotherapy also had advocates among nineteenth century Euro-Americans. Genoa, the earliest settlement in Nevada, had Genoa Hot Springs where its waters cured rheumatic, cutaneous, and scrofulous affections. The spring, a short distance south of Carson City, offered hot or cold mud and vapor baths supervised by a physician who helped the healing process along with proper drugs and concoctions.

Another form of hydrotherapy involved the use of the sweat house by the medicine shaman.

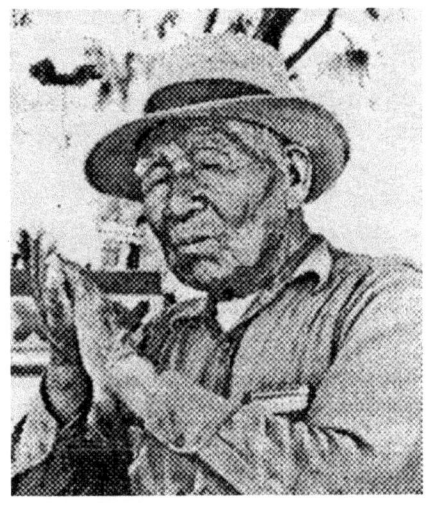

Shaman Johnny Shoshone

A small brush hut was made air-tight with mud and the shaman placed the patient inside. Water thrown on hot rocks produced steam while the shaman, with an assistant, sang and smoked a pipe. Sometimes, he buried the disease beneath hot rocks, at other times he buried it in ashes under a fire by thrusting his bare hands through the hot ashes, thereby producing a cure. Again, there are similarities in western culture. North European cultures used the Finnish sauna or steam room for healing or cleansing of the body. The difference between native American sweat houses and the old-world sauna is that the former stressed cleansing of the soul or spirit while the latter stressed cleansing the body.

## SOUTHERN PAIUTE MEDICINE

The territory of the Southern Paiute extended from a corner of California across southern Nevada, southern Utah and into northern Arizona. Many of the Southern Paiute's medical practices were the same as the other Great Basin tribes: disease-object-intrusion, soul-loss, sorcery, and power-from-dreams. To remove a disease producing object, the shaman lay beneath the patient and removed the object by sucking. Both Southern Paiute and Northern Shoshone used chanting, drums, and dancing by the medicine man in the healing ceremony. Various paraphernalia used by the medicine doctor was contained in his medicine pouch. Although most were crude or simple items—a cane, body paint, eagle claw, deer dewclaw, pipe, rattle, or even a stone—that gave great power to the healer and were indicative of supernatural powers.

Tobacco, when smoked by the Native American was used for ritualistic, medicinal, and religious purposes. Limited to small amounts on infrequent occasions, it is doubtful there were any harmful effects to the natives who inhaled the smoke through their noses.

It remained for the new immigrants to abuse and spread the tobacco habit throughout the world. The World Health Organization (WHO) estimates approximately 750 million individuals will have significant health problems from the use of cigarettes. This is true revenge for the introduction of the many infectious diseases by the new inhabitants to the native Americans.

## KAWAIISU MEDICINE

The Kawaiisu placed magic and curative powers in the use of tobacco. Kawaiisu, located totally within California in a small area on the southwestern edge of the Great Basin, were more closely associated with their California neighbors than with the Great Basin tribes. Two species of tobacco grew in their area: *Nicotiana attenuata*, native of the Great Basin, and *N. bigelovii*, native to California. Mixtures of these tobaccos and herbs were believed to have magical and medicinal powers. They were used both as an emetic and soporific. Externally, they relieved pain, cured skin conditions, and stopped bleeding. Like other Indians of the Great Basin, they smoked tobacco during some healing ceremonies.

The Kawaiisu used three other primary medicines: jimsonweed, nettles, and red ants. A ball of live red ants mixed with eagle down was swallowed to cure gastrointestinal, kidney and blood disorders. To cure other diseases the Kawaiisu utilized counter-irritation, a principle of treatment also used in western and oriental cultures.

Beside these forms of treatment, Kawaiisu medical practice included the use of a shaman. Their name for shaman was *huviyagadi* (one who has a song). Like other tribes of the Great Basin, laying on of hands, blowing smoke and removal of a foreign object were prominent methods in the shaman's healing process.

Owens Valley Paiute Medicine Like the Kawaiisu, the Owens Valley Paiute lived on the southwestern rim of the Great Basin in a small stable community. In their culture, the shamans had a dual role. They figured prominently in the social structure of the community and were called to give advice and to arbitrate disputes.

The practice of medicine was a more important duty, and like other Great Basin tribes, they were held accountable by the threat of death for the undesired results of disease. *The Inyo Independence* poignantly emphasized the shamans' accountability in 1876 when measles killed many in the Owens Valley Paiute community. The tribe, in turn, killed more than eighty of their medicine men and their sons for practicing witchcraft. Thus, many of the traditions died and little is known of their medical practices.

During the epidemic, Dr. Washington Matthews from nearby Fort Independence offered help, but the Owens Valley Paiute were suspicious of non-native medicine. The following year a smallpox epidemic hit the Owens Valley. By then, they would accept help, and Dr. Matthews provided vaccination. Ten years later in 1887, there were 716 Native Americans in the county, a reduction by a third of their number before military presence.

## Northern Paiute Medicine

In contrast to the stability of the Owens Valley Paiute, the Northern Paiute consisted of seminomadic groups who seasonally occupied parts of the western Great Basin in an area extending from the Owens Valley in the south, across Nevada to Oregon on the north, and west to the Humboldt River. Their territory consisted of the western half of Nevada, and in this area the Army established most of its larger military installations: Forts Churchill, Scott, McDermit, McGarry, Bidwell, Warner, and Harney together with several dozen smaller temporary encampments.

Military Surgeon George Martin Kober described some of the Northern Paiute practices at Fort Bidwell, California. Paiute used internal and external herbs, dry cupping, and scarification for some inflammatory conditions. He witnessed the application of hot, dry stones on the umbilicus to treat hysteria. The Indians treated rattlesnake bite with sucking, ligature, and a poultice of chopped lupine. These treatments were used by ordinary Indian doctors, while the shaman practiced on a higher plane, rescuing the soul. An individual could become a shaman in the Northern Paiute culture by all three of the methods used by Great Basin tribes.

Power (*puha*) to heal could be inherited from a parent (either sex) and usually deceased, (2) acquired in a dream, or (3) deliberately sought by visiting designated caves considered to hold *puha*.

After spending a night in the cave, the neophyte shaman spent two or three years in preparation, usually apprenticed to a practicing shaman to learn the secrets and methods of curing. The process of curing took two days from the time relatives of the sick person visited the shaman, usually in the morning. He smoked and meditated, then he or an assistant placed an eagle feather on a willow shaft outside the dwelling of the sick person to inhibit evil influence. That evening, the shaman placed the head of the patient and the eagle feather to the south. At dusk, he sang to acquire *puha* and sometimes he chose a person to dance throughout the night. The shaman prescribed a second night of treatment or called another shaman if the cure didn't work. The ceremony often involved the medicine doctor sucking the affected part and disposing of the disease producing object. To finish the healing process, he might prescribe food or herbs. His fee was an animal hide or beads. Which was a token to establish a relationship.

Furthermore, contrary to what many local people say, shamanism was still alive and well among the Fort Bidwell Paiutes in the late 1940s. The drumming-singing rituals were clearly audible to the white community.

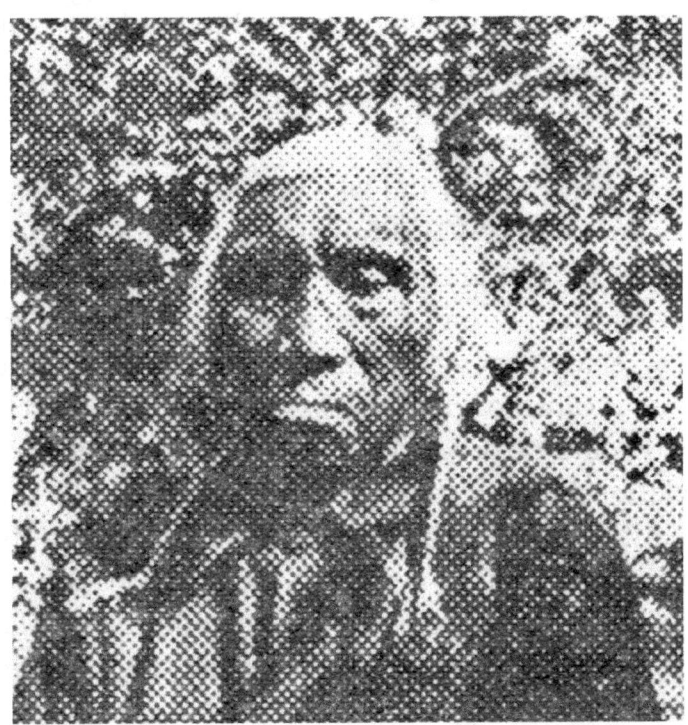

Shaman Tayoni

As with other Great Basin Indians, repeated unsatisfactory results might result in the death of the doctor. Patricia Barry whose family has lived for over a hundred years in Northern Modoc County in the village of Fort Bidwell recalls, "Sometime in the late 1800s or early 1900s, the Warner Valley-Surprise Valley Paiutes' Sing Doctor, Doc Noah, or Doc Noey, failed in a cure and lost his patient. Noah fled in fear of his life, but the patient's relatives pursued him into Warner Valley and attacked him with knives. According to the oral tradition among both Indians and whites, Noah was cut across the abdomen from hipbone to hipbone. Some whites found Noah lying alongside the road and took him to the Adel store.

"He was placed upon the store counter and some sympathetic men cleansed the wound, then proceeded to sew up the damage with a needle and sack twine. Noah recovered and lived to be a revered old man. In the end, losing the patient only added to his charisma, because no one was supposed to be able to survive an abdominal knife wound."

**WASHOE MEDICINE**

The Washoe occupied the lake area of the Sierra Nevada to the north and south of Lake Tahoe and neighboring valleys on the western slope of the Great Basin. Though they predated the other tribes in the region and belonged to a different language group, they shared many beliefs, including sorcery and object intrusion as a cause of disease. Sorcery was the cause of most disease and could be produced by evil doctors. A shaman had a special relationship with the spirit power (*wegeleyu*). The power manifested itself to an individual and it took three to five years under a senior shaman to become a shaman. Healing objects of the profession were cocoon rattles made under the guidance of a dream, eagle feathers bound with buckskin, various items such as miniature baskets, stone mortars, bird-bone whistles, tobacco pouches, and stone pipes. It also included elaborate costumes used with red and white body paint, decorative headdresses, and personal ornaments worn by the shaman.

For a healing ceremony, the family paid in advance with buckskin, ornaments, or baskets. (The Washoe were the expert basket makers of the Great Basin.) The ritual took four nights and was open to the public. With the patient's head to the west, the shaman blew smoke over the body.

He then danced and sucked the object out or blew a whistle to invoke the cure. Sometimes he passed out and then coughed up the object holding it out for all to see. The patient was washed and rubbed with sage. At the end of the cure, a feast was held. If the patient was not cured or died the pay was returned. They then hired another shaman to neutralize the sorcery of the first shaman. If too many patients died after treatment, they killed him.

## UTE MEDICINE

The Great Basin territory of the Ute comprised a small part of the middle of Utah, extending south of the Great Salt Lake. Most of their territory extended further east into Colorado. Utes, like the other Great Basin tribes, relied on shamans for treatment of serious illness. Thus, there was a strong reliance on the supernatural as a cause and treatment for disease. Also, like their Great Basin neighbors, the Utes permitted both men and women to practice as shamans. For less serious disease members of the tribe were treated with herbs and concoctions.

**NOTE:**

Washoe lived in the Great Basin for at least 6,000 years—since 4000 BC. (ref. Wikipedia/Washoe People). This description of the medical practices of the various tribes of the Great Basin demonstrates many similar practices. Their white neighbors also borrowed from them. Some of their herbs, such as valerian, ephedra, and ergot, have been incorporated into the modern pharmacopeia. Chemical analysis has found pharmacologically active ingredients and led to isolation and synthesis of related compounds. In a new industry, "chemical prospecting," current researchers are studying plants in the Great Basin that were used by native inhabitants. Ronald Pardini PhD, at the University of Nevada School of Medicine investigated the antineoplastic properties of the Greasewood or creosote bush (*genus Larrea*). This plant is the oldest known plant form growing in the southern Great Basin.

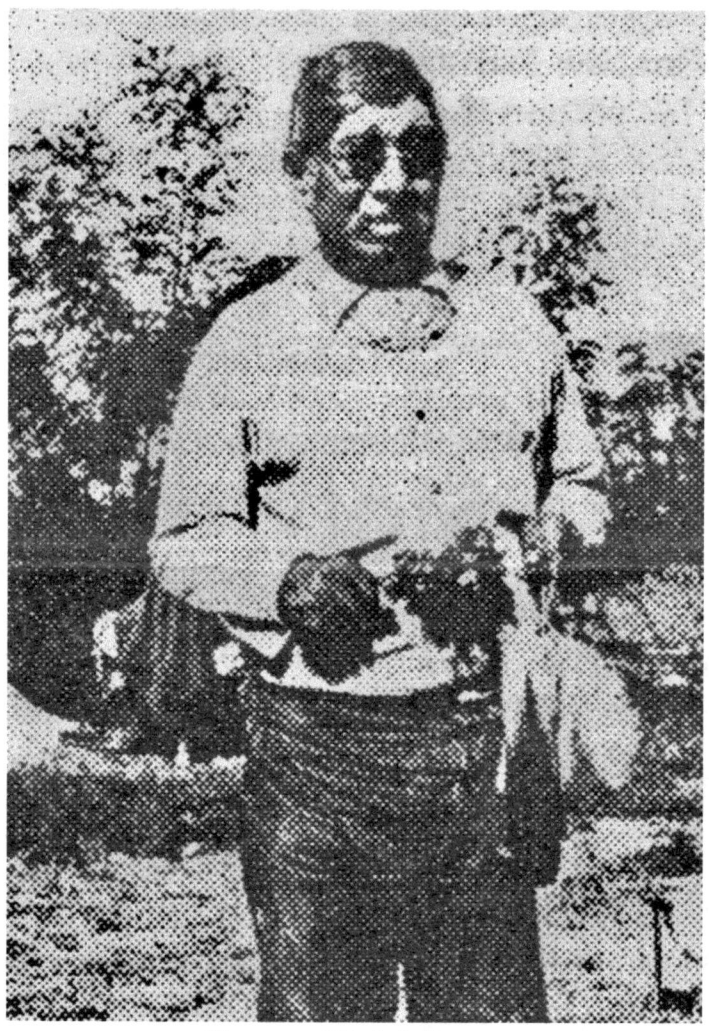

Shaman Dick Mawee
with Doctoring Paraphernalia

The herbal methods used by the Native American Doctor worked for many diseases. Conversely, many cures sold to the American public by doctors or purveyors of patent medicine in the nineteenth century had no efficacy. Also, Native American medicine placed a strong emphasis on the psychology of healing, a potent ingredient in the healing process.

With some exceptions, such as techniques in surgery and vaccinations, the Native American shaman provided a service to his patient that compared favorably to medicine delivered to the average American during "Frontier Days" in the West.

# II

# AMERICAN DOCTORS
## "FIRST DO NO HARM" HIPPOCRATES
## "PRIMUM NON NOCERE" AD 275

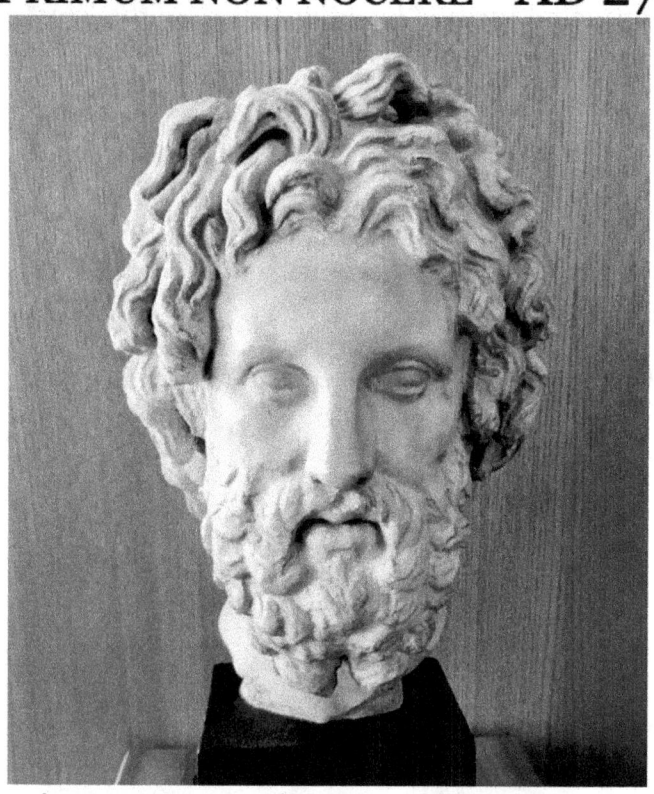

*ASCLEPIUS, GOD OF MEDICINE*
(EXHIBITED IN THE GREAT BASIN
HISTORY OF MEDICINE MUSEUM)

## Dr. Frederick Hiller, Virginia City, 1866-67
### Kitchen Table Surgery and Neurosurgery

Alfred Doten, August 22, 1866: "This PM I assisted Dr. Frederick Hiller to operate on a leg of John Tookey or Tuohig, which was broken in the Ophir Mine some 5 weeks ago. Dr. Wakeman Bryarly has had the case and discharged the patient. Dr. Hiller was sent for—right leg not set at all—we sawed off the end of tibia and picked out lots of small pieces–5 or 6. Sawed off about an inch–set leg in iron frame prepared for it, fixed up and left it–took just two hours to do the job–may lose leg yet–very bad job to undertake–All done under chloroform <u>on the kitchen table</u>.

"I went with Dr. C.C. Green and helped him to perform an operation on the head of Mr. C.R. Gates—Near Summit Mill—He was hit with a stone playfully thrown at him, at American Flat some eight months ago—has hurt him ever since—Dr. now raised his scalp just over the left temple and took out several small pieces of bone and some granulations that had formed, sewed up wound, and put him to bed—He stood it like a major, taking no chloroform–suffered much pain however—Dr. gave me $5.00 for assisting him—I put item in the paper about it—"

**NOTE:**
Information from *Journals of Alfred Doten, 1849-1903*, edited by Walter Van Tilburg Clark, University of Nevada Press, 1983. Joseph Lister published his landmark article, *On a new method of treating compound fractures, Abscesses, etc.* (with antisepsis) in *Lancet* between March and July 1867. It is unlikely that antisepsis was practiced in Virginia City in August 1866.

## Dr. Vinton A. Muller (1892-1975)
### Nevada's First Blood Transfusion, 1920

### By Dr. Anton Sohn

Dr. Vinton A. Muller writes in his brief biography about performing a blood transfusion, which he felt was the first ever done in Nevada. Dr. Muller, the son of a pioneer physician in Nevada City, California, and a 1917 graduate of the University of California School of Medicine in San Francisco, took his surgical training under Chairman Dr. Wallace I. Terry.

Dr. Vinton Muller opened a surgical practice in Reno in 1920. Soon after he had arrived in Reno, Dr. Muller gave a paper on blood transfusion at a meeting of the Washoe County Medical Society. A short time later, he received a call from Dr. James Wiggins Gerow in Verdi, asking him to treat a woman who was critically ill from a post-partum hemorrhage. Dr. Muller packed up his Kelley bottle set, some group II and group III typing serum (in those days blood was classified according to the Moss Classification), his microscope, hanging drop slides, and all the other equipment that might be needed. Rushing along in his Stutz Automobile (one of two in Reno), he drove to Verdi on the only road, which at that time was south of the Truckee River. He typed the patient's blood, and then tested three of her relatives before finding a suitable donor. Using #6 needles on the patient and #8 needles on the donor, he performed the transfusion. The entire procedure required between four and five hours and was successful.

**NOTE**

Although various forms of transfusion had been attempted off and on for some 600 years, it wasn't until Karl Landsteiner's discovery of the four major blood types: A, B, AB, and O in 1901 that there was a scientific basis for transfusion of whole blood. Dr. Vinton Muller was a founder of Reno Surgical Society and president of Nevada State Medical Association. He died in Reno in February 1975.

## 1939 CARLIN CANYON TRAIN WRECK
### By Dr. Leslie A. Moren

It must have been just after 1o:30 PM on the evening of August 12, 1939, because I can remember the folks were just coming out of the movie theater when we got the word there had been a train wreck west of Elko.

The wreck involved S.P.'s Stream Liner, *The City of San Francisco,* which had roared through Elko west-bound only an hour or so earlier. I had only been in practice in Elko for about a year, having graduated from the University of Minnesota in 1938, so I really hadn't had very much experience in the care of trauma patients. As the youngest man in the group of Drs. Hood, Roantree and Secor, I was on weekend call as usual. Dr. R.P. Roantree was on vacation that week, so we were already shorthanded.

Dr. Hood (A.J. Hood II) called me by telephone informing me of the accident and asked me to assemble whatever emergency supplies and equipment I could gather and meet him at the railroad station in Carlin, 21 miles west of Elko.

In Carlin, a relief train was being made up since the site of the wreck could not be reached by road. I really didn't know just what supplies to bring along, but took my stethoscope, a sphygmomanometer, morphine, and lots of bandages, together with some bass wood splint material, which turned out to be very useful. We carried flashlights. It was a very dark night.

In Carlin, I met Dr. A.J. Hood II and Dr. Fred Poulson, who was another young physician practicing in Elko. Dr. Charles Secor, the senior member of our group, stayed in Elko to care for things there. The relief train which had been assembled in Carlin consisted of cabooses, pulled behind the locomotive. It had to proceed westward on the east bound track since the west bound tracks had been blocked by the wreckage. The east bound tracks was 1/4 mile away from the wreck, so we had to walk cross country in the dark to reach the scene.

The situation at the site of the wreck was horrifying. The derailment had occurred just as the train was crossing a trestle across the Humboldt River. Fourteen of the train's 17 cars had left the tracks, with Pullman cars strewn everywhere—on their sides, up-ended, across the tracks and in the canyon. The Club car was lying on its side, partially submerged in the river.

The impression that remains etched in my memory now, some 50 years later, is of the darkness lit only by the feeble light of a few flashlights, and the silence broken only by distant moans and cries for help.

I remember a young woman dressed in a pretty-blue gown. Both of her legs were gone, and she had long since exsanguinated.

Crossing the river, I remember seeing the arm of a porter wearing a white jacket protruding from a window of the club car. He had been trapped beneath the waters of the river and was, of course, dead of drowning.

We did whatever we could at the scene; bandaging wounds, splinting fractures, and administering opiates.

With the help of many volunteers from Elko and Carlin, we extricated the injured from the wreckage and carried them to the relief train for transport to the Elko General Hospital.

The choice of the caboose cars for the relief train was a poor one, for when we tried to carry the litter onto the car, we found the safety railings on the ends of the cars made it necessary to negotiate a sharp 90º turn into the door at the end of the car.

Twenty-three persons were pronounced dead at the scene, and 69 injured were transported to Elko General Hospital for care. Since the hospital only had 52 beds, and 35 beds were already occupied, it was necessary to put many of the injured on spare beds and mattresses in the hallways. A surgeon from San Francisco, Dr. Ward, who was visiting friends in the Elko area, volunteered his help, and the operating room was busy for some 24 hours. As I recall, we only lost one patient after arrival to the hospital. I think was a person with crushing injuries of the chest and could not be stabilized. Not a bad record for a bunch of county doctors!

The locomotive engineer, who survived the wreck, reported

the train had been travelling at about 70 mph. when the accident occurred. He had walked from the scene to get assistance, which accounted for a delay of almost one hour before help was sent. Investigators later determined the accident was caused by a missing tie plate. The Federal Bureau of Investigation stated it had been an act of sabotage and posted a $5,000 reward for the person or persons who caused the wreck. However, they were never found.

## Dr. Mary Fulstone's Recollections in Smith, Nevada

"I was married my last year when I was in medical school in San Francisco, and then, I came up here and moved to this house and have been here ever since, fifty-three years. When I came up here it was kind of nice because they'd never had a doctor here before. So, there was no discrimination between a woman and a man doctor.

"I think they were so happy to have a doctor right in the community. Before I arrived, they had to send to Yerington for a doctor.

"And you know that was a horse and buggy drive up here, which was kind of long, and they had all gone through that influenza epidemic without having a doctor here. I think they were very happy, because there were a good many deaths and very serious illnesses, and they were happy to have one. But of course, there were probably some who think, 'Oh, a woman doctor, how terrible!' (Laughs)

"But I always said the Indian people were my saviors. They took to me right away; that is, they were going to try me out right away. So many of them worked on our ranch right here.

"In those days, before we had 'new' ranch machinery, you know, you'd have twenty men working, where maybe now there'd be five. And they all came and got little things—cuts and bruises and sickness. So they took to me right away and I always said, 'Well, I think they were good advertisers.' (Dr. Mary

Laughing) And I have been very friendly with the Indians, with the Indian population here throughout the years.

"I have (had) lots of funny experiences. I was even asked to consult with an Indian medicine man at one time, which was quite an idea. I went up to the camp and walked in and the room was all decorated in different things, like little feathers and a little bow and arrow and things like that.

"The patient had a little band on her head and a feather or two up. And we had a consultation, the Indian medicine man and me. He said, 'Well, I thought it might be well to consult with you because I could help you a little bit by telling you what the Indians took as laxatives and things like that, you know.'

And I said, "Oh, I think you could, you'll be a great help. We had quite a little conversation. Come to find out, he was an Indian man that had worked on this very ranch and just lately, had gone into being an Indian medicine man.

"I travelled all around this area. In the beginning I used to go to Bridgeport, Coleville, Sweetwater, and all around. In fact, I had a contract for a while with the government in taking care of those patients. I got to know them very well. We became great friends.

"But one little story—I went up to Sweetwater one night to deliver a baby.

They said this woman was having a great deal of trouble having her baby.

"Indians usually didn't have a doctor when they had their children. They seemed to get along all right. But this baby was a cross presentation and an arm had come down in the deliverance area.

"The other Indian woman had been pulling on the arm, you know, thinking if they pulled hard enough, they'd get the baby out, not realizing that they couldn't do it. So finally they sent for me. The baby was dead, of course, but I went up.

"It was—we'd been away someplace and had just come back; it was quite late in the night Fred drove me up, and here she was in a little tent, you know, right on their little beds (which) were always on the floor. So we had to get one of the neighbors up and get a kitchen table and get her up on that. So, I had one Indian woman giving a few drops of ether to kind of ease off the pain, two other Indian women kind-of assisting me. And those two Indian women kept saying, 'Now Mary, you wouldn't leave us, would you? You're going to stay here, aren't you? You wouldn't go away and leave us?' And I said, 'No, I wouldn't leave.' The sweat was rolling down; I was working hard.

"The other Indian woman kept saying, 'Do you think you can make it; do you think you're going to get the baby; do you think you can make it?' So finally, anyway, after quite a long siege, I got the baby delivered and the woman back in her bed and comfortable. I was just terrified that she'd have an infection, but she got better.

"Finally, about two months later, we were having dinner out here and there was a rap on the door of my office and the housekeeper went. She opened the door and there was a big, tall Indian there and she says, 'Oh you want to see Dr. Mary.' He says, 'No, I want to see Fred Fulstone.'

"And so Fred went to the door and the Indian man said, 'Oh, hello Fred,' and Fred said, 'Hello.' He says, 'Oh, Fred, your wife came up and took care of my wife and now she's all better, and I've come down to pay you. Now what do you charge?' (Laughing) That was one of my best stories."

**NOTE:**

This story was abstracted from an oral history by Mary Ellen Glass, between July 5, 1973, and February 7, 1974. The title is *Recollections of a Country Doctor in Smith, Nevada*.

## DR. MARY FULSTONE, NEVADA'S DOCTOR FOR THE AGES
### By Dr. Anton Sohn

Dr. Mary was a full-time physician, but she was also a full-time housewife. Exactly when she first met Fred Fulstone is not mentioned in the book, but his family had been in the territory since 1858. Mary and Fred married in 1919, a year before she finished her medical training. Fred understood his wife's demanding schedule and helped with household chores in addition to becoming a leading rancher in Smith Valley. Fred and Dr. Mary Fulstone eventually had five children.

In the early 1950s, Congress passed the Hill-Burton Act, which made money available to remodel, enlarge, and build new hospitals. Most of Nevada's hospitals were recipients of Hill-Burton Funds, and they provided an opportunity to construct a new Lyon County Hospital. County bonds provided $150,000, and the federal government came up with the rest of the money to build the $350,000 hospital, but there is no question Dr. Mary was the driving force behind the campaign to build the hospital and improve healthcare in her community.

Besides serving the hospital in various capacities, Dr. Mary was active in the community and state. Civic duty was a way of life for the busy physician.

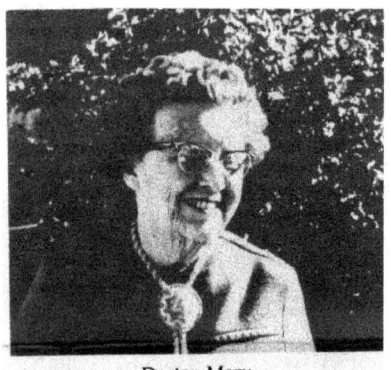
Dr. Mary Fulstone, 1987

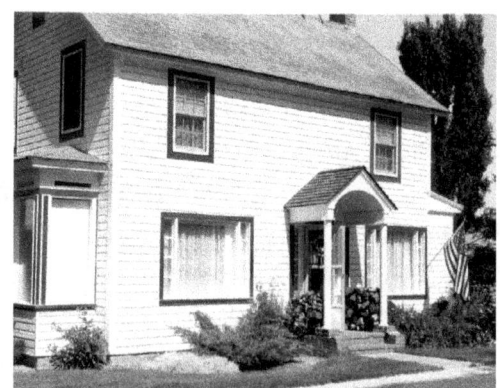
Residence and Office

**NOTE:**
Sierra Pathology Associates did all surgical pathology for Smith Valley Hospital, and I was assigned to visit the hospital's clinical laboratory once a month. On each visit, Dr. Mary asked me to make rounds with her on patients. She introduced me as a

"Consultant" from Reno.

On occasion, I visited her office and clinic in her home. Each fall Dr. Mary hosted a turkey shoot on her farm. I have lots of memories attending the event with my family. It was my honor to be pallbearer at Dr. Mary's funeral.

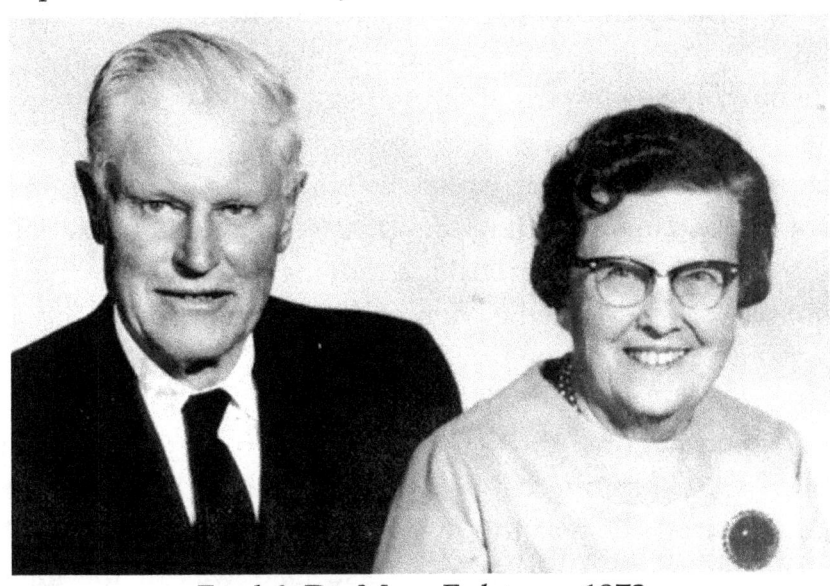
Fred & Dr. Mary Fulstone, 1973
(Great Basin History of Medicine Achieves)

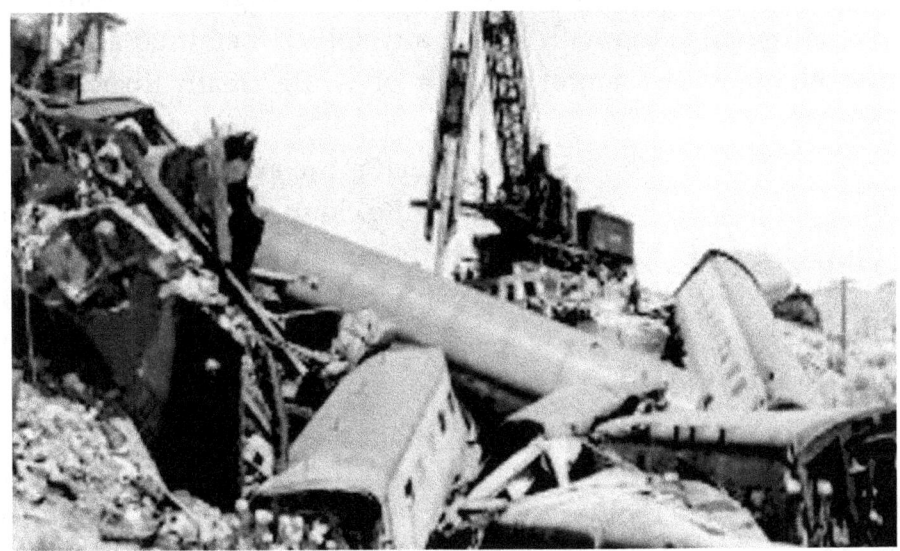
1939 Carlin Canyon Train Wreck

## Dr. James W. Gerow
## "Call in Indian Country"
## By Dr. Lynn Gerow

One morning my father, Dr. James Wiggins Gerow, was awakened by a persistently ringing telephone. On the other end was the Indian agent from Nixon, Nevada, saying one of the Winnemucca squaws was about to have a baby—could he come immediately.

How my father had any responsibility for treating Indians, I do not know. However, it seems that went with the position of Washoe County physician. All the Indians in the county thought of him as "Chief Medicine Man" and every Indian in the area knew him on a first name basis.

That name was "Doc." There were many good friends in the area's Indian nations. Dad quietly awakened me and asked if I would like to help him deliver an Indian baby. I sprang out of bed as eager as if it was the first day of fishing season. While I dressed and had a hurried breakfast, Dad was in the garage steaming up his Stanley Steamer for the trip.

The Steamer was a long black seven-passenger open touring-car that moved along with ease at any speed. It emitted a hissing noise along with a small amount of white steam through its exhaust.

On cold days the steam was much more evident, and the car would sometimes appear to be a white cloud as it silently moved through traffic. One of the notable things about the car that rather fit my father's sense of humor, was that the car developed a charge of static electricity when it was being steamed up to a head of pressure sufficient to move the large pistons.

If one was in the car, he would not notice the electricity generated, but if one was standing on the ground and touched the car or put his foot on the running board, he would receive a charge of static electricity that would make all the hairs on his head stand up.

Many times, I was in the car while the boiler was being steamed and someone would pass by making smart remarks about the steam buggy. My father would call out "Hey, George, come here a minute." When the "wise-cracker" came over, he would put his foot on the running board to hear what Dr. James Wiggins Gerow had to say; all his hair would stand on end.

A shocked expression would appear which was always followed by ugly blasphemy and a loud chuckle by my father. Soon everyone in town knew it was dangerous to touch "Old Stanley" at such a time. After an hour and a half drive, we arrived at Nixon. The Indian agent directed us to an 8 x 12 white army tent. On entering, we found a young squaw, lying on a deer hide, obviously in labor.

Her *Aye, yi, yis* were heard throughout the camp with each labor pain. Surrounding her were four older squaws administering to her needs with cool sips of water, fanning with a chafing fan, giving words of encouragement and going *Aye, yi, yis* with her every contraction.

My father cleared the tent of all but one squaw and me. Following an examination to determine the stage of labor, she was given "twilight sleep" and prepared for delivery.

During the next forty minutes and many subdued *Aye, yi, yis,* Dad remarked, "Do you smell something burning?" He directed me out of the tent to investigate. About fifty yards away, the ground was mounded up along a 30-foot-long-trench and smoke was coming up through the soil. It smelled something like burning hair and fat. Several bucks were in attendance, but they were unable to tell me what was going on.

Back to the maternity ward I went. After giving my father a report, he retorted, "Burning garbage, I guess." At that moment, the baby's head came into view and a yelling baby girl was brought into the world to a happy mother. Following delivery of the after birth, the squaws were summoned into the tent to attend the needs of mother and child, which they did with much chatter and deliberation.

After leaving the tent, we were met by a group of happy men who told us they had been preparing a feast to celebrate the occasion. Directing us to the smoldering pit, we saw the men unearthing dozens of smoking, steaming puldoos. Puldoos are mud hens, which had not been dressed. The feathers remained on the skin, the entrails were in the body cavities, and the heads and webbed feet were still present.

The master of ceremonies insisted we remain for dinner to celebrate the arrival of the new princess.

My father tactfully declined stating that there was another woman in labor in Reno who needed his attention. They accepted this explanation. The "Old Stanley" was steamed up to half a head and we made a hasty getaway.

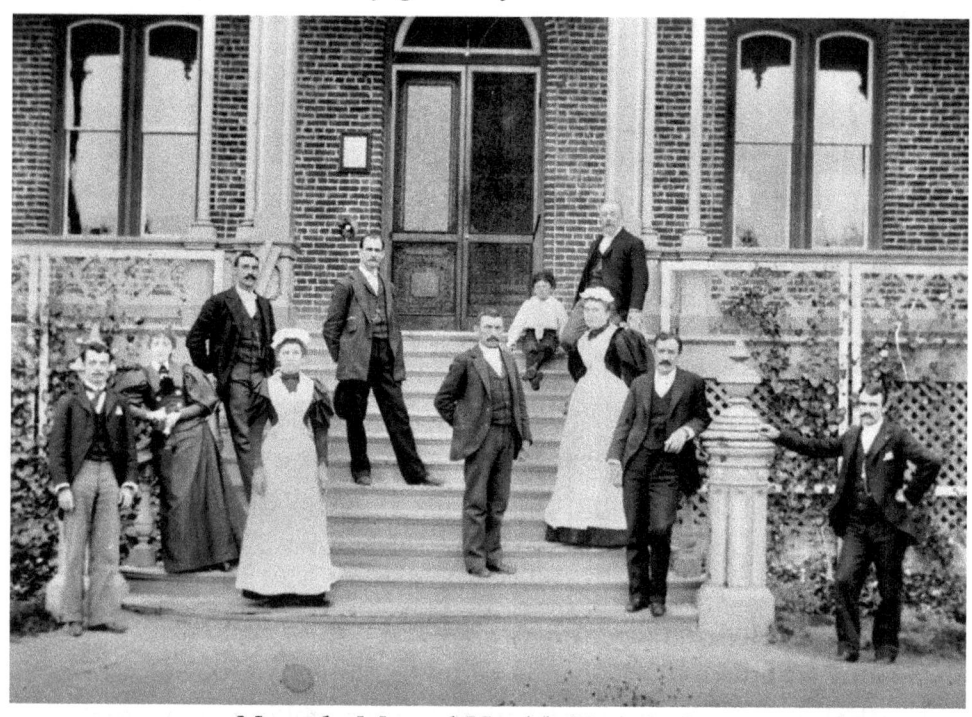

Nevada Mental Health Hospital
Sparks, Nevada, late 1890s, Back Right: Dr. Henry Bergstein

About two weeks later, a committee of Indians brought my father a gift of appreciation. There were seven arrows, the shafts made of tagemite (a reed which grows wild along the Truckee River), colorful goose feather flyers and beautiful obsidian points. Appreciation was gratefully shown, and the committee returned to Nixon. These arrows were later given to Dorothy Smith, wife of Harold Smith Sr., who displayed them in Harold's Club for several years. Mrs. Smith has since returned them to me, and they remain as one of my most cherished possessions, recalling one of my most pleasant and exciting memories.

**NOTE:**

Dr. James Wiggins Gerow, "Call in Indian Country" was taken by the late Dr. Lynn Gerow from his autobiography *First Opinion*, an unpublished manuscript given to us by his son. Dr. Lynn Gerow, Jr. The manuscript contains many other fascinating stories about life and the practice of medicine in Dr. James W. Gerow's early years.

## DR. HENRY BERGSTEIN
## 1874 NEVADA MEDICAL PRACTICE ACT

Fancy, if you will, a city surgeon accustomed to the elegance of a well-equipped hospital with its corps of trained assistants and nurses, performing operations without a single trained assistant and his patient lying-on-the-floor. Yet such was a common experience of the early surgeon in Nevada.

Having anaesthetized his patient, he handed the anesthetic to any one at hand and proceeded with his operation. Cutting an artery, he seized it with a tenaculum, or forceps, while any bystander held the instrument for the hemostatic forceps, which was unknown in those days. He proceeded to ligate it, and thus step by step, watching the patient, the anesthetic, and his unskilled assistant, he completed the operation and had a fair modicum of success, not altogether due to his skill, but more likely due to the hardy manhood he had for subjects. As for gunshot and knife wounds, no surgeon except during war times had the experience of early Nevada surgeon. Pioche in 1872 had in its graveyard one hundred and eighty denizens and only three died a natural death.

The crack of the revolver was heard, knife-wounds were seen, and to the sorrow of many surviving friends, their companions frequently died "with their boots on." The average bravo had a great horror of dying with his boots on and, when wounded, before priest or surgeon were called, his boots were pulled off.

Pioche is in Lincoln County in a ravine on the side of a mountain in the Ely range, at an elevation of 5,942 feet. The principal mines being located above the town, close to its peak, the mills for the reduction of the ores were located at Bullionville, eleven miles distant.

Owing to the absence of water at or near the mines, the latter being dry until a depth of 1,200 feet was reached, the ores containing a large amount of galena oxidized rapidly upon being exposed to air. Consequently, this led to many cases of lead colic, both in the mines and at the mills. I am, thus, particular in describing these conditions because they lead up to the first medical legislation west of the Rocky Mountains.

There was no resident physician at Bullionville, and when aid was needed, it was summoned from Pioche.

**NOTE:**

Information from *The History of Nevada*, published in 1915, chapter xxv, page 610. Dr. Bergstein ran for and was elected to the Nevada State Assembly in 1874. Because of the below events involving a pharmacist, he sponsored legislation entitled *An Act to Prevent the Practice of Medicine or Surgery by Unqualified Persons* in the 1875 Legislature.

# Dr. Henry Bergstein
## An Important Jewish Doctor in Early Nevada

Most of the information in this article is taken from research by John P. Marschall PhD, Professor Emeritus at UNR, for a book on a comprehensive history of Jews in Nevada. According to John Marschall, no physician in Nevada's early history was more influential than Dr. Henry Bergstein. His years of service to the state as a physician, legislator, organizer, and superintendent of the State Mental Hospital spanned the period from 1872 beyond 1920. Although he had left the state briefly in 1900 upon his second marriage to the widow of his political associate, Dr. C.C. Powning, he returned to Virginia where he struggled to make a living. Sam Davis called upon Bergstein to contribute his book, *History of Nevada*, with an essay on the history of medicine in the Nevada.

Dr. Bergstein was a natural choice for the project in view of his long tenure as a physician and his several administrative positions. Henry Bergstein was born in Virginia in 1847 to German speaking parents. At an early age he came west and enrolled in the Medical College of the Pacific in San Francisco. He graduated in 1872, and that same year he moved to Pioche, Nevada, where he helped form an association of physicians, which later became the Nevada State Medical Association.

It appears the primary reason for their meeting was to set or control fees. Some of the fees they agreed upon were as follows: office visits $5, night visits $10, delivery $100, and operations $100 and up.

Bergstein astutely observed most Pioche citizens died from accidents, gunshot wounds, and knife injuries. He noted that of 108 denizens in the local graveyard, only three died of natural causes.

Henry Bergstein was even more alarmed that a local druggist treated miners with quicksilver (mercury) when they presented with constipation due to lead poisoning. The druggist succeeded in giving them a quick passage to the grave. At that time there were no licensing laws in Nevada, and because of an everyman is his own doctor attitude, few of these laws had been passed anywhere in the nation. To remedy the situation, Bergstein ran for the legislature in 1874. After being elected, he moved to Virginia City in 1875 with the intent of initiating legislation to limit the practice of medicine to qualified persons, which was passed.

His law had several sections, but most importantly, it required doctors to have a diploma from a chartered medical school and have it recorded with the county recorder. Not only did Nevada not have a method to verify the diplomas, but there were no uniform requirements for medical schools in the U.S. Anyone could start a medical school and issue a diploma. Furthermore, many doctors graduated from foreign schools, which could not be verified. This included a plethora of Chinese doctors with diplomas written in Chinese script.

Governor L.R. Bradley forced through a 10-year grandfather clause that permitted unqualified doctors to continue practice.

Doctors Bergstein, John Van Zant, and Benjamin Robinson were the leaders in forming the Nevada State Medical Society, which enforced the new law. The law was short lived, as it was later declared unconstitutional by the Nevada Supreme Court.

Medical practice aside, in 1880, Bergstein married Pauline Michelson in San Francisco. Later that year he became entangled in a lawsuit with D.L. Brown, editor of *Footlight*, a Nevada newspaper, for an article that Bergstein claimed was derogatory to him as a physician. The case was dropped, but Bergstein continued to be controversial.

In 1883, he was associated with Dr. Simeon Bishop, the second superintendent of the Nevada Hospital for Indigent Insane in Sparks. He accused Bishop of misappropriation of funds.

On the political side, Dr. Bergstein was lifelong member of the

Democratic Party, but in 1892, he stepped down as chairman of the Washoe County Democratic Party to join the Silver Party.

Bergstein was instrumental in re-establishing the Nevada State Medical Society in 1894. As a result he was elected president of the society and state delegate to the American Medical Association. After 1895, the state society met regularly, and members presented scientific papers. Bergstein's contribution was a paper in 1912 on *Criminal Abortion from a Moral and Business Standpoint*.

His next controversial episode resulted after he succeeded Dr. Simeon Bishop as Superintendent of The Hospital for Indigent Insane in Sparks. Bergstein held this position from 1895 until 1898, when his term of office expired. Psychiatry was in its infancy, but Dr. Bergstein was in the forefront of humane care for the mentally ill.

He stopped the custom of placing the inmates on exhibit for the amusement of and to gratify the morbid curiosity of visitors, and he changed the name to Nevada Hospital for Mental Disease. Bergstein would have been held in high esteem for these actions, but his feisty nature continued to get him in trouble.

In 1897, Dr. Bergstein fired his business manager, who retaliated by charging him with performing unauthorized autopsies on patients, then throwing parts of their bodies in the nearby Truckee River. At a hearing of the State Mental Hospital Commission, Bergstein defended himself by arguing that the patients were deceased and without families, and what he did with their bodies made no difference. It appears from witnesses and by his statement that he disposed of human remains, including brain tissue, in the Truckee. The Board of Commissioners dismissed the charges.

By this time, his domestic life was becoming chaotic. He deserted and abandoned Pauline and divorced her two years later. She was to receive $100/month for support of their three children and a dwelling at Second and Chestnut (Arlington) in Reno.

It is now the site of St. Thomas Aquinas Cathedral. Court fights between the two would continue for years and were remarkable for Bergstein's lack of paying support. Bergstein was unable to establish a successful practice in Reno after his 1900 marriage to Clara Poor Powning, so the couple moved to San Francisco. Despite the move, financial problems continue to plague Henry. In 1907, hotelier J.M. McCormack seized his surgical instruments (worth $275) for an unpaid bill. By this time, he was separated from Clara, and he described himself as ...an old and broken man, with his earning capacity very much limited, and without any resources except his practice... He also noted his three sons had assumed the name Michelson, his ex-wife's maiden name. That year her brother, Albert, received the Nobel Prize for Physics.

Apparently, Henry was paying some alimony, but Pauline accused him of being addicted to gambling, resulting in his inability to pay support.

By 1908, Bergstein was practicing again in Reno, and the 1910 census listed him as widowed. His private life difficulties apparently did not damage his professional reputation, and he became prominent in Nevada's medical circles.

Dr. Henry Bergstein responsibilities included Reno City Physician, Reno City Health Inspector, and member of the Reno City Board of Health. His knowledge and position in the medical community prompted Davis to ask him to write Nevada Medical History which was published in 1913. In 1920, Doctor Henry Bergstein was practicing at 117 North Virginia, but in 1921, there is no mention of him in the city telephone directory. Apparently, he died in 1920 or 1921, but there is no record of his death in Nevada vital statistics.

## Dr. Laurence D. Nelson
### Adventure in the High Sierra, 1951-'52

## By Dr. Owen Bolstad

During the winter of 1951-52, a fierce storm hit the Sierra Nevada. Recorded at Donner Summit, the temperature was near zero. It snowed heavily for almost a month. Winds were over 100 miles per hour and snow had completely blocked U.S. highway #40. The little town of Truckee had been snowbound for some time.

On Sunday morning January 13, 1952, the west bound streamliner, *The City of San Francisco*, an extra-fare luxury train carrying 226 passengers plus its crew, became stalled west of Donner Summit in a snow avalanche. Many of the passengers aboard the train were delegates to the National Republican Convention, which was to be held in San Francisco the following week. Rescue units with rotary snowplows were dispatched. Rotary plows sent to rescue the train were stalled or broken down. Passengers aboard the snowbound streamliner passed the first night in relative comfort with heat provided by the diesel engines and with plenty of food on board the dining car. There was no panic, and most regarded the adventure as a lark, confident they would soon be rescued.

On Monday afternoon, Dr. Laurence D. Nelson was asked if he would try to reach the scene to assist those aboard, and Nelson readily agreed. After a brief prayer, Nelson donned his winter clothing, grabbed his medical bag, and set out. An ambitious 29-year-old, healthy and confident, he felt up to the challenge. He went into Truckee and contacted Lloyd VanSykle, a well-known dog sled racer. VanSykle agreed to help him, and they boarded a locomotive and steamed up the grade to Norden. They unloaded the rig in the Norden tunnel and assembled the team and sled. With Dr. Nelson snugly tucked into the vehicle, they started out.

Moments after they emerged from the tunnel into the fury of

the blizzard, the lead dog completely disappeared into the deep powdery snow. Soon the entire team was floundering about in the powder, and it quickly became apparent that proceeding by dog sled was impossible.

Dr. Laurence Nelson then set out alone by snowshoe, passing Soda Springs to reach Donner Summit Lodge. With snow so deep that the entrance to the lodge was blocked, he entered the lodge on the third-floor level and stopped there to rest and have a bite to eat. Reevaluating his situation over a cup of coffee, he decided to snowshoe down US highway #40. By then, dusk had fallen.

Huge drifts surrounded the road, and over-hanging cornices of snow threatened to avalanche at any time. Along the highway there were tall stands of Ponderosa pine that protected the road from winds.

Larry relates that, at times, the moonlight would break through the clouds revealing a scene of incredible beauty around him. He describes an awesome silence, broken only by the rustle of wind in the tops of the tall pines.

Trudging on through the night, he became increasingly fatigued, and at one point, fell face forward in the powdery snow. With his snowshoes buoying up his feet, and unable to gain any purchase with his hands, he floundered about for some time. He said he lay there in the snow, warm and comfortable. Realizing how easy it would be to lie there and die peacefully, he renewed his efforts, and finally was able to stand upright and continue the journey.

Continuing throughout the night, he arrived at Nyack Lodge at daybreak. Entering the lodge, he had breakfast and slept for several hours. When he awakened, he found that Mr. Jay Gold, a supervisor for Pacific Gas and Electric, was at the lodge. Best of all, he had a Sno-Cat capable of negotiating the deep snow. Gold had been working without rest for 36 hours ferrying supplies and personnel to and from the site of the stranded train. He agreed to take Dr. Nelson to the scene, and, as they approached the train,

Nelson saw an indescribable scene. Huge drifts surrounded the cars and large icicles hung from the corners of the cars.

About thirty-five section hands from nearby Crystal Lake were valiantly trying to keep the ventilators beneath the cars clear of snow and maintain a foot path beside the cars. Entering the train, he met the train master, who briefed him on conditions.

Making rounds in the train he found no serious illnesses. Later, he was approached by one of the Mexican section hands. The man's one year old child was desperately ill at his home in Crystal Lake and needed attention.

Although by that time he was completely exhausted, Nelson agreed to see the child.

Again, he set out on-foot for Crystal Lake, some 2 or 3 miles distant. He found the child had severe tonsillitis and administered medication. He asked for a pillow and a blanket, lay down on the floor and slept for eight hours. Returning to the train, Dr. Nelson found the situation there was rapidly becoming more tense.

The only food remaining on the train was beans, which were being served at every meal, much to the distress of all.

The sanitary facilities had been overwhelmed, and conditions were bad despite a bucket brigade organized by the train master. The prolonged internment was getting on the nerves of everyone. They began to show increasing symptoms of stress. Dr. Nelson, together with the conductor and train master, began to plan for the evacuation of the passengers.

The train was stalled not far from a place where the railroad bridged highway #101, about five miles from Nyack Lodge. On January 16, word came that the highway department had finally been able to clear US Highway #40 to the intersection with 101. Skies were clear and winds were calm, so they began detraining the passengers. Group by group they hiked down the path that had been kept open by the section hands and were driven to Nyack Lodge by five automobiles owned by lodge employees.

There they were fed and cared for until a relief train from San Francisco arrived to transport them to their destination. Jay Gold, who did such heroic work with the Sno-Cat was stricken by a massive coronary occlusion brought on by sheer exhaustion. He died on the way to Colfax.

Another fatality was recorded when the engineer of one of the rotary snowplows was buried by an overturned engine. The Republicans reached San Francisco in time to attend the convention and nominate Dwight D. Eisenhower for President.

**NOTE:**

The foregoing story is an excerpt from an audiotaped interview with Dr. Larry Nelson by Dr. Owen Bolstad as part of an oral history project. Not long after this story was related, Dr. Nelson died of a self-inflicted gunshot wound on June 3, 1991, after being told he had an uncurable cancer. This story is told with permission of his widow, Mrs. Alberta Nelson RN.

## LIFE HISTORY OF DR. LAURENCE D. NELSON
### By Dr. Owen Bolstad

To supplement the details of his life in Truckee additional interviews were recorded by some twenty-two former patients who lovingly provided reminiscences and additional photographs.

This is the story of a remarkable man who practiced medicine in the Reno and Donner Lake areas for nearly forty-five years. He was dedicated to his patients independent of their position in society. Unfortunately, he died before his life story could be completed, and it may have remained incomplete were it not for his former patients in Truckee, who came forward to complete the story of the man who was devoted to them.

Life presented a challenge for Larry Nelson from the day he was born. He came into this world as an orphan and lived with a family who couldn't legally adopt him because his birth mother could not be located. When he reached twenty-one years of age, he officially changed his name to Nelson in honor of the couple who had raised him as their own child.

As a result of his compassion for people, he went to medical school and finished an internship before starting a general practice at the age of 26. When he moved to the small mountain town of Truckee, California, he was the only physician in the community, practicing without any hospital facilities. As the only physician, he was on call twenty-four-hours-a-day, seven-days-a-week. During his time in Truckee, he made many trips over snowy passes to treat his patients. As mentioned, he risked his life as he snow-shoed to a stranded passenger train, *City of San Francisco,* because the snow was too deep for a dog sled team.

During the Korean War from 1952 to 1954, he served as a medical officer in the United States Navy, performing forty-eight major surgical procedures while aboard a troop ship. After military service, he served as assistant medical director during the Eighth Olympic Winter Games in Squaw Valley, California.

Returning for additional training as a resident in surgery at St. Joseph's Hospital in San Francisco he moved then to Sparks, Nevada, in 1968, where he served as Sparks Police Surgeon and medical advisor for the Drug Enforcement Agency and the Nevada Narcotics Bureau.

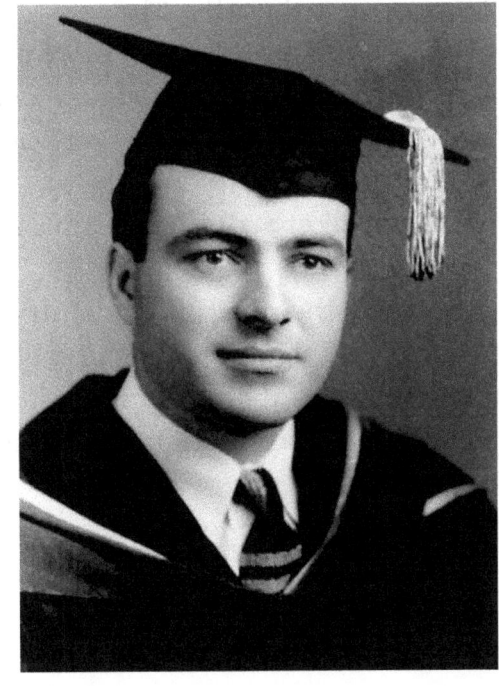

Dr. Laurence Nelson, 1949

**NOTE:**

The following four articles are devoted to brief biographies and interesting anecdotes about the early-day horse-and-buggy physicians of the Great Basin. Many of these physicians were poorly trained, ill-equipped, and did what they could to ease pain and suffering.

## DOCTOR MORRIS R. WALKER, "SINK OR SWIM, 1901"

After graduating from the College of Physicians in San Francisco in 1901, Dr. Morris Rollin Walker immediately moved to Reno, Nevada, and located his practice there. Reno at that time was a bustling western town of 4,000. The unpaved streets were well dotted with saloons and gambling houses. There were uneven board walks in front of the businesses. There were several churches, several school buildings, and a promising State University just north of town.

Downtown there were three drug stores, an old opera house, and three prospering banks. Only five or six doctors were actively practicing. There were no hospitals, so only emergency surgery was attempted.

Dr. Walker writes in his autobiography about how he began his practice:

"It was the practice, some fifty or sixty years ago, for medical colleges to send their graduates out to <u>sink or swim</u> with, generally, no intern training.

I had already bought my medical and surgical cases, also a few textbooks.

"At this time examinations for a state license were not required. I took the train for Reno at 7:00 PM, knowing full well that I was "ill-prepared" for the work, responsibilities, and the uncertainties of the near future. However, I went with a determination to make good: I must survive or perish; I, no longer would have a friendly professor to advise me.

"I was not long getting settled in my office. It was a tiresome and discouraging experience, waiting, waiting, for sadly needed patients.

"Finally, one evening about five o'clock a call came from an old Englishman (a druggist). There had been a runaway girl who was thrown out of a cart and was badly hurt. Would I come at once? I grabbed my medicine case and ran. I found the young woman unconscious but could find no outward marks of serious injury. The young woman was taken to the nearby home of a relative for the night.

"I proceeded to put on an appearance of professional seriousness and to do watchful waiting, at the same time keeping relatives and friends doing all sorts of errands.

"Towards morning the girl revived and before night left for her own home. The "strange doctor" became the subject of comments and inquiries, (Advertising?) I received profuse thanks from the family. No cash. However, the ice was broken. The family later gave me many calls.

"Late one afternoon, a week later, a row and robbery took place in one of the many saloons. The chief of police, who constituted the entire police force, was called. The robber made a break, ran into the willow thicket that lined the riverbank. Shots were exchanged. The chief was shot through the lower abdomen. As usual on such occasions, all the known doctors were called.

"While everyone was engaged with this affair, one of the older doctors, Doctor Jay Gibson, received an urgent call to go out to the mines some five or six miles from town. As he was busy, he called the new man (myself) to make the call for him. I had not bought a horse. I borrowed a bicycle.

"I found a woman desperately ill with pneumonia She was living in a miner's shack. I gave emergency treatment and returned to report to Dr. Gibson, who promptly turned the case over to me as he had no time to attend the patient. Later, I learned he regarded it as a charity case.

"I, of course, was eager to take over. I found a kindly

neighbor, who was also a graduate nurse, to take over the nursing and on the side, look after the woman's five little children. Dr. M. Rollin Walker, stuck around counting out a few tablets, giving many orders, trying to look wise and professional.

"The nurse with consummate skill brought the woman through to recovery. There is an interesting history connected with this patient. Her husband was a miner. About a week before, he had been killed in a mine accident, leaving his family all but destitute.

"The death and the widow's sickness aroused the sympathies of the entire camp. Some six months earlier John Sparks, Governor of Nevada, purchased the mine. He and his wife were noted for their charities and neighborly acts. Mrs. Sparks visited the sick woman, often bringing substantial aid. Mrs. Sparks asked me to spare no effort or expense and to keep her informed as to the progress of the disease. Some four or five weeks later she handed me two twenty-dollar gold pieces."

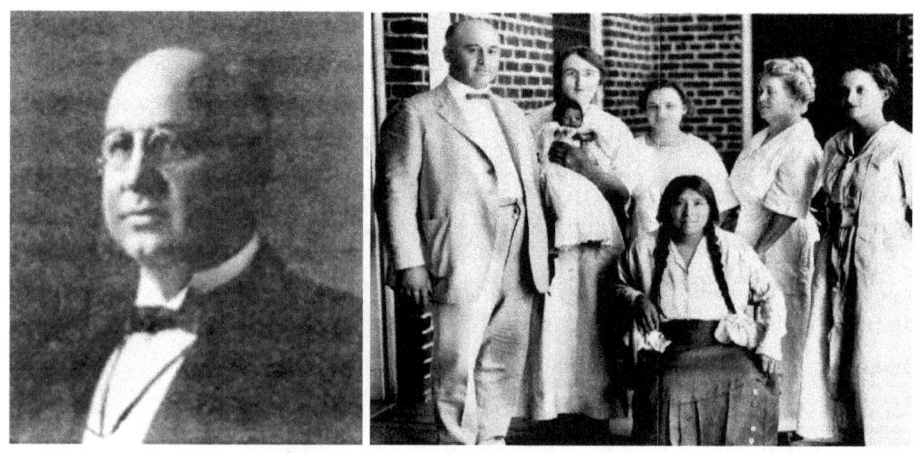

Dr. James Wiggins Gerow
with Indian Mother, Nurses, and Indian Baby, 1928
(Great Basin History of Medicine Achieves)

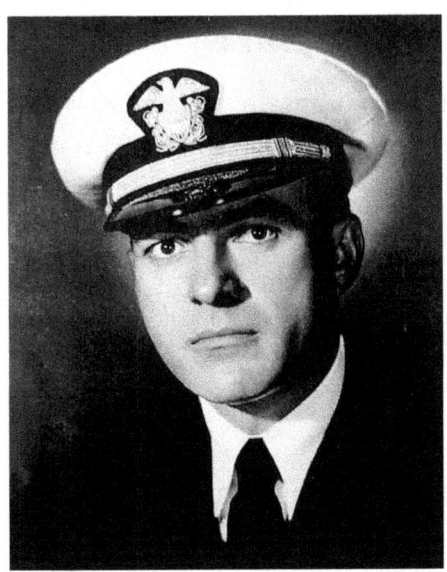 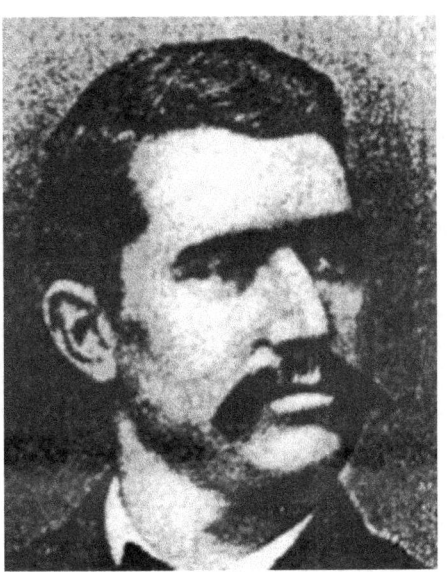

Dr. Laurence Nelson, 1953     Dr. Morris R. Walker, 1900

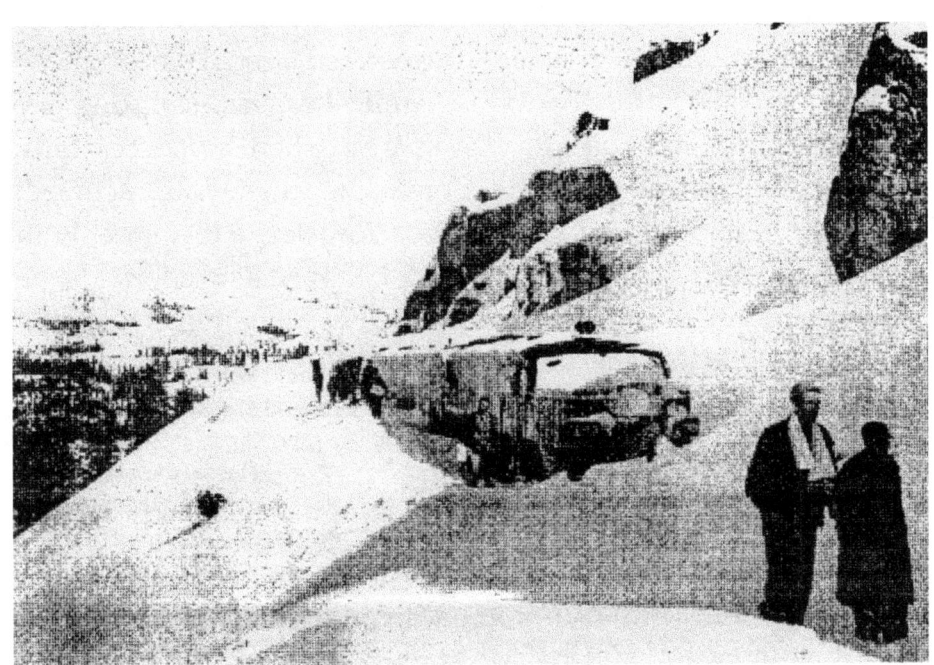

1951 Snowbound Train near Donner Summit

## Doctor John Marsh, "Practice in the Old West"

It is not known if Dr. Marsh came to Nevada, but the name of Doctor John Marsh is often seen in accounts of events in the very early development of the West. He received a Bachelor of Arts degree from Harvard University. When the United States Army built a fort at the junction of the Minnesota and the Mississippi rivers in 1819, to protect the northern reaches of the recently purchased Louisiana territory, John Marsh moved west, and took employment as a schoolteacher for Colonel Josiah Snelling, the first commandant of that fort.

While tutoring Colonel Snelling's children, John Marsh "read" medicine with the first physician in Minnesota, Dr. Edward Purcell. Leaving Minnesota, Marsh embarked upon a checkered career of mail carrier, and then Indian agent in Wisconsin. Accused of selling arms to the Indians, he fled to Independence, Missouri, where he operated a retail store.

Moving down the Santa Fe trail, he was captured by Comanche Indians. His life was spared when he successfully treated an arrow wound the Comanche chief had incurred. Escaping the Indians, he reached Los Angeles, a tiny pueblo in Mexican territory. Using his BA from Harvard as credentials, he requested a license to practice medicine. Since no one in the pueblo was able to translate the Latin of his diploma and because they desperately needed a physician, his license was granted by Mexican authorities in 1836.

Despite his rather sketchy medical education. Marsh developed cleverness with the scalpel and had enough confidence to attempt any kind of surgical case, from amputation to difficult obstetrics. With quinine in his pharmacopeia he treated chills, ague, and fevers. He knew how to vaccinate for smallpox and possessed the cowpox virus to do it.

Smallpox was widespread in California at that time, and he had many such cases to deal with. While he was still in southern

California, there was an outbreak of hydrophobia (rabies).

This epidemic of rabies was so serious that Mexican authorities issued a decree forbidding any man to keep more than two dogs and requiring that all dogs be kept tied securely.

It is difficult to know just how Dr. Marsh treated rabies since the Pasteur treatment was unknown, but he had plenty of brandy (aquardiente) and quinine, which was considered a panacea. He sometimes encountered medical problems that he did not know how to deal with. He was called to see a patient with amaurosis (blindness) and was most perplexed.

He heard the Man-of-War USS St. Louis was in Monterey harbor, and that there was a surgeon, a Dr. B.R. Tinslar, on board the ship. Marsh sent Tinslar a letter requesting literature on the subject, an opinion regarding treatment and sufficient strychnine to treat the patient. He received a rather terse reply. Dr. Tinslar would not render any opinion without examining the subject, and he was unwilling to share any of his meager supply of strychnine. Marsh made no further reference regarding the outcome of the case.

He soon moved northward into the San Joaquin Valley. where he practiced medicine, traded cattle, and prospected for gold. He became wealthy selling cattle and prospecting for gold. eventually finding a bonanza on the Yuba river. Never popular with his neighbors, he was accused of extorting money from the starving immigrants. Before he could enjoy the benefits of his considerable wealth, he was murdered by three of his Mexican ranch hands in a dispute over wages.

## DR. ELIZA COOK, NEVADA'S FIFTH FEMALE MD, 1884

Although Dr. Cook was the fifth female MD, she was the second woman to hold a regular MD degree and practice medicine in Nevada. Hydropath Dr. Ada Weed came in 1864, but Dr. Post Van Orden in 1879 was the first with a regular MD.

Eliza Cook was born in Salt Lake City on February 5, 1856.

She was the daughter of English immigrants who were well educated. The Cook family, with their intelligence and education, was unusual in the Frontier West.

Eliza developed an interest in medicine early in life, and soon became an apprentice to Doctor H.H. Smith of Genoa. With the encouragement from Dr. Smith, and with her family's support, Miss Cook enrolled at the Cooper College of Medicine (now Stanford SOM). She received her MD degree in 1884, at the age of 28 years. After six years in practice, Dr. Cook spend a year of post-graduate study in Philadelphia and New York City.

Several years later, Dr. Cook travelled abroad, visiting the British Isles, Europe, and the Holy Land. Upon her return, she became a popular lecturer in Carson Valley, giving many entertaining talks about her travels.

Eliza Cook was a dedicated physician, answering calls by horse and buggy to care for her patients as far away as Markleeville, California. She practiced obstetrics, orthopedics, surgery, and internal medicine, compounding many of her own pharmaceuticals. She had a reputation for courage and discipline. She was stern, yet gentle and kindly. She was known as an accomplished cook, baker, seamstress, and home maker. Dr. Eliza Cook died quietly in her sleep at the age of 91 years, truly a pioneer.

## "Unverified Doctor" A.P. Lagoon, Early 1900

Dr. A.P. Lagoon came to Ely in about 1900. With his peg leg, the result of a Spanish-American War accident, he hunted, fished, climbed hills, cursed, and could drink anyone under the table. He claimed he could do more with his peg leg than most men could do with two normal ones. Dr. Lagoon performed operations on kitchen or library tables.

One night in the saloon, several men were boasting about how much weight they could carry. The doctor claimed he could carry 500 pounds of sugar across the main street from corner-to-corner, over chuck holes, mud, all obstacles, and never falter. The saloon keeper took bets and banners were made for the event. Five hundred pounds of sugar were delivered from the big mercantile store at Lane City and the contest was on. Ten other men tried and failed. Doc's turn came and he won and collected the money.

In 1908, he bought a new car for trips to Ruth, Reipetown, and Kimberly. About a month later, coming down from Ruth, he stopped on the railroad tracks while he and his three friends made a comfort stop. An ore train came around the curve and smashed the car. Nevada Northern Railroad refused to pay for the car, since it was stopped on the tracks, and no one occupied the car at the time of the impact. Doc claimed the engineer would have had plenty of time to see them had he not been asleep. Railroad officials met with their lawyers and informed Doc that he had no case.

Doc's lawyers said he would tell his story in court. Then Nevada Northern Railroad's lawyers asked, "What about the other three men involved? What would they say?"

Just then Doc piped up and said, "They'll swear to anything I say—they were drunk!" He so charmed the railroad investigator that they awarded him money for a new car and some damage, and he promptly spent his new fortune entertaining them all.

**NOTE:**

This story was taken from *The Nevada Bicentennial Book*, by Elgas, Paher, et al. A search of the files at the Nevada State Board of Medical Examiners, shows no evidence of licensure for Dr. Lagoon in the years between 1900 and 1908. No mention can be found in Si Ross' book, *Physicians and Surgeons of Record Who Have Practiced Medicine in the Territory and State of Nevada from 1855 to 1957*. Search of other sources also came up blank. We cannot verify Dr. Lagoon existence.

# "Irregular Doctor" Simeon L. Lee
## By Dr. Anton Sohn

One hundred and twenty-five years ago, after the Civil War, the practice of medicine was not performed by a cohesive medical profession in the sense we recognize it today. A percentage of the population depended upon unorthodox medical practitioners known as "irregulars."

"Irregulars" includes botanical healers, homeopaths, water-cure proponents, religious healers, chiropractors, Indian doctors, charlatans, and many more. Regular physicians or allopaths, on the other hand, were not uniformly trained and many had marginal skills. Such was the scene in Nevada when Dr. Simeon L. Lee left Illinois in 1870 for Carson City.

Simeon L. Lee was born in Vandalia, Illinois, on September 4, 1844, and in his early twenties became a lieutenant-colonel in the 8th Illinois Infantry. After the War of Retribution, he went to Cincinnati, Ohio, and for two nonconsecutive years attended the Physio-medical Institute, an irregular school of medicine. In his words, this school was chosen because

"I was a lad, comparatively, when I matriculated in the school from which my father's family physician graduated. Of course, I then thought it the only college. I have, I think, grown wiser since."

Physio-medical schools were an outgrowth of Thomsonism which popularized botanical remedies. These schools were established from 1839 to 1850 in Ohio, Georgia, Alabama, Tennessee, Virginia, Massachusetts, and New York by Alva Curtis, a professional botanical healer, who split off from Thomsonism.

As can be seen from Dr. Lee's statement, he tried to distance himself from "irregular" physicians who practiced what is known as "eclectic medicine." He appeared to be successful in this attempt and was accepted by the regular physicians. His advancement in professional status in Nevada is documented by his application and letter quoted above on letterhead from the Board of Registration and Examination to the US. military requesting appointment as surgeon in the Nevada National Guard. He was the first president of the Nevada State Board of Health and at one time, was secretary of the Board of Registration and Examination. According to his letter he was voted into this position by his associates, of which all but one were regular physicians.

After arriving in Nevada, Dr. Lee was in-charge of the Pioche, Lincoln County Nevada Hospital from 1875 to 1879, in-charge of the Carson City, Nevada Hospital from 1879 until at least 1901 (except 1893-4) and a railroad surgeon for the Virginia & Truckee and Carson & Colorado Railroads for 20 years.

Military service was always a part of Dr. Lee's career. After his military service in Illinois, he was commissioned in 1877 as a major and inspector general in the Nevada National Guard and later advanced to the rank of colonel. In his letter he stated he was the only surgeon with Nevada National Guard in [the] war with Indians in what is known in history as the White Pine Indian War. Interestingly, no mention is made of the White Pine Indian War in Nevada history books.

Dr. Lee also was an avid collector. He collected stamps, arrowheads, baskets, stones, ceramics, fossils, guns, and other rare objects that he found. His collection was given to the state of Nevada in 1934 by his widow.

This material became a cornerstone in the state collection in Carson City. As a result of military and community service and dedication to his adopted state, Dr. Simeon Lee was an important Nevada physician and citizen until his death in 1927.

**NOTE:**

Some information used were obtained from *Simeon L. Lee Papers*, Box 3, MS C 142, History of Medicine Division, The National Library of Medicine, Bethesda, Maryland. Many of Dr.

Lee's instruments and his microscope, the first microscope in Nevada, are in the Great Basin History of Medicine Museum at UNRSOM.

## Doctor Harris S. Herrick
## Letters to his Daughter, 1869-1891

During the fall of 1867, rich silver deposits were discovered near Hamilton, Nevada. At that time, Hamilton was the county seat of White Pine County, and with the rapid influx of miners that city soon became a real boom town. It was estimated that the population of Hamilton and the surrounding mining camps reached upwards of 30,000 people at its height.

The mining bonanza soon played out, and the transient miners and their followers began to leave for other places. Within a period of 20 years, the once bustling city of Hamilton was fast becoming a ghost town, and after a disastrous fire burned down the County Court House in Hamilton, the county seat was moved to Ely.

Dr. Harris S. Herrick was a native of New York and had received his medical education at an eastern medical school, possibly Yale. He began the practice of medicine several years before he moved to Hamilton, Nevada, in 1869. For some unknown reason his wife and family had remained in the east when the doctor moved out west to seek his fortune.

During this long separation from his family, he maintained communication with his family with a series of letters to his daughter. These letters, covering the period from 1814 to 1891 were preserved, and are now available in the Nevada Historical Society. A study of these letters gives a look at the practice of medicine in rural Nevada during the late 1800s. Nothing in his letters indicates whether Dr. Herrick's family ever joined him in Nevada, or if he returned to New York. Dr. Herrick played an active role in his community, acting as county physician for many years and served several terms as county superintendent of schools. He also owned and operated a drug store, where in addition to drugs and medicines he sold groceries and other sundry items.

In a transcript of the letters to his daughter published by Russell R. Elliott in a Nevada Historical Society Quarterly are references to Dr. Herrick's medical practice: "....You speak about smallpox. I was vaccinated when a child and then about 20 years ago, have been a great deal exposed since, but have never taken ill although it does not hurt to be vaccinated once in 10 years.

"It has been terrible in Troy (New York) during the past winter, hundreds have died. It has been very bad in San Francisco and in Virginia City, Nevada. It has been here since 1869. I have attended persons with all diseases in which flesh is heir to but of all loathsome, which caps the climax, I must say smallpox takes the preference."

Dr. Herrick had suffered a paralytic stroke some time in 1881, and reports on his own health: "I feel very much better to think I am again able to be around and see to my affairs. I can't write yet with that facility I could before I was taken sick, still I am gradually gaining under numerous tonics. I was not out for New Years to take any dinners, lots of eatables were brought to me. I have many good- hearted friends in these regions.

"Everybody called when I was sick. I did not want for anything. It cost me $8 per day, for help to be on hand. It is very expensive to be sick here, at the best. Still it doesn't trouble me if I fully recuperate..."

After a vacation trip he writes: "I ought to have remained longer in practice but was obliged to come back on account of more patients in the hospital. The doctor I left in charge did not give satisfaction, consequently, I was obliged to return or resign, which I did not want to do if I do business in Hamilton. We must ride in wagons 45 miles over hills and mountains before arriving at the narrow gage railroad, then go ninety miles on the Central Pacific, then 600 miles to San Francisco.

"It costs heavily to travel in this country. My passage down and back was $108. While at the Bay City I took Turkish baths every other day, it wouldn't do to take them every day. They are too weakening.

"The first operation is to sit in an easy chair in a hot room till the perspiration flows freely. Then go into another room and perspire still more freely than in the first, this takes an hour or more, then a man goes through manipulations with water and soap by rubbing and brushing. Then one is put under a shower bath of tepid water after which another rubbing is given then one is wrapped in woolen blankets and sleep as long as-you-please, on rising another shower bath is given and rubbing, then dress and sit in a comfortable room & read papers ½ hour."

In June 1883, he writes: "…I have had more mountain fever than any spring since I came to Hamilton. Some days I have had as high as 8 or 10 patients with mountain fever, which is a nervous, low type of bilious fever. If a physician understands it is easily treated. The fever lasts from 12 to 24 hours under proper treatment and while under it they generally think they are going to die. Women, if on the order of hysterical are to *die,* certain, but I have never lost any by this complaint. It is a pandemic disease. Several New York gentlemen and ladies are out here at present.

"All have had the fever & I have brought all of them safely through. The first one taken sick was the president of the company. I was sent for; he began by giving orders. I interrogated by asking him if he or I was the physician, he said that was his custom. I informed him that it was not according to my practice, he said that he did not want my attendance.

"I left about 15 hours after I was sent for. He had got a quack doctor, who had 3 or 4 things to give. The gent begged for me with his wife and daughters to take his case, and in two hours the fever began to go down from 108 degrees to 98 degrees. It took a week to get him around as he was a man hard on 70 years."

**NOTE:**

Dr. Herrick died from a stroke in 1891, without ever returning to his home in the east. The entire transcription, commentary, and notes done by Russell R. Elliott is titled *Letters from a Nevada Doctor to his Daughter in Connecticut* (1881-1891) was found in *Nevada Historical Society Quarterly*, Volumes 1, 2, & 3, summer and fall 1957.

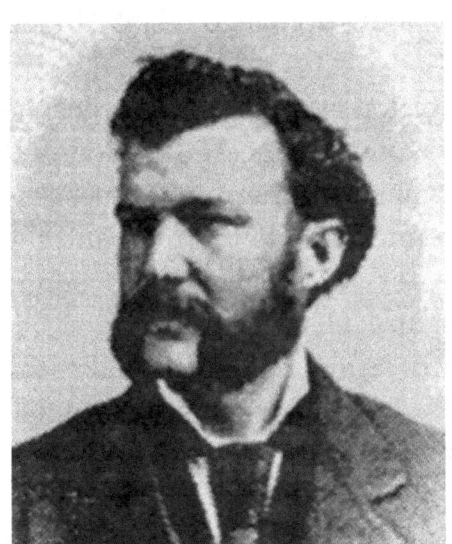 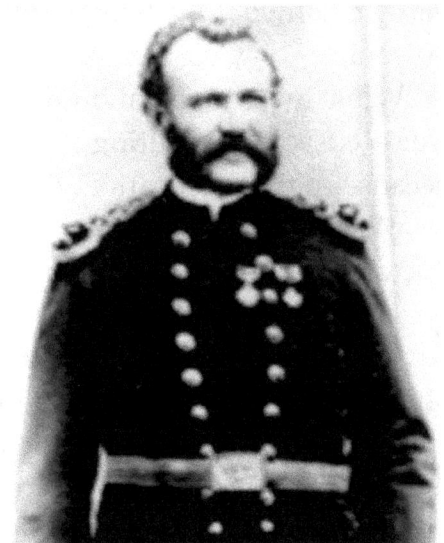

Dr. Simeon L. Lee

## "COLORFUL DOCTOR" FRED H. WICHMANN, 1905

Perhaps one of the most colorful physicians ever to have practiced in Nevada was Dr. Frederick Hugo Wichmann. Born in St Louis, Missouri about 1874, he worked his way through the University of Illinois, graduating in 1902. After obtaining his degree, he enlisted to serve with the insurgents in Cuba, and helped them fight their battle for independence. When American forces invaded Cuba during the Spanish-American War, he befriended General Frederick Funston.

After that war, General Funston became the commandant of The Presidio in San Francisco and served there during the great earthquake and fire of 1906.

Dr. Wichmann followed the rush of gold prospectors to the far north during the Alaska Gold Rush. He practiced medicine in the arctic region, then returned to California when an unhappy patient shot him because he was enforcing sanitary regulations. He practiced medicine in Lovelock, Nevada, in 1905, moving later to Reno where he soon got into trouble. On September 10, 1906, he was accused of performing an illegal operation on a patient named Lily Benson. The poor woman died of "blood poisoning" on October 14, 1906.

While awaiting trial on the abortion and murder charges, he was accused of assaulting another woman named Ethel Fine, and because of that accusation, the woman's brother, Fred Fine, shot Dr. Wichmann in the arm. The wound became infected, and the doctor's life hung in the balance for some time when "septic poisoning invaded his entire system." His attending physician advised amputating the infected arm, but eventually the physicians decided to remove two inches from his ulna, while authorities awaited the outcome of Dr. Wichmann's life-threatening infection.

On December 5, 1906, the State of Nevada indicted Wichmann for the murder of Lily Benson. By March 1907, following a trial during which the stepmother of Lily Benson testified as to Lily's "wild ways," Dr. Wichmann was acquitted of the charge. Within a year, Dr. Wichmann was continuously in trouble with the law.

There was another abortion charge. He threatened his tailor with a gun. He was involved in street fights and named in assault charges. In May 1910, following a charge of disturbing-the-peace and carrying an unlicensed firearm, Dr. Wichmann signed a deposition admitting to excessive gambling and drinking, and promised to keep-the-peace in the future.

On October 6, 1910, Dr. Wichmann was arrested on a charge of murder, following the death of yet another patient, Mrs. Emma Ross, after an alleged abortion. The first-degree murder trial, which began on February 1, 1911, was sensational.

It was prosecuted by District Attorney William Woodburn and Assistant District Attorney M.B. Moore, with Judge French presiding. The defendant's attorneys were Judge W.W. Jones and a young Patrick A. McCarran, who would later become a powerful United States Senator.

Numerous well-known citizens of Reno were called to testify at the trial. Dr. Sidney King Morrison, the county physician was called to give expert testimony, as were Drs. George McKenzie, Albert Heppner, Mulchyor Wise, Charles Edward Mooser, and A. Parker Lewis. Dr. A.W. Wullschleger and Dr. O.J. Johnstone, Mr. William Cann, of Cann's Pharmacy testified regarding a prescription for ergot and quinine. Nurse J.A. Talbot, of the Talbot Sanitarium was called, as was the Reno Chief of Police Burke. Mr. J.P. O'Brien of the Groesbeck and O'Brien Undertaking Firm testified. Mrs. Rosalie Saunders, manager of the Nortonia Apartments on Ridge Street where Mrs. Ross had resided after her arrival from Los Angeles, was called to the witness stand. Dr. Johnstone, from the bacteriology department at the University of Nevada, to whom Dr. Benjamin King gave the body organs removed from Mrs. Ross for his examination gave his opinion. Mrs. M.A. Lissak of St. George's Hospital also related her experiences.

Dr. Wichmann was not without support in the community, for he was considered handsome, quite affable, as well as having considerable medical ability. Many of his friends testified in his behalf. The trial came to a sudden conclusion when the Assistant District Attorney, in his closing argument, asked for a conviction of involuntary manslaughter, rather than the original charge of murder. After adjournment, the jury went to dinner at the Riverside Hotel, returning to the jury room at 7:30 PM. It took just two hours and forty-seven minutes before the foreman of the jury, Mr. E.H. Roctor, read the verdict of guilty. Sentenced to eight years in prison, Dr. Wichmann served just eighteen months of his term when five hundred petitioners were able to get the parole board to release him in September of 1912. His Nevada medical license was revoked on May 1, 1911, and Dr. Wichmann promptly left the state. On April 14, 1916, the *Reno Evening Gazette* reported that Dr. Wichmann had gone to Mexico to serve in the army of Francisco (Pancho) Villa.

It was further reported he had created a sensation when he appeared half dressed in the streets of El Paso, Texas with the story that he had been sentenced to be shot at sunrise by Villa but had made his escape. Nothing further is known concerning the fate of this colorful character from early Nevada, a man who seemed to attract trouble wherever he went.

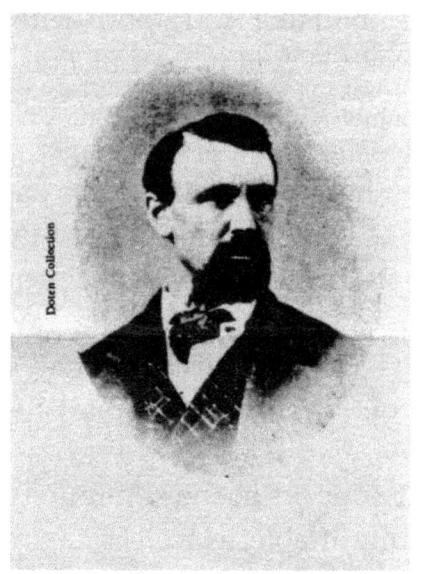

Alfred Doten, 1866

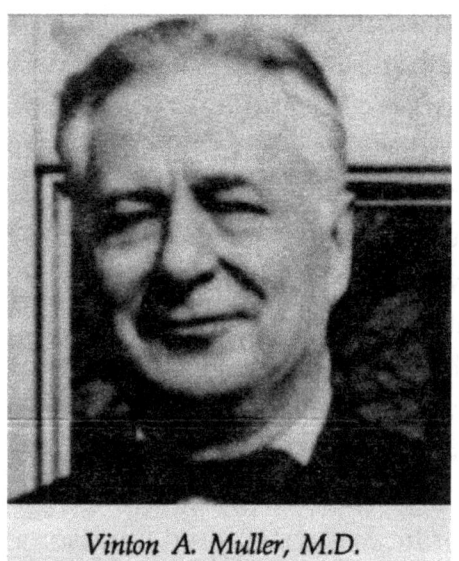

*Vinton A. Muller, M.D.*

Dr. V.A. Muller, 1920s

**NOTE:**

This story is the result of extensive research done by Eileen Barker, office manager of pathology, UNSOM.

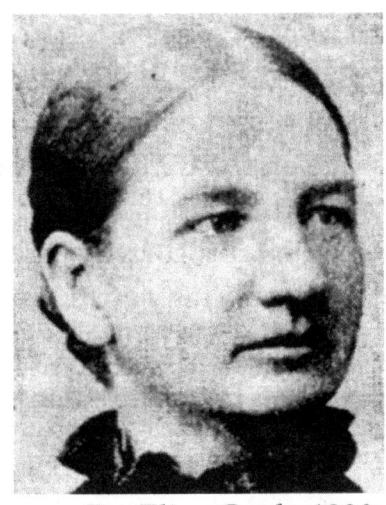
Dr. Eliza Cook, 1900s

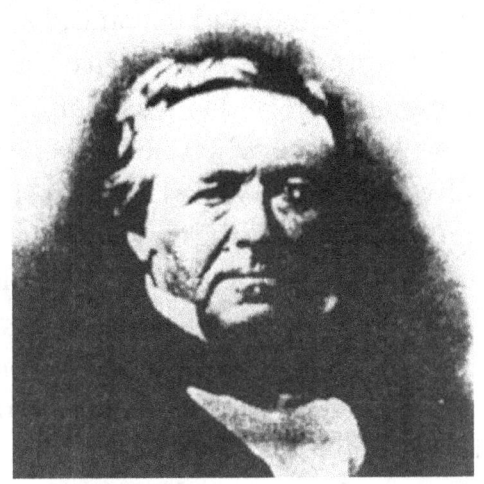
Dr. John Marsh, 1900s

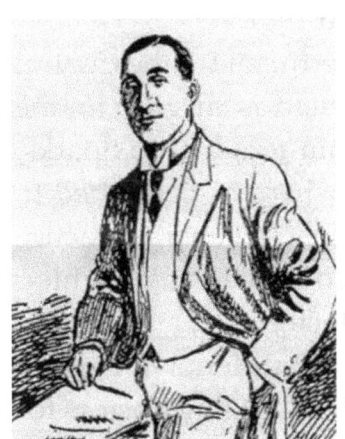

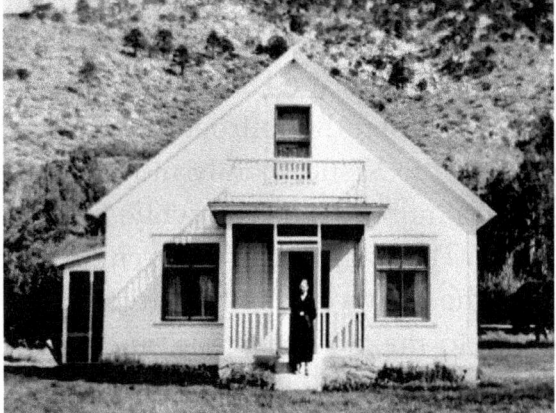

Dr. Frederick H. Wichmann, 1900s
Dr. Eliza Cook in Front of her Home in Carson Valley

## DR. WASHINGTON L. KISTLER
### "A MOST ROMANTIC DOCTOR, 1901"

Washington Lincoln Kistler, the youngest of thirteen children, was born in Pennsylvania in 1863. He developed an interest in medicine at an early age. At the age of eleven years, he mastered the Morse code used by telegraphers, and in 1876, he became the youngest telegrapher employed by the Pennsylvania Reading Railroad, where he worked to earn money for his goal of going to medical school and becoming a doctor.

Attending the University of Buffalo in New York, he graduated in 1896. He was planning to set up a medical practice in San Francisco when he booked passage on the Central Pacific Railway headed West. The train stopped at the railroad division point in Wadsworth, Nevada, for fuel and water, and while he was stretching his legs on the station platform, he noticed the legs of a lovely young lady standing near the station.

Dr. Kistler was smitten the moment he saw the young lady, and turning to his brother and traveling companion, he said, "That is the girl I am going to marry!" After a short visit to San Francisco, he returned to Wadsworth, found the young lady, Pearl Patience Pike, set up a practice in Wadsworth, and after a whirlwind courtship, he married the girl in 1901.

Wadsworth at that time was the main terminal for the Central Pacific Railroad, and Dr. Kistler was appointed as Surgeon for the railroad. When the railroad moved its main terminal to Sparks, Nevada, the Kistler family moved there, where he continued to serve as railroad surgeon while he developed a general practice as well. The Kistlers had three children, two sons and a daughter.

In the early years of his practice, the doctor used a horse and buggy to make house calls, and later used a Model T Ford to make his rounds, It is said he was one of the founding doctors for St. Mary's Hospital in Reno.

While he was in general practice, Dr. Washington Lincoln Kistler developed a deep interest in the practice of anesthesiology and became quite adepts at using ether anesthesia. He was often asked by other doctors to provide anesthesia during surgical operations.

He died a premature death, reportedly from kidney failure due to ether exposure. In retrospect, it seems much more likely that his early demise was the result of liver failure from chloroform exposure, an anesthetic agent known for its liver toxicity.

**NOTE:**

Material about Dr. Kistler was provided by his granddaughter, Mrs. Gay Metcalf, who is associate librarian at UNR Learning and Research Center. Photograph of Dr. Kistler is from Mrs. Metcalf's collection.

## DR. JOHN A. FULLER
## FROM LAS VEGAS TO RENO, 1910-69

This monograph by Dr. Fuller was preserved by Dr. Joseph C. Elia. Dr. Elia gave the document to Dr. John Dooley, who gave it to Greasewood Tablettes. Born in Massachusetts in 1883, John Andre Fuller MD, received his pre-medical education in the Omaha, Nebraska school system. He was granted an MD degree from the University of Nebraska in 1906 and interned at the State Hospital in Glenwood, Iowa. Licensed to practice medicine in Nevada in 1910, he practiced in Las Vegas, Nevada from 1910 until 1917 and in Reno where he practiced from 1917 to 1949.

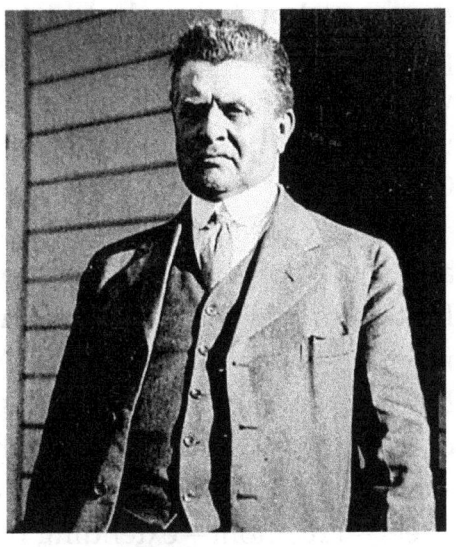

Dr. Washington Kistler, 1910

## DR. JOHN A. FULLER, LAS VEGAS YEARS, 1910-1917

Dr. John Fuller: "Never will I forget my first impression of Nevada. I arrived on an evening train in the spring of 1910, after slogging it out in muddy roads and snow in a horse and buggy practice in a small Nebraska town for three years. As I got off the train in Las Vegas there was a full moon, and the desert seemed to pulsate with violet light glowing against the surrounding mountains.

"I was met by my future associate, Dr. Hal Hewetson—as picturesque looking a character as I have ever seen. He was dressed in khaki pants which were stuffed into high leather boots, a woolen shirt and dirty sombrero, and a full beard. He had just returned from a prospecting trip in the mountains.

"My new job was assistant railroad surgeon for the *Los Angeles and Salt Lake Railway*, and the main shops for the road were located here in Las Vegas. We had a small dispensary with four beds. There was no other hospital except a small private mine contract establishment kept by Dr. Royce Martin. We had no trained nurses-only male attendants trained by ourselves, no X-ray nor laboratory-only test tubes and a few reagents. It was primitive. We did not have a decent surgery. All our major work we referred to Los Angeles, and we often accompanied the patient ourselves, hoping to keep him alive until we reached the City.

"Las Vegas in those days was a small town of between 1,500 and 2,000 persons. We had one school and two churches-a Protestant and a Catholic, one hotel-the 'Las Vegas', and several rooming houses over saloons. At that time there was a peculiar law that allowed only hotels to have bars. Naturally, the downstairs was occupied by the bar, with usually an outside stairway to the rooms above. There was only one main business street—Freemont—extending from the depot for five blocks and ending in the residential district. Standing on Fremont Street one could look down a side street, (Second Street, I believe) and view Block Sixteen, a very prosperous Red-Light District. More of this later. There were no paved roads in those days, only wagon trails. (Later, when I had acquired an automobile, it took me two days to drive to Los Angeles). Our medical practice was largely limited to Railroad men and their families.

"A trip out of town had to be made by train, although I made many a call by gasoline speeders, and even by railroad velocipedes if the distance were not too far!

"I even delivered a woman on a train. I was called to the train to see a very sick passenger and found her in the last stages of labor.

"I could not take her off the train as I had no place to put her. The only alternative was to get her into a 'stateroom' with the help of passengers and the porter, so I could deliver her. Everything went off fine, except that the people never remembered to pay me, and it was thirty-six hours before I got home.

"Speaking of our obstetrical practice, and there was plenty of it, as we had no hospital it was necessary to deliver a woman in her own home. Usually we had a neighbor to help, but not always. We had no pre-natal care. Perhaps we would be engaged for such and such a time, but more often we were not consulted until the patient was in labor. If the patient lived some distance away, it meant 'camp' on the job until it was over, maybe all day. I recall one nerve wracking case. I was called to see a patient in active labor and puerperal eclampsia. I had no help. Between Chloroform and Chloral hydrate, I delivered her by forceps, and both the mother and child recovered.

"Another case, and I had no help this time, was one in which the delivery had been normal. I was attending the baby when I thought I heard a peculiar dripping sound. Turning to the mother I discovered the bed full of blood and she was hemorrhaging profusely. I will not mention my procedure, but I stopped the bleeding, and the woman made a slow but uneventful recovery. I mention these cases to show what the doctor had to contend with in those early days.

"Automobiles were extremely scarce and I used a bicycle to get around. One time I had three cases of labor going at the same time. Remember, we had no hospital, so I was kept busy pedaling from one house to another keeping track of their progress. I managed to confine two of the patients, but by the time I could get around to the third, I was greeted by a squalling new baby, and I was out ten dollars. That was the fee in those days.

"At that time it was an unwritten law that a newly delivered woman remain flat on her back for nine days. I remember one healthy young woman whom I allowed to get up on the fourth day. She was so strong that I could see no reason for keeping her immobilized. I thought for a while that older women were going to run me out of town!

"Before I return to Reno, I want to refer back to a statement regarding the Red-Light District. There were no more charitable and public minded people in town than the 'girls down on the line'. If a townsman were down on his luck, they were always ready to pass the hat to help him out. I was returning from Goodsprings, a town about 35 miles away from Las Vegas, and I picked up a woman hitchhiker. I knew what she was, but this was desert courtesy. When we reached the edge of Vegas, she insisted on getting out. She said it would hurt my reputation to be seen in her company.

"While I was in Las Vegas we had a real gold rush. Someone came in with a report of a rich strike in the mountains near the Colorado River. In no time at all, anything with wheels or four legs was commandeered.

"Everyone who could get away started out for the hills, some on foot. One woman, a waitress in the Railroad beanery was picked up about eight miles out in the desert, exhausted. She had no provisions; not even a canteen of water-an example of what hysteria could be caused by GOLD. The strike proved false, but there was plenty of excitement while it lasted.

"And another example of mass hysteria: One day a prisoner in the local jail knocked out the jailer when he came in to feed the prisoners and escaped. He was reported headed for the Colorado River. A large crowd started out after the man, who was reputed to be a dangerous horse thief. The self-imposed posse was armed with everything from old shot guns to .22 caliber rifles. Fortunately none of them caught up with the fugitive. I do not recall if he were ever captured.

"The weather in Las Vegas used to get 'pretty warm' in summer. That was in the days before air-conditioning. I was called to Moapa one evening to attend some railroad workers who had been overcome by the heat. When I arrived, I found one man dead and another still breathing faintly, although rigor mortis had already set in. The temperature was 135 degrees!"

## Dr. John A. Fuller, Reno Years, 1917-1969

"Although I was in general practice in Las Vegas, I encountered many eye injuries and infections, and it was through Dr. Hewetson's interest that I went east for a post-grad course. When I moved to Reno in 1917, I dropped general medicine and associated myself with Dr. M.A. Brown. I took over his eye, ear, nose, and throat practice.

"I cannot recall more than fifteen or twenty physicians in the community at that time. There were old Drs. John Pickard, W.H. Hood, George McKenzie, D. Maclean Jr, J. Gerow, Sullivan, Bath, T.C. Harper, Horace Brown, William West, Martin A. Robinson, John LaRue Robinson, S.K. Morrison, George Servoss, R. St. Clair, G. Gardner, and Parker Lewis.

"Most of these men were real characters. Dr. Pickard was said never to have given a bill to a patient. Dr. Hood was never seen without his pipe. I have been told he once carried it to the operating table, but I think that was an exaggeration. McKenzie was said to be one of the finest surgeons in the west. Dr. Bath gold-plated all his instruments, and it was quite a sight to see gold clamps protruding from an abdomen! Dr. Sullivan was one of the most picturesque; in those days he wore a full beard. He was a very outspoken and perhaps profane man, but his profanity was never offensive, and he could swear at a patient and the patient enjoyed it. I was once operating on one of his young patients for tonsillectomy. The patient, a small boy had an unusually redundant foreskin. I suggested he should have a circumcision. Looking at the nurses out of the corner of his eye, he replied, 'Oh Hell, let him wear it off'

"Dr. Horace Brown was the Executive Secretary of the Nevada State Medical Association the year that I served as President.

"We had three small hospitals. St Mary's was the largest and was open to all the doctors. The Reno Hospital was a private institution ow(n)ed and operated by Dr. Parker Lewis. The Mt. Rose Hospital, an old, converted residence, was Dr. McKenzie's surgery, although occasionally others had patients there, including myself. I was sort of a protégé of Mac's. He took me under his wing when I arrived in Reno and was largely responsible for my taking root-roots that have held all these years.

"St. Mary's was in the old building across the street from the present hospital and is now a convent for the Sisters. The old Sister (I cannot recall her name) who had charge of the drug room, used to take the key to bed with her. It was said-and if any supplies were needed during the night, we had to wake her up. The Washoe General was only a county institution.

"We had no trained anesthetists. Anyone could pour ether. I recall one harrowing experience. One old doctor, whose name I shall withhold, was etherizing a patient for a tonsillectomy. The Patient was a rather husky man. The doctor himself went to sleep before the patient, who was just reaching the excitable stage. The patient suddenly rose, jumped off the table, knocked over the instrument stand, and nearly wrecked the surgery before he could be subdued.

"Another time, Dr. Frank Samuels, Jr., who was really a very fine anesthetist was working with me. The machine, a little old pump operated by an electric motor, caught on fire. With quick thinking, Frank grabbed a sheet and threw it over the machine, while I pushed the table out of danger, and a near tragedy was averted.

"Some of our doctors can remember the annual Nevada State Medical Society meetings. We had some notable sessions at Elko, and at Ely when Dr. Ralph Bowdie was alive. But the real sessions were held in Reno and out at Bower's Mansion. We never lacked for essayists from the Bay region and Salt Lake City. Many of them came every year. Pop Gossi, of the Riverside Hotel, was the caterer. The day before the meeting he would go out to Bowers and build his barbecue pits, and we would have roast beef, lamb, and pork. Being prohibition each member was assessed two pints. The only difficulty was to get an audience for the speaker. Most of the sessions were held around the improvised bar. Sometimes we had difficulty locating the essayist. But I truly believe we got more out of the informal discussions, and the old friendships rekindled, than from the most learned lectures of our modern meetings.

"In 1946, when I was president of the Nevada State Medical Association, we were just beginning to feel the pressure of Federal interference in medicine. I almost had to throw a government man out of my office one day who was insisting on making the State a Federal loan for Public Health, with the government, of course, telling us how to spend it.

"During the first World War, several of us old men were considered essential to the local medical needs. We acted on draft boards, giving a good half of our time without pay. The same conditions prevailed in the Second World War, but by that time, we were deemed too old for service.

"The only recognition we ever received was a rubber-stamped signed certificate, thanking us for our services. We were not looking for reward or glory—we were only doing our part, as many others did who were unable to take part in actual combat, and we suffered the same deprivations of rationing.

"It was rather galling to call on the family of a 'civilian war worker' and find sitting at the dinner table with a steak apiece.

"Reno has progressed vastly from the time I describe. We have a fine modern medical center, with specialists that can be surpassed nowhere. Our hospitals have advanced enormously, with their modern laboratories and other conveniences. As I look back to the old days, a feeling of nostalgia grips me, and I wonder if we were not actually happier under the old regime. They are all gone now, the old timers, and I guess I am the only one left, and I am expecting to read my obituary most any day!" Dr. Fuller died November 14, 1969, at 86 years.

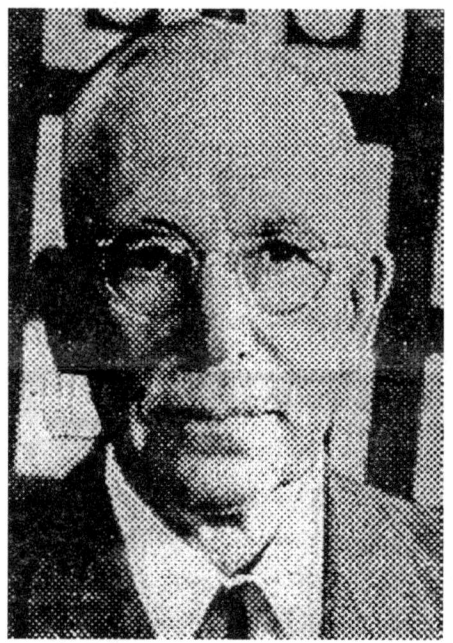
Dr. John A. Fuller

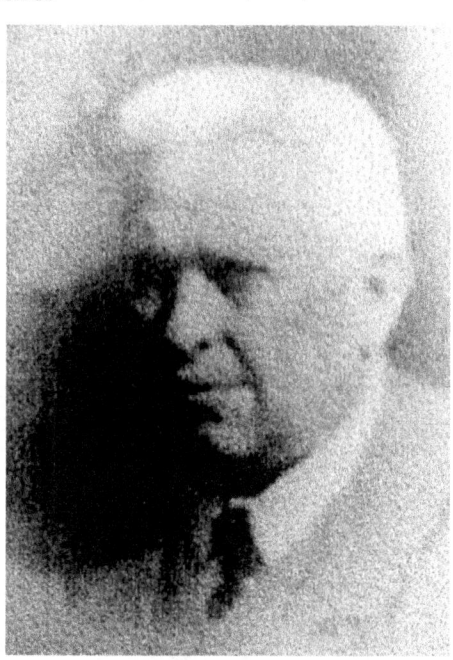
Dr. John Pickard

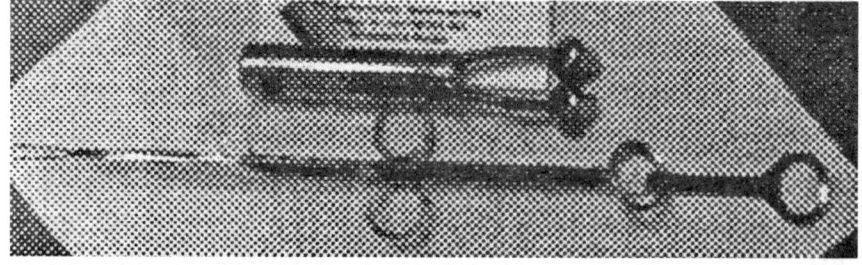
Dr. Fuller's ENT Instruments
(History of Medicine Museum)

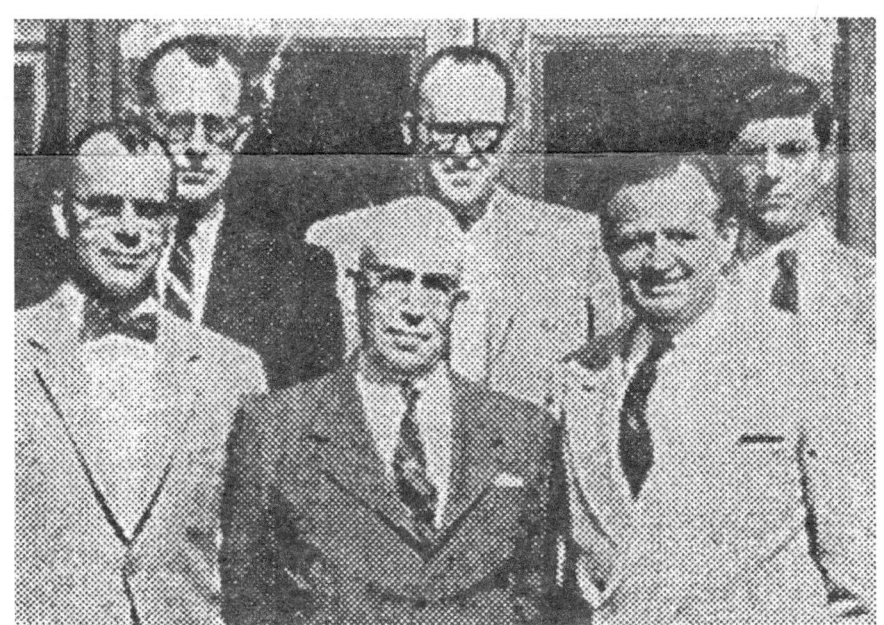

1958 St. Mary's Staff,
Front: Dr. John Detar, Dr. John Fuller, Dr. Henry Valenta,
Back: Dr. John Scott, Sr., Dr. Walter Quinn, Dr. Leslie Gould

## DR. ZETUS SPALDING
## SUSANVILLE, CALIFORNIA, 1852-1898

### By Dr. Anton Sohn

Researching history can be exciting because now and then a bit of information appears that will shed light upon a subject that had been at a dead end. Such is the case of Dr. Zetus Newell Spalding, who was only a name, until one of his relatives, Gene Sofie of Washougal, Washington, saw his name in my book on frontier military medicine and contacted me.

Until then, there was no face or information to go with the name. Dr. Zetus N. Spalding was listed in the records of Fort Scott (near Paradise Valley, Nevada) as acting Assistant Surgeon during 1865, but his personal military records were missing from the National Archives in Washington, D.C. (Only in recent years has increased government security prevented pilferage of historical records from the National Archives.)

The following is the story of Dr. Zetus Newell Spalding as related by Mr. Sofie. The earliest known ancestor of Zetus Spalding was Edward Spalding, who came to America in 1619 with Sir George Vardley. Descendants of Edward Spalding lived in Vermont, were Zetus was born August 13, 1819, in Albany, Orleans County, Vermont.

When Zetus was seven years old the family moved to Ohio, finally settling in North Norwick on the Sandusky and Mansfield Railroad. After elementary education, at the age of twenty-one, he commenced the study of medicine at the Norwalk Academy under the preceptorship of Dr. Hugh F. Prouty in Monroeville, Ohio. He completed his medical degree six years later at the Cleveland Medical College in 1846 under Dr. Moses C. Sanders and moved to Roxana, Michigan.

Zetus was restless, and like thousands of Americans, he headed west to pursue his golden dream. He arrived in Sierra County in California, August 12, 1852, and worked in the mines for three years before going into the mercantile business in Sierra County.

In July 1857, he lost everything he owned in a disastrous fire. He married seventeen-year-old Mary Ann Brown from Sussex, England, in August after the fire. With a new wife to support he found a way out of his financial predicament by volunteering for the U.S. Army. The Indian Wars in the West were heating up, as was the Civil War, and the U.S. Army was searching for doctors at an attractive salary of $100 per month. (At that time, a laborer in the mines made about $20 a month.)

After his military service Dr. Spalding returned to Susanville, California, where he became county physician, coroner, and public administrator for Lassen County. He established a pharmacy called Spalding's Drugs in Susanville with another relative, A.C. Neal. The Pharmacy was still in existence until recent years. Dr. Spalding had eight surviving children, losing several to diphtheria.

At least two great granddaughters still live in Susanville. His brother, Noah, lived at Eagle Lake in Sierra County from 1873 until 1880.

Dr. Zetus Spalding died on May 17, 1898, apparently drowning while fishing in the Susan River. He is buried in the old cemetery in Susanville. Much was unknown about Dr. Spalding's life and career in Susanville, but slowly the pieces of the puzzle came together.

**NOTE:**
Stephanie Ernaga researched Dr. Spalding for this article.

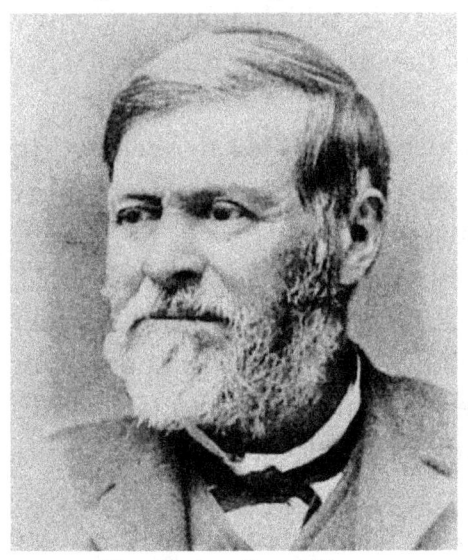 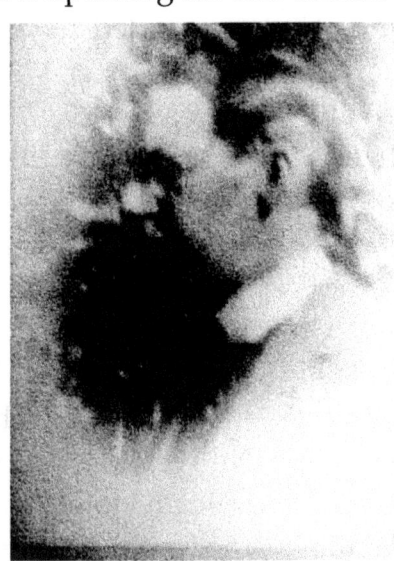

Dr. Zetus Spalding          Dr. Martin Robinson, 1918

## DR. T.P. TYSON, "SERIOUS-OVER-STUDY, 1923"

The following is the story of an incident in 1923 in Wadsworth, Nevada, involving the shooting death of Dr. Thomas Parry Tyson. (Various sources indicate his name was J. Perry Tyson, but we are using Nevada Board of Medical Examiners' records that indicate his name was Thomas Parry) My thanks to Dr. Tyson's grandson, Jerry Tyson of the San Francisco Bay Area for permission to share his thoughts on this event and to Pierre Hathaway, Jerry's shirttail relative, of Carson

City, who provided interesting details and valuable newspaper clippings of this incident.

Dr. T. Parry Tyson, a well-known and respected Reno physician, became a raging madman and maniac when he went on a shooting rampage while holed-up in the Wadsworth Bazzini Hotel in 1923. Tyson was born in 1866 and received his medical training at the University of Pennsylvania School of Medicine. He was licensed in Nevada in 1905 and became chief autopsy surgeon for Washoe County.

In a front-page headline dated February 17, 1923, the *Reno Evening Gazette* reported the tragedy in which Washoe County Under Sheriff J.W. Carter killed the doctor with a .45 caliber automatic pistol.

It was reported that Dr. Tyson had traveled to Wadsworth from San Jose for the expressed purpose of encouraging Paiute Indians in the area to revolt against white settlers.

*Reno Evening Gazette* headlines on February 16 and 17, 1923, states: "Crazed Man is Killed in Gun Battle With Posse—Former Nevada Physician Dies in Pistol Duel— Maniac Endangers Lives of Citizens—Arrest Sought When Attempt Made to Get Piutes (sic) to Wipe Out Whites —T. Perry Tyson Holds Force of Officers at Bay in Wadsworth Hotel."

While it is not entirely clear why he wanted to do this, Jerry Tyson speculates he apparently was distraught because Indian fishing grounds were being deprived of valuable water due to the 1915 Newlands Reclamation Project and construction of the Lahontan Reservoir and Derby Dam. Dr. Tyson's grandson also suggests the doctor may have become disturbed at the numerous Indians he suspected had been murdered by white settlers. 'Dr. Tyson may have had good reason to be sympathetic to the Indian cause, said his grandson in a recent letter to Mr. Hathaway.

There were numerous attempts by Washoe County Sheriff J.D. Hillhouse, Deputy Sam Kearns, Deputy J.W. Carter, Justice of the Peace W.D. Ingalls, and the owner of the Bazzini Hotel to persuade the doctor to surrender, but nothing worked. Kearns and Carter were thought to have used tear gas but were not successful in getting the doctor to give up. They injected chloroform through the keyhole into Tyson's room, a tactic suggested by Physician S. Lees Joslin who was on the scene. The tear gas and chloroform worked to make the disturbed physician vacate the room, but it led to him being shot and killed by Carter. Evidently Carter spied Tyson through a knothole taking dead aim at Kearns and shot first, possibly saving Kearns' life.

Earlier in 1917, Dr. Tyson had moved from Reno to the San Jose area, but he returned to northern Nevada yearly. On one of his visits in 1922, he was arrested on a "lunacy charge" and was paroled into the custody of his son, Howard Tyson, who took him back to the Bay Area.

The doctor returned to northern Nevada on February 12, 1923, and stayed at the home of a long-time friend, Mrs. Zeigler, who saw him off to Wadsworth two days later. She later commented to investigators that he appeared normal at the time.

The *Gazette* commented that Dr. Tyson had been studying psychiatry and was planning on writing a book on the subject. He became "unbalanced because of studying psychiatry which pertains to healing mental diseases and to which he was devoting his energies in writing."

*Reno Evening Gazette* headlines on February 18, 1923, state: *"Tyson's condition was a result of over-study."*

The *Nevada State Journal* reported that Dr. Tyson's body was sent to the Ross-Burke Mortuary in Reno on February 17 to await instructions from the family in San Jose. *"Tyson became mentally deranged and endeavored to have the Indians at Wadsworth annihilate white settlers,"* commented the writer of the article. *"He had been of unsound mind for a long period... although at times he appeared lucid."*

Howard Tyson interred his father in a "beautiful columbarium in Oakland." It is possible that all the facts of his father's death may never be known. There was a brief investigation, but no evidence was ever presented to disprove anything other than Dr. Tyson being shot in the line of duty by Under Sheriff Carter.

Jerry Tyson states the family will continue to think of our ancestor as an eccentric but good person, who was sincerely trying to help our Native American brothers.

**NOTE:**

Richard Pugh, who wrote this article, was raised in Charleston, South Carolina. After graduating from the University of South Carolina, he served in the U.S. Public Health Service as a field epidemiologist advisor. Later, he was assistant CEO and lobbyist for the South Carolina Medical Association. In 1973, Pugh moved to Reno to head the Nevada State Medical Association (NSMA). He retired in 1987 and died in 2019.

## DR. EDWIN CANTLON'S MEMORY OF DR. T. PARRY TYSON

A few days after we published the article on Dr. Tyson, we received a call from Dr. Ed Cantlon a longtime Reno surgeon. Ed vividly remembers the day Tyson was killed February 1923 in the Nevada House. Ed was twelve at the time and living in Wadsworth on the family ranch. He was sent down to get the mail from the Columbus Hotel, which is across the railroad tracks from the Nevada House. Authorities would not let anyone cross the tracks because a "crazy man," in the Nevada House, wanted to kill white folks for what they did to the Indians. Joe Bazzini owned the Nevada House, also called the Bazzini Hotel. Ed was in the post office when Tyson was shot

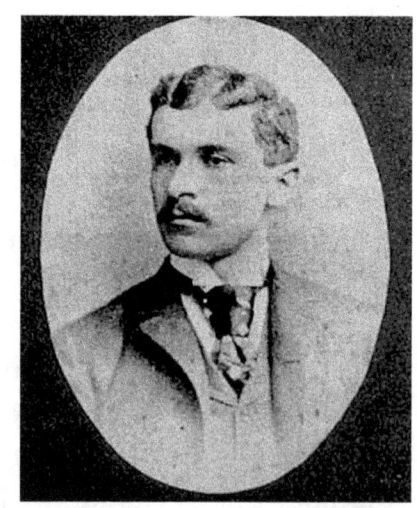

Dr. T. Perry Tyson, 1920s

so, he didn't hear the gunshots. According to Dr. Cantlon, the hotel was eventually sold to Joe Bianchini who became a longtime patient.

## DR. SAMUEL WEAVER, PARADISE VALLEY, NEVADA, 1884

Greasewood Press published in *The Healers of 19th Century Nevada* by Dr. Anton Sohn the names of over 700 doctors, who practiced in the territory or State of Nevada between 1857 and 1900.

Obviously, this list is not complete because in the early days, for various reasons, doctors came to the state, stayed a short time, and left no records.

Prior to 1899 when the Board of Medical Examiners was created by the legislature, some county records were incomplete and even destroyed. Furthermore, only names and dates of some doctors survived. Others left only their name. Therefore, when we were alerted to a new name or more information about an individual, we will record the information in our history of medicine archives and alert our readers who might have more information.

Samuel Weaver was born in Canonsburg Pennsylvania, on January 9, 1853. He attended a local academy before graduating from the College of Physicians and Surgeons in Baltimore in 1882. After two years of practice in his home state, the young bachelor moved to Paradise Valley, Nevada, in 1884, where he remained for two years. No information is recorded as to why he left Nevada. Maybe the mines played out, maybe there were no eligible young women, or maybe he moved on for better economic opportunities.

At any rate, he settled in Hubbard, Oregon, where he married and spent the rest of his life. In that community, he served on the city council and played first violin in the Hubbard Symphony Orchestra. According to the Journal of AMA, he died of heart disease October 10, 1924.

In 1884, when Dr. Samuel Weaver came to Nevada, there were minimal laws in the state governing the practice of medicine. In fact, the only requirement was to pay a fee and attest to being a physician. Even doctors from China registered their diplomas, written in Chinese. On the other hand, Dr. Weaver had undergraduate training at a private school, had graduated from a recognized and leading medical school and was an educated individual.

**Note:**

In 1999, we received a letter from Richard A. Sumin of Battle Mountain, a relative of Dr. Samuel A Weaver. Mr. Sumin sent us a capsule history of Dr. weaver from the 1912 Centennial History of Oregon. He also noted the Weaver's arrival was announced in The Silver state, Humboldt County newspaper in 1884.

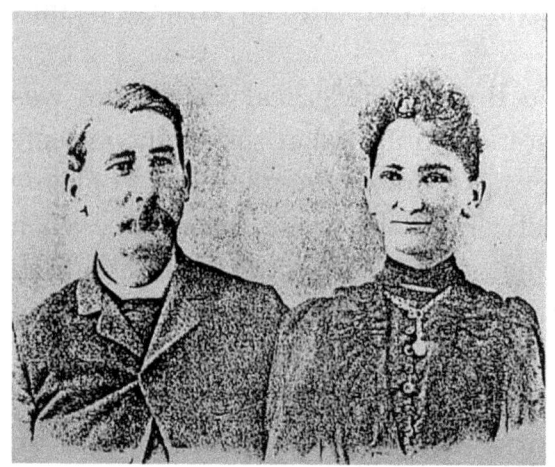

Dr. Samuel and Mrs. Weaver

## "Extraordinary Doctors"
### Dawson, Bergstein, Thoma, and Lewis
### By Ryan Davis

Drs. Alson Dawson, Henry Bergstein, George Thoma, and John Lewis were "extraordinary doctors," who were lost in time because they practiced one hundred years ago. In the following article, we will describe the importance of these four doctors, not only to the development of surgery in Nevada, but as leaders in medicine in the nineteenth century. Many physicians in Nevada condemned surgical operations in 1888.

On March 22, 1888, these four men set the standard in Nevada for medical advancement by performing a surgical procedure, which had never been attempted in this state. This procedure, known in the medical profession as an ovarian serous/mucinous cyst adenectomy, was regarded as a dangerous operation. The first doctor in America to perform removal of this kind of an ovarian tumor was Ephraim McDowell (1771-1830). He operated on his patient on a kitchen table in Kentucky in 1809.

Many physicians in Nevada condemned the operation in 1888, performed by Dr. Alson Dawson and assisted by Drs. Henry Bergstein and John Lewis, as a disastrous venture. They believed the state simply did not have the adequate medical facilities or people with adequate training to master such a daunting challenge.

In both McDowell's and the present case, the tumor was so large that pregnancy was considered. Furthermore, if the tumor was malignant or the contents of the benign cyst spilled in the abdomen, it could seed throughout the intestines and cause bowel obstruction and death.

The patient who became the first Nevadan to undergo the procedure was fifty-year-old Louise Ancker, who resided in Washoe City. Dr. Alson Dawson diagnosed the plight of Mrs. Ancker four months prior to surgery. He thought the cyst was benign, but by its mere size threatened the healthy function of other internal organs. Mrs. Ancker was informed of the procedure's dangers and elected to have the operation done despite its risks.

On that March day, the surgery was accomplished in one and a half hours in the old two-story Washoe Hospital building at Kirman and Mill Streets. Done with great precision and delicacy was the main reason for its success. Careful preparation went into the endeavor. Most of the instruments used were sterilized using a carbolized spray, and every nurse involved in the operation was required to take an antiseptic bath. Routine as it may appear to many physicians today, these preparation techniques were all new and key to the procedure's success.

Many of these men accomplished more in the field of medicine than most doctors could hope to accomplish. Dr. Alson Dawson, besides being a prominent physician for over twenty years, was also one of the founders of the Nevada State Mental Hospital (NSMH) and was its first superintendent. Though no longer referred to by this name, the institution is still in service as the Northern Nevada Adult Mental Health Services on Galetti Way in Sparks.

Alson Dawson, born in New York in 1844, left no record of where he received his MD. He was removed from his position as NSMH superintendent for an unknown reason shortly after the start of 1883. He died at the age of fifty-one from injuries sustained when his horse lost control on September 15, 1895, in Reno.

Each of Dr. Bergstein's assisting physicians served as superintendent of NSMH as well and was a founding member of the first medical staff at Saint Mary's Hospital. Dr. Henry Bergstein, in addition to serving in the Nevada Legislature in 1875, was the father of the Nevada Medical Law of 1875, which required all doctors to present a medical license to the county recorder before they could practice in Nevada. Bergstein was one of seven members who formed the first organized medical society in Nevada in 1897. He attended Cooper Medical College (now Stanford School of Medicine) in 1872 and again in 1905. He died in San Francisco in 1918.

Dr. John Lewis served as president of the Nevada State Medical Society in 1909. He also served on the Nevada Board of Medical Examiners and was a member of the AMA until his death in 1924.

Dr. George Thoma came to Nevada from New York after being an Assistant Surgeon in the Union Army. After settling in Eureka, Nevada, in 1867, he served in the Nevada Senate, before moving to Reno to practice in 1887. Before his death in Reno in 1907, he served as president of the Nevada State Medical Society.

Pioneers and trailblazers in the field of medicine, these men proved Nevada had the resources to accomplish what many believed was impossible. They formed the basis of Nevada's healthcare.

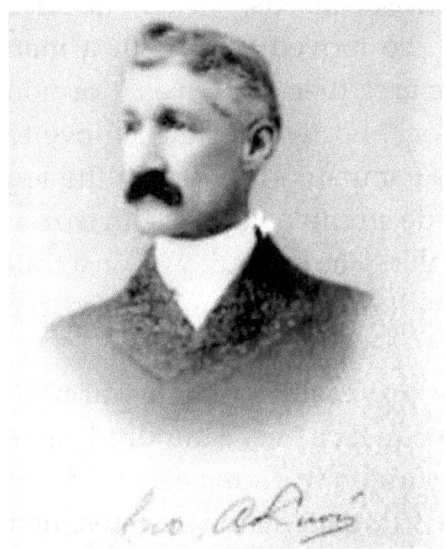
Dr. John Lewis, 1909

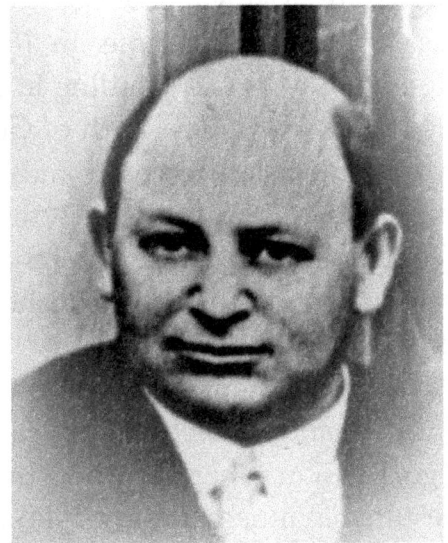
Dr. A. Parker Lewis, 1913

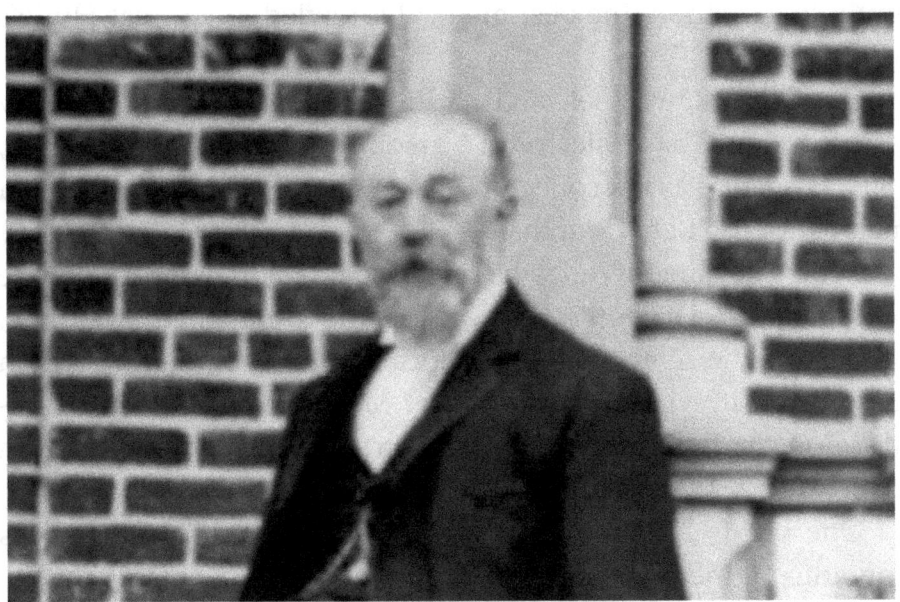
Dr. Henry Bergstein, 1890s

# Dr. Charles Daggett, Nevada's First Doctor, 1851
## By Ryan Davis and Guy Rocha

Born in Vermont in 1806, Charles Daggett graduated from the Berkshire Medical College in Massachusetts, where he also received his law degree. In 1851, he moved west with a man known only as Gay, settling in the area then known as Mormon Station, a few miles south of Genoa. Shortly after their move to Mormon Station, Daggett and his companion settled in the log cabin where LDS leader Orson Hyde stumbled upon with frozen feet. Kingsbury Road, where the cabin was located, was on a trail that had been established shortly before they moved to the community.

The treatment of frostbite is a process of gradual warming rather than sudden heat application. In fact, over a hundred years ago, Russian fishermen knew that sudden warming of frozen fish resulted in mushy flesh, while slowly warming the flesh resulted in firmer more normal meat. What is remarkable is that a doctor who lived nearly one hundred and fifty years ago was able to apply this method, the best medical knowledge, to treat Hyde's feet frozen feet.

Dr. Daggett was selected as Prosecuting Attorney, County Assessor, and Tax Collector of Carson County on September 20, 1855. His value as tax collector was enhanced by him not being a member of the LDS Church.

People in Carson Valley had never paid taxes before and were outraged. Dr. Daggett's life was openly threatened over this. Because of the reluctance of the locals to come under "Mormon Law", almost everyone on the first Mormon Ticket was a non-Mormon. Dr. Daggett became Nevada's first resident-attorney on November 2, 1855, before he tried his first case.

One of his last known distinctions occurred when he was appointed a member of the Committee of Arrangements for the formation of the Second Convention to form a separate territory out of the Utah Territory. With Dr. Charles Daggett's persistence, this territory became the State of Nevada. After his political career he settled down in the Genoa area and there are no surviving document attesting to the year he died.

**NOTE:**

The first lawyer in Nevada was L.A. Norton, a temporary resident from Placerville. Unfortunately, no photo of Dr. Daggett is known to exist.

## Dr. Jack Gilbert, Twenty-six Years Of Devoted Service In Cedarville, California, 1955-'80

### By Patricia Barry, Fort Bidwell

Born October 27, 1919, in Manhattan, California, Jack Clinton Gilbert was the oldest child of Roy and Ella Gilbert. When Jack was a child, the family moved to Whittier, California. His mother died of cancer when he was ten years old, and his father raised the three children.

Jack graduated from Whittier High School where he was valedictorian of his class. He continued his education at UCLA, but his schooling was interrupted by World War II when, in 1943, he joined the U.S. Army. During Jack's time in the service, he completed a course for medical corps candidates. While on duty in England, he met a nurse named Rosalind Robertson, and after his honorable discharge from the army, Jack returned to England where he and Rosalind were married.

Upon return to the states, Jack continued his medical education and graduated from the University of Southern California with BA and MA degrees. He received his MD degree in 1951, from Hahnemann Medical College in Pennsylvania. (Hahnemann was a homeopathic medical college.) In 1952, Dr. Gilbert completed internships at Seaside Memorial Hospital in Long Beach and LA County General Hospital.

He also completed residencies in surgery and anesthesiology at Seaside Memorial Hospital and contagious diseases at Los

Angeles County General Hospital. He received fellowships in radiology and nuclear medicine at Santa Ana Community Hospital. A two-year assistantship was accomplished in general practice, serving as radiologist for a group practice.

In 1952, Dr. Gilbert's first private practice was with a group in Sierra Madre which lasted three years. Hearing of a vacancy in Northern California, Dr. Gilbert applied for and was accepted as Modoc County's health officer.

Dr. Gilbert arrived in Cedarville on August 6, 1955. His first office in Cedarville was in Modoc Medical Center, and he practiced there until 1958. Then he moved to an office in the old Cressler-Bonner Building on Main Street. An x-ray unit was installed, so that his patients could have access to both lab and x-ray facilities.

Dr. Jack Gilbert was on-call for twenty-six Modoc County Fairs. The first one was in August 1955, and one day there was an automobile accident with serious multiple injuries and another patient with a cervical fracture.

He turned no one away. This initiated him into the work pattern he would follow for the next twenty-five years.

On September 1, 1968, ten years after the death of his first wife, he married Patricia Dagsen. Each of them had three children, so they had the formidable task of raising six teenagers.

Recognizing the need for more office space, Dr. Gilbert's employees started a building fund in 1971, which was augmented by numerous personal as well as business donations and became the nucleus of what was later to become the Surprise Valley Medical Building Fund. Work was started on the building in 1974 and completed in June 1975. With the help of many volunteers on a weekend, the office equipment was moved into the new space, and Dr. Gilbert opened for practice on the following California morning, July 1, 1975. Today this building, which has undergone various remodeling, is home of the busy Surprise Valley Medical Clinic.

During the first ten years in Cedarville, Dr. Gilbert was only away for a brief period of two or three days.

Until July 1980, he had been the only doctor in Cedarville. Many of his family outings or special occasions had to be cancelled because of an emergency.

Dr. Gilbert's habit of working at night became legend. He didn't mind working late, often until 2:00 AM, as he turned no one away. His dedication came from a deep love of his work and the needs of his patients. Dr. Jack Gilbert not only addressed the physical needs of his patients, but also took care of their mental and emotional well-being.

Many a youngster who left home for college or an older person leaving the area often called back home, sometimes collect or late at night, for reassurance from Dr. Gilbert.

When the original ten-bed Modoc Medical Center in Cedarville overflowed, the county planners approved twenty-two beds, which, at times, were still not enough.

One reason for this was that the doctor's patients were not just from Modoc County; they were also from adjoining Washoe County, Nevada, Lake County, Oregon; and as far away as Winnemucca and northeastern Nevada. Besides being a very compassionate and caring individual, he was known as an exceptionally gifted diagnostician, and his advice was sought by patients and doctors, as well. If he couldn't fix the problem, he researched until he found someone who could and referred the patient to that physician.

Dr. Gilbert was always interested in the community, serving for many years as Modoc County's health physician. It was during this time in 1957 that the first pilot project for a Visiting Rural Nurse Program was initiated. This program was widely used throughout the county, including California reservations, and proved to be very successful. The program was recognized throughout the State of California and subsequent visiting nurse programs were patterned after it.

As part of his health physician duties, Dr. Gilbert held monthly immunization clinics in Newell, Adin, and Canby. He also developed a Civil Defense disaster plan, which was approved countywide.

Dr. Gilbert always gave freely of himself despite his busy work schedule.

He provided school physical education exams free of charge, spoke at graduation ceremonies, gave Medic Alert memberships to graduating seniors, and didn't charge many needy patients for his services. Dr. Gilbert delivered 1,014 babies, some of which were second generation, and treated as many as five generations of the same family. He was honored by a Jack C. Gilbert MD Appreciation Day, at which many of his patients and friends appeared to say, "Thank you."

He was also honored in 1980 by being selected as Grand Marshal of the Modoc County Fair Parade. Dr. Gilbert died of cancer on California Day, 1980, at the young age of sixty-one. He had died without knowing he had been named the 1981 recipient of the prestigious Frederick K.M. Plessner Award. Dr. Gilbert knew he was one of the three finalists but did not live long enough to know he was the recipient. The notification that he was a finalist for the award, from Brad Cohn MD, California Medical Association, read, "I am pleased to inform you

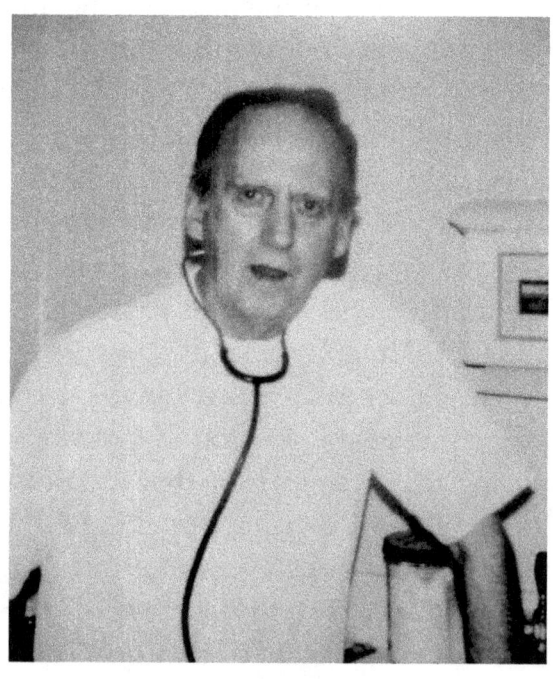

Dr. Jack C. Gilbert, 1980s

that Doctor Jack C. Gilbert has been selected as one of the three finalists for consideration as the 1981 recipient of the Frederick K.M. Plessner Award. This award goes to a candidate that best exemplifies the practice and ethics of a rural country doctor." All his patients knew that. (Submitted by Pat Barry, Fort Bidwell, information from the *Modoc County Record,* 1/8/81.)

## "POLITICIAN DOCTOR" SELDEN MCMEANS, 1859-1876

Dr. Selden McMeans was known to *Greasewood's* editor because of his high profile in Nevada, where he lived until his death in California on July 31, 1876.

The presence of the painting of McMeans by S.A. McLellan in the Nevada Historical Society's collection was brought to our attention by a direct descendant, Walter McMeans of Sugar Land, Texas.

Selden Allen McMeans was an important civic-minded doctor who was present at the birth of Nevada, but he was also a rabble-rouser for the South during the war between the states. He was born in July 1806 near Knoxville, Tennessee, and later moved to Greenville, South Carolina, where he married and began his career in medicine. When the war with Mexico began in 1846, Dr. McMeans left his plantation to volunteer for military service. In July 1849, he was in Mexico City, but he was planning to move to California. He ultimately settled in Sacramento, where he jumped into politics.

The Democratic State Convention elected McMeans one of twelve vice-presidents in 1852, and on January 1, 1854, he was installed as Treasurer of the newly formed State of California, a post he held for two years. In November 1855, the State Council of the American Party in California, which supported the South's position on slavery, elected Dr. McMeans president. In fall 1859 the cry for secession from the Union was growing, but the cry of silver in the Nevada Territory was louder, and McMeans moved to California City. Here, he and a friend from California, Judge

California Terry, organized support for the Confederacy by forming the Knights of the Golden Circle in John Newman's house, the first 'permanent' structure in California City.

Besides being a politician and maybe a part-time miner, McMeans practiced medicine. Drs. McMeans and Edmund Gardner Bryant (cousin of poet William Cullen Bryant and married to Mary, who later married mining mogul John Mackay) treated most of the miners in town for drinking water contaminated with arsenic. Julia Bulette, a well-known Virginia City prostitute, is also alleged to have provided health care for the miners, but there is no historical evidence to verify this.

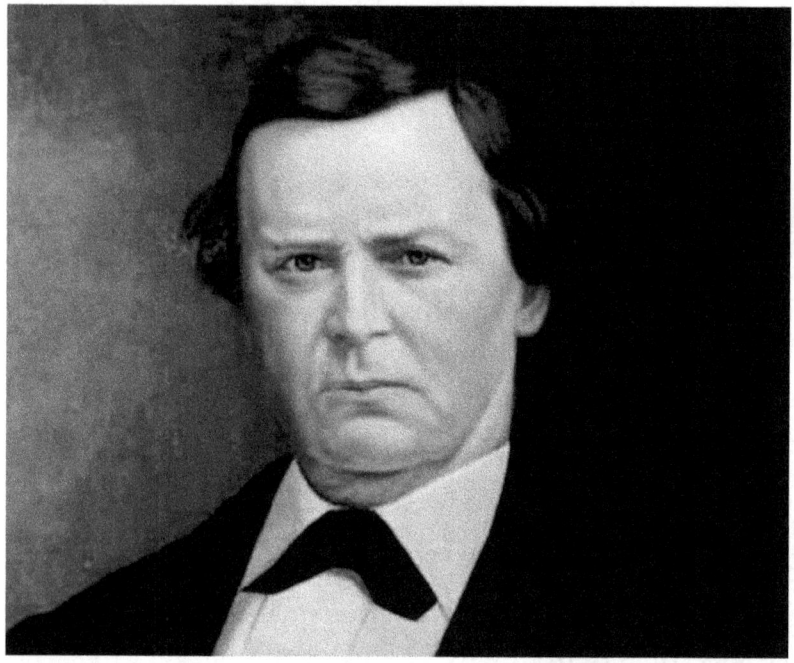

Dr. Selden McMeans (Nev. Hist. Soc. painting by S. McLellan)

April 12, 1861, brought news of the South firing on Fort Sumter, its surrender, and the secession of South Carolina. McMeans sprang to action for the South and announced his plans to capture Fort Churchill and claim the territory for Jefferson Davis. The Confederate flag was raised over Newman's saloon, and Dr. McMeans organized 200 members of the Knights of the

Golden Circle to defend the building. With the news of a detachment of soldiers from Fort Churchill being sent to Virginia City, Dr. McMeans and his supporters evaporated. During the Civil War, McMeans organized the Democratic Party in Nevada and was its first chairman.

After the war, Dr. McMeans continued his political activities, and on June 22, 1872, he organized the Pacific Coast Pioneers in Virginia City. To be eligible one had to be male or a direct male descendent of a resident in one of the Pacific Coast States on January 1, 1851. The Society acquired a building and had 400 members. Dr. E.B. Harris was president of the Society in 1881.

Dr. Seldon McMeans eventually relocated his practice in California. He died at the age of 70 in his California office on July 31, 1876.

**NOTE:**
Source of information was Sonoma County Historical Society's *The McMeans Family* by Connor and *The Saga of the Comstock Lode* by Lyman and Thompson and West's *History of Nevada*.

## "CIVIL WAR HERO" DR. ELIAS B. HARRIS, 1860

Elias Braman Harris was born September 13, 1827, in Otsego County, New York. He attended Fairfield Academy and Geneva College where he studied medicine under Professor Frank Hamilton. In 1845, he enrolled in the two-year course in medicine at New York Medical University, one of the top medical schools in the country. After practicing in New York for two years, he eventually made his way to California by way of Panama and arrived in San Francisco in 1850.

He settled briefly in Calaveras County, which is now known for its vineyards and Mark Twain's humorous story about jumping frogs. Disgusted with frontier justice and witnessing a lynching, he stayed only a few months before moving to Ione in Amador County. There, he became involved in politics, opened a hotel, and leased a mine, the Oneida Mill and Mine. Dr. Harris is credited with building the first Nevada Territory steam quartz mill in 1860.

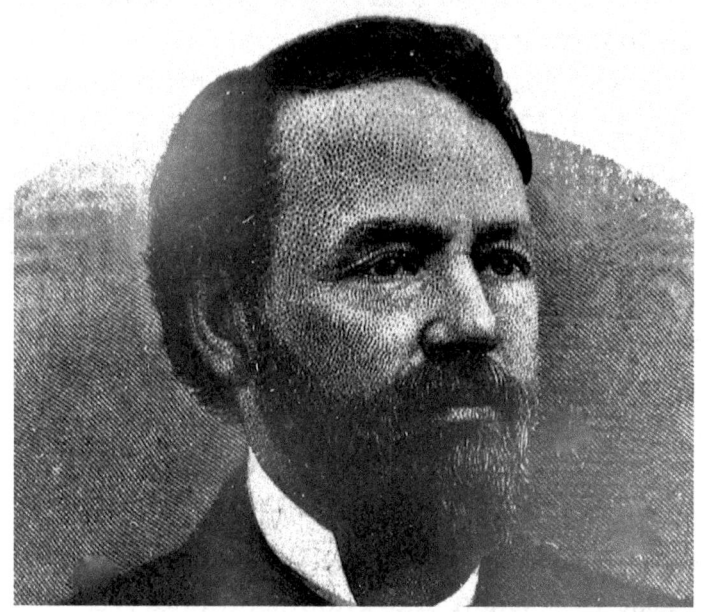

Dr. E.B. Harris, late 1800s

When the Civil War broke out, he returned East and joined the Union Army as a surgeon with the rank of Major. After the war, he married and returned to California City where he practiced from 1875 until 1881. He also had a practice in Sacramento. He died in San Francisco on 8/7/1900.

**NOTE:**

Source of information is Thompson and West's *History of Nevada* and Bancroft's *History of Nevada, 1540-1888*.

## DOCTORS HUFFAKER, GRISBY, AND HEWETSON, 1800S

### By Dr. Anton Sohn

**DR. ANTHONY A. HUFFAKER** was born in 1863 and graduated from Cooper Medical School in San Francisco. It was later bought by Stanford University and became Stanford University School of Medicine.

He came to Carson City in 1896, where he is said to have been the first pediatrician in the area. Dr. Huffaker was president of the Nevada State Medical Association in 1907. He was also a physician for the State Prison in Carson City.

Dr. Huffaker decided in the early part of the century that he should buy an automobile to use on his routine of daily visits to patients. He bought the car, studied his book of instructions, and boldly took it out on his rounds.

Several hours later, Mrs. Huffaker was in the front yard watering his prize dahlias (his hobby) when the doctor came driving down the street. He called out to her but drove on past; in a few minutes he came back around the block, and with an agonized look on his face, drove past again; the third time around he leaned out and called to his wife, "Go get the instruction book and throw it to me the next time around- I've forgotten how it says to stop the blamed machine!" Huffaker Lane is in South Reno. (This story is from the Nevada State Historical Society records.)

**DR. EDWARD SHEPARD GRIGSBY** graduated from Hahnemann Medical College, a homeopathic school, in 1894. Like many doctors he was attracted by mining excitement and the need to supplement his income from medicine. He went to Nome, Alaska, and later to various locations in Nevada (Bullfrog, Rhyolite, and Tonopah). He was licensed in Nevada in 1905. He formed a partnership with Dr. Patrick J. McDonnell, a graduate of Johns Hopkins Medical School, who arrived in Tonopah in 1910.

While practicing in Rhyolite, he was called to attend Jim Arnold's lynching by the citizens of a mining camp, in Skidoo, California, near Death Valley. Arnold was tried by the mob for killing Joe Simpson.

The doctor's car got stuck in the sand and he didn't get to Skidoo in time to save Arnold but was associated with one of the most famous lynching stories of the West. Simpson's dead body was 'strung up' several times, as everyone in the town wanted a picture of the lynching and the citizens obliged by a re-enactment of the incident, including for the sheriff when he arrived. The story is a favorite "western," and no doubt the doctor told it as many times as other spectators of the "reenactment." (This story is from the Nevada State Historical Society records)

**DR. HALLE L. HEWETSON** was born in Clarisville, Ohio, April 1, 1864, and graduated from the prestigious University of Pennsylvania, Department of Medicine, in 1886. That year he joined the U.S. Army where he organized the chair of pathology and bacteriology in Omaha, Nebraska. This gave him the opportunity to become railroad physician for the Union Pacific Railroad. Because of poor health he moved to Kemmerer, Wyoming, and in 1903 he became the physician for the Los Angeles and Salt Lake Railroad.

He arrived as the railroad doctor in 1905 and was the first to pitch a tent on the site that is now Las Vegas. The tent was in the middle of an alfalfa field in the vicinity of Fremont Street. At the time there were only two ranches, Kyle's, and Stewart's, in the valley. When Las Vegas town sites were auctioned with prices of twenty-five-foot lots going above the thousand-dollar mark, Hewetson attended the auction.

He established the first hospital in Las Vegas...which was in a tent. This hospital later became the Las Vegas Hospital owned by Doctors Ferdinand Ferguson and Balcom. During World War I, Dr. Hewetson was assigned to Fort Lewis, Washington, in the medical corps.

At the end of the war, he returned to Las Vegas and was county physician until his retirement. He died in 1930. (This story is from the *Las Vegas Evening Review Journal*, March 28, 1930.)

## DR. ANTHONY HUFFAKER'S JOURNALS, 1896-1907

Reno Surgeon Dr. R. Thatcher Dilley came into possession of a priceless historical artifact. Ruth Thom of Carson City gave him seven volumes of Huffaker's hand-written journals (3/22/1896 to

8/9/1907). These journals by Carson City Dr. Anthony Huffaker contain patient records.

Dr. Huffaker developed a personal form of "shorthand" with numerous abbreviations that make the entries somewhat difficult to decipher.

The entries include the patient's name, date treated, age of patient, and place of birth. Some family and past medical history is usually included. Many of the patients are easily recognized as Nevada pioneers. There are short descriptions of the patient's complaint, physical findings and treatment prescribed. Volume VIII skips a two-year period during the time Dr. Huffaker engaged in post graduate studies in Germany. There is also a small volume (with only a few entries) concerned with a gold mine-possibly one of Dr. Huffaker's investments. Dr. Huffaker practiced in Reno during his later years and owned a ranch in South Reno-the present day Huffaker Hills. These leather-bound books are remarkably well preserved, and as far as we can determine are the only known physician's journals from that time.

### DR. JOHN ALLEN VEATCH, VIRGINIA CITY

John Allen Veatch was born in Kentucky on March 5, 1808, the first of eight children in a growing frontier family. In 1822, his mother died, and the family moved to Spencer County, Indiana. At nineteen he was back in Kentucky where he began his medical studies, and it is thought he got his diploma by studying under a practicing doctor. Unfortunately, we do not have definitive information about his training. Two years later, in 1929, his restless nature led him to Louisiana, where he taught school and had two children with his first wife, Charlotte Sheridan Edwards.

In 1834, the family moved to Texas, where Dr. Veatch acquired land and became involved in politics. He was elected delegate from the community of Bevil to the Consultation of 1835, which met to consider autonomous rule for Texas a year before the Texas Declaration of Independence. In the 1840s, Veatch practiced medicine in Town Bluff, Texas. During 1846-47, he served as first lieutenant in the Independent Volunteer Company, and later he served as surgeon in the Texas Mounted Volunteers. After Charlotte's death, Dr. Veatch married Ann Bradley and they had two children. By 1850 he had acquired property and his intellectual interests led him to the study of botany and mineralogy. By all accounts, Dr. Veatch was a brilliant man.

Veatch also once owned what would become some of the most valuable land in Texas at Sour Lake and Spindletop, where oil was discovered fifty years later.

Still restless for adventure, he went to California and Ann sued for divorce based on abandonment. During his explorations in California, Veatch discovered borax in Lake County. He explored and surveyed Carros Island off Lower California, was curator of conchology at the California Academy of Sciences from 1858 to 1861 and authored several scientific papers.

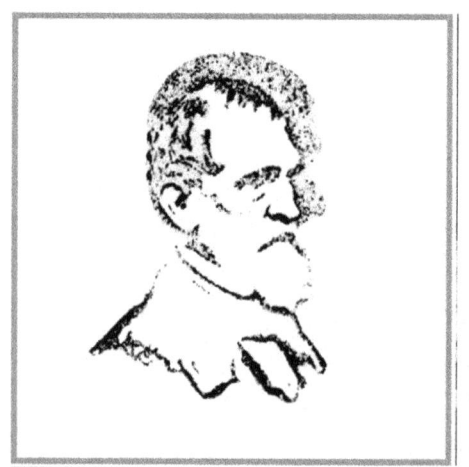 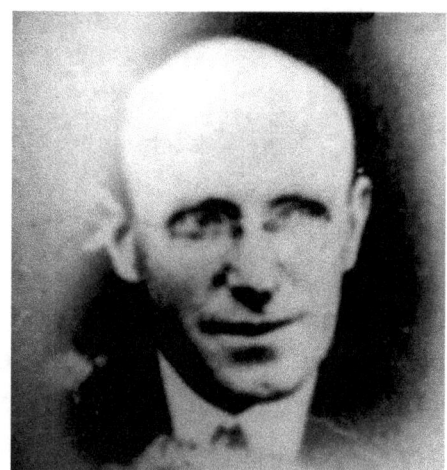

Dr. John Allen Veatch          Dr. Anthony Huffaker

The Comstock Lode discovery of June 1859 and the growth of Virginia City drew Dr. Veatch to the mining district where he practiced medicine and was involved in geology from 1862 to 1863. The Nevada Census shows he was a resident of Clifton, Lander County, in 1863.

In 1865, he married his third wife, Samantha Brisbee, and moved to Oregon. After an unsuccessful attempt to become state geologist of Oregon in 1868, he took a position as professor of chemistry, toxicology, and materia medica at the newly founded Willamette University Medical School. Willamette was Oregon's first medical school, and in 1913, it became the University of Oregon School of Medicine. Dr. Veatch died of pneumonia in Portland on April 24, 1870. His obituary listed him as an officer of the Ancient United Order of Druids.

## Sixteen Outstanding Homegrown Doctors of Northern Nevada

### By Dr. John M. Davis

In the 1930s, there was a cadre of remarkable men native to northern Nevada, who entered the study of medicine and returned home to become the foundation of the excellent medical community that materialized in the Reno area in the last half of the twentieth century.

This group of men included 1. Fred Anderson (surgeon & Father of the Univ. of Nev. School of Med.), 2. Donald Atcheson, 3. Edwin Cantlon (surgeon & pres. of NSMA, 4. Vernon Cantlon (surgeon & pres. of NSMA), 5. Lynn Gerow (family practice), 6. Arthur J. "Bart" Hood II (surgeon), 7. Dwight Hood (internist & pres. of NSMA), 8. Louis Lombardi (surgeon & regent of the Univ. of Nev.), 9. Kenneth Maclean (surgeon & sec. of Nev. Board of Med. Exam.), 10. Leo Nannini (surgeon), 11. Ernest Mack (neurosurgeon & chairman of WMC Trustees, 12. Frank Samuels (OB/GYN), 13. George Cann (internist), 14. James Herz (founder of Reno Orthopedic Clinic), and 15. William Arbonies (radiologist). Dr. Davis failed to mention 16. Robert Locke (pulmonologist).

These men attended the University of Nevada and came under the influence of Peter Frandsen, who stimulated their interest in science, guided them into medicine, and helped admission to medical school, including McGill, Michigan, St. Louis University, Harvard, Stanford, Cornell, Johns Hopkins, Northwestern, and Washington, St. Louis—some of the most prestigious institutions.

It is quite remarkable and a tribute to Professor Frandsen and the educational system at the University of Nevada that a small community fostered such an array of outstanding physicians. These men were instrumental in the development of St. Mary's Hospital, Washoe Medical Center (now Renown Regional Medical Center), and the ascension of medicine in northern Nevada. Their knowledge, skills, ethical standards, and influence served as a nucleus in attracting physicians to the area.

## DRS. ADA AND GIDEON WEED, 1860
## DR. ADA WEED, NEVADA'S FIRST FEMALE MD
### By Dr. Kristin Sohn Fermoile

Guy Rocha brought Dr. Ada Weed to my attention. She may be the first woman doctor to practice in Nevada, although she was not a regular doctor. Her husband's practice is extensively documented, but I could not find any information on her in our archives. Since they went to the same medical school before they came to the state, one can assume they shared information on patients, and she may have had an active practice.

Doctors Gideon A. and Ada M. Weed brought eastern hydropathic medicine to the western frontier in 1858. The couple met while enrolled in Dr. Russell T. Trall's Hygeio-Therapeutic College in New York City. In 1857, they both received irregular diplomas as the institution did not yet have a charter. Dr. Trall's college taught the principles of hydrotherapy, also known as the "water-cure," which was considered an alternative to allopathic medicine. Supporters believed drug therapies were unnecessary and, in fact, detrimental to successful medical treatment. Instead, practitioners of hydrotherapy relied on principles of hygiene, diet, rest, and the therapeutic value of water.

Dr. Trall established hydrotherapy as a medical system in the United States during the 1840s. Admission requirements to his school included a common school education and possession of common sense. Most students were from the working class, and Dr. Trall advocated training women, despite the societal restrictions of the time. In fact, a third of Trall's graduates were female, during a time when it was extremely difficult for women to gain admission into traditional medical schools.

A few months after graduation, Ada (1837-1910) and Gideon (1833-1905) were married in the school's lecture hall. The couple quickly departed the east coast for the western frontier. They arrived in San Francisco in early 1858.

Unlike many who migrated during this time, the Weeds did not plan to make a quick fortune and return east. They planned to settle in California.

They dreamed of opening their own Hygeio-Medical Institute. Unfortunately, unforeseen professional competition existed in San Francisco, and the Weeds decided to continue their migration into Oregon.

Oregon proved to be a state with abundant opportunities for the Weeds. The territory lacked hydropathic physicians, and furthermore, there existed a great demand for their services. Oregon citizens wrote to the editor of *The Water Cure Journal* asking for a hydropathic physician and a hydropathic institution in their area. The Weeds rented an office in Salem and advertised in the *Oregon Statesman*. They began plans for a water-cure establishment, which included bathing facilities, a gymnasium, and boarding rooms. Ada focused on the female populations, advertising a specialty in obstetrics and pediatrics.

Soon after their arrival, the Weeds began eliciting criticism and stirring controversy. Being irregular practitioners, they were subjected to criticism by those who believed in traditional medicine. The women mistrusted Ada because she was the first female in Oregon with a medical degree. The couple was also suspect because they actively advertised. Lastly, the couple stirred controversy because they advocated social change. In addition to curing people of their ills, they desired to cure society of its problems.

Ada strongly pushed for social reform. She gave a series of lectures to Oregonians, in which she espoused woman's rights and the need for improved conditions for frontier women.

Although her efforts produced no significant changes or advancements among women in Oregon, she did succeed in eliciting controversy and gaining opposition. Perhaps her strongest and most publicized opposition was from Asahel Bush, editor of the *Oregon Statesmen*. After hearing one of Ada's first lectures, he published several lengthy critiques in his newspaper. Ada issued rebuttals, but her reputation had been permanently damaged.

The Weeds continued their reform efforts despite this opposition. They traveled among various settlements in the Oregon region and gave talks in churches and courtrooms. Some lectures were free, and others required a fifty-cent admission fee.

In lectures, her topics expanded to sex and birth control. Portions of the public soon began to view her as a woman's rights zealot.

Despite the negative publicity, the Weeds outwardly painted their crusade as successful. They believed they were making headway in converting the public towards hydrotherapy. In correspondence with Dr. Trall, they claimed the people of Oregon were in a transitional state. They opposed traditional medicine and its drugs but did not yet fully support hydrotherapy. Additionally, they believed the traditional doctors in Oregon, who initially denounced hydrotherapy, were beginning to claim they had always used water therapy in their treatments.

After their second lecture tour, they wrote accounts of receptive audiences, many of whom were already practicing their principles. They described the success of their practice and claimed they had as many patients as their house could hold.

They failed, however, to divulge their financial hardships. As the economy in Oregon was depressed, many patients were unable to pay. The Weeds took on a partner to help finance the outfitting of their treatment house. Although their lectures were well attended, their profits did not cover their expenses.

Unable to get ahead in Oregon, the Weeds returned to California in the spring of 1860. A year later, they opened a Hygeio-Medical Institute in Sacramento. Even though this was their unfulfilled dream while in Oregon, the Weeds were still unable to settle down and prosper. That fall, they followed the silver rush to Washoe City, Nevada. A few years later, they returned to California, settling in Vallejo. It seems they remained restless.

In 1869, at the age of 36, Gideon returned to school and received 18 weeks of allopathic training at Rush Medical College in Chicago. This marked a turning point for the couple, as their success and status greatly improved, and they were no longer met with strong opposition. In 1870, they moved to Seattle, where Gideon practiced as a physician and surgeon. He enjoyed a lucrative practice and refocused his reform energies on improving healthcare conditions. In 1874, he founded the Seattle Hospital to improve medical care for those injured in the logging camps.

He provided medical care to indigent, was active in various medical societies, assisted in creating the State Medical Board, and helped secure funds to start a medical school. During two terms as mayor, he was able to pass many reforms and earn respect from fellow citizens. In fact, he was the first mayor to succeed at reelection.

Dr. Ada Weed did not continue to practice medicine after their move to Seattle. Furthermore, neither Dr. Weeds advertised their hydropathic degrees or continued lecturing. Gideon's medical practice, along with wise real estate investments, allowed the couple to maintain a high quality of life. They built a mansion in 1876 and raised two children, Benjamin, and Mabel. Ada became somewhat of a society lady.

She hosted social events at their mansion, served as director of the Library Association, represented the Plymouth Congregational Church, and supported charities. She continued to push for women's rights, but she allied with the local temperance movement and shunned the more dramatic suffragists. Additionally, she assisted her husband in his medical reform activities.

While in Seattle, the Weeds were very successful in their medical and social reform activities. Their newfound traditional methods were in stark contrast to the previous methods they had utilized while in Oregon and California. They garnered significant respect from the citizens of Washington, and they avoided the criticism and opposition they had received during previous crusades. A detailed article ran in Seattle's *Pacific Tribune* on October 25, 1877, which described their twentieth wedding anniversary. They received valuable china pieces as gifts from other prominent citizens, which testified to their important position in their community.

In 1890, the Weeds moved to Berkeley, where Gideon continued to practice traditional medicine and the children attended the University of

California. The couple's nephew, Dr. Park Weed Willis, an allopathic physician trained at the University of Pennsylvania, took over Gideon's Seattle medical practice. Ada continued to be active in social causes, and she assisted victims of the San Francisco earthquake. In her final years, she nursed her paralytic husband and continued to practice.

She suffered from a variety of physical ailments and continued to drink large amounts of water, self-treatment of which her nephew approved. She died of cancer in 1910.

**NOTE:**
Various sources list Gideon Weed as practicing in Nevada from 1860 to 1867. Unfortunately, Ada is not listed in any of the same sources. If she was practicing in the state in 1860, she would be Nevada's earliest known woman doctor. Edwards, Thomas G. (1977). "Dr. Ada M. Weed, Northwest Reformer," *Oregon Historical Quarterly*, 78 (1), 5-40.

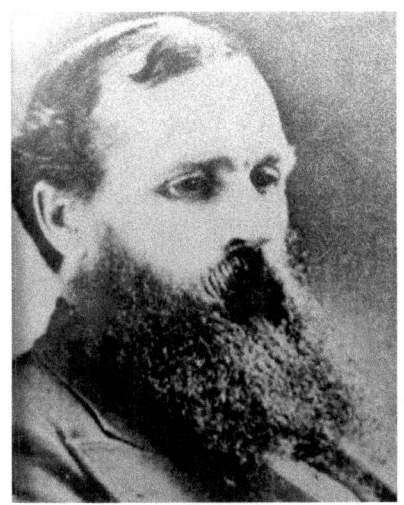

Dr. Gideon Weed        Dr. Ada Weed, 1860s

## "A Doctor's Doctor"
### Dr. Kenneth Frazer Maclean
## By Dr. Robert Daugherty

1. "A tremendously interesting curmudgeon"
2. "He was very, very, rude, abrupt, and abusive"
3. "Yes, he was abrupt, but one always knew exactly where one stood with Ken"
4. "He was one of my physician heroes in Nevada"
5. "He wasn't in the business of medicine for money — he was really a good doctor — A Doctor's Doctor"
6. "The Board of Medical Examiners was run by the seat-of-the-pants of Ken Maclean"
7. "His importance didn't stop at the door of the Board"

8. "Ken cared deeply for the well-being of his patients and of his peers"
9. "Ken demanded quality of care for Nevada's citizens"

All the above quotes from fellow physicians describe Kenneth Maclean, an important physician who practiced surgery in Reno from 1946 until his retirement in 1983. He was a Reno native whose medical legacy began in Scotland with his grandfather, who pioneered academic surgery in the United States, continued with his father, Donald Maclean Jr. an early Carson City doctor. He practiced in the "Golden Age of Medicine."

Ken Maclean's grandfather, Donald Maclean Sr., was born in Canada in 1839, received his medical education in Scotland where he was a student of Joseph Lister, the father of aseptic medicine, and served in the Northern Army during the Civil War. Returning to civilian life in 1872, at the age of thirty-four, apparently because of his success and popularity among his patients and students, he was appointed professor and chair of surgery at the University of Michigan SOM in Ann Arbor.

William Mayo, who graduated from the University of Michigan School of Medicine in 1883 noted: "In 1882, Dr. Maclean began to practice asepsis and antisepsis while teaching about the work of Joseph Lister. In my first year, I remember him being fastidious to operating room routine. Before surgery, he would roll up his sleeves and carefully wash his hands before beginning an operation and again a couple of times during the operation." Dr. Mayo went on to say that one of the most important concepts he acquired as a student and assistant to Ken Maclean's grandfather was: 'The sick man was the hub around which the entire education turned" and "the application of the art of medicine is based on the science of medicine" a concept that to this day, we admire and strive to instill in our students.

At the time of Donald Maclean, Sr.'s appointment at the University of Michigan, not only did the University of Michigan not have a teaching hospital, but no other medical school in the

United States had one. In fact, hospitals were not a part of medical care in this country until late into the nineteenth century when scientific discoveries advanced medical care. Individuals who could afford medical care were not treated in a hospital.

At the start of the nineteenth century, there were only two significant hospitals in the United States, located in Philadelphia and New York City. Massachusetts General became the third hospital in 1821.

The first hospitals were originally established as infirmaries to provide for the poor, disabled and the infirm. For example, Philadelphia General, Bellevue, and Baltimore General evolved from almshouses or pest houses-to care for those suffering from an epidemic. The county hospitals of Nevada evolved in 1860 from a pestilence—smallpox.

Thus, when the University of Michigan finished its hospital in 1877, there were fewer than two hundred hospitals in the country and none were university teaching hospitals. Ken's grandfather was the chairman of surgery in the first university teaching hospital in the United States. However, his seventeen-year tenure ended abruptly in 1889 when he advocated the relocation of the university clinics to take advantage of a larger teaching population in Detroit. This was against the opposition of both the board of Regents and the president of the university. The regents instructed the president to request Dr Maclean's resignation, which, of course, he provided. As further proof of his importance, in 1894, Donald Maclean was elected president of the American Medical Association. He died in Detroit in 1903, where he lived since 1883.

Ken's father, Donald Maclean, Jr., was a graduate of the Royal College of Surgeons in Scotland. Dr. Donald Maclean, Jr. came west and served as a doctor in Hawaii during the Boxer Rebellion.

After the service, he came to San Francisco, and in 1906, moved to Reno. In 1910, he moved to Carson City, where he was the physician for the Nevada State Prison. After ten years in Carson, he moved to the Riverside Hotel in Reno, where the family lived, and his practice was relocated. He died in Reno on January 4, 1939.

**KENNETH F. MACLEAN** was born in Carson City, March 9, 1914. He graduated from Reno High School and the University of Nevada in Reno and received his medical degree from McGill University School of Medicine in 1939. His surgical training at the University of Michigan was interrupted in 1942 by World War II.

From 1942 until 1945 he served with the University of Michigan Unit 298th General Hospital in the European Theater of Operations. Over twenty years later, Dr. Ken Turner, an obstetrician from Las Vegas was appointed to the Board of Medical Examiners. Dr. Turner had been a private as a medical aid on a glider assault team and had suffered serious injuries requiring several operations. In talking about his war injury surgeries with Dr. Maclean, Dr. Turner recalled Dr. Maclean had been one of the first surgeons to operate on him after his evacuation from France to Liege, Belgium, where Maclean was stationed.

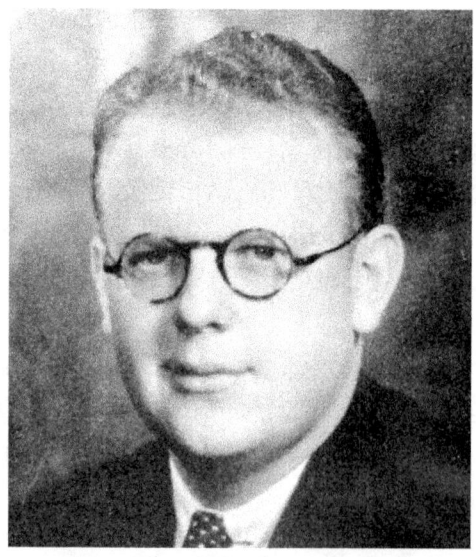

Dr. Ken Maclean, 1950

After the war, Ken continued the legacy of his grandfather and father by returning to the University of Michigan to complete his surgical training. At the completion of his training, he and his wife, Margaret, returned to Reno in 1947 to begin practice. Two years later, he was appointed by Nevada Governor Vail Pittman to serve on the Board of Medical Examiners.

Ken Maclean was the leader of the Nevada Board of Medical Examiners for over thirty years, and thereby directly influenced the standards and quality of the practice of medicine in Nevada over three decades. It was during these three decades (1950-1980) that Nevada truly "burst" onto the national scene, going from a population of less than 200,000 to more than one million people.

Some say it was without question, the "Golden Age of Medicine" with technological and scientific advances beyond anyone's dreams. During Maclean's tenure, the physician population increased from less than 1,000 to over 4,000 in 1980. The Board established standards that determined the quality of medical care in Nevada into the twenty-first century.

These new standards ranged from recognizing and licensing physician assistants, defining the criteria for legal abortion, establishing rules for professional conduct, setting up procedures for investigating and disciplining physicians, and enumerating punitive actions the board could impose on a physician found guilty of misconduct. These changes led to a much more precise extensive document that served as the under pinning for the current Nevada Medical Practice Act.

The above description and accounts of Dr. Ken Maclean tell us a bit about the man known as the czar of Nevada medical licensure.

He was considered a doctor's surgeon; a physician that other physicians would seek for their own personal surgical care. The legacy continues in Nevada through the standards of practice enabled by the actions of the Nevada Board of Medical Examiners under his thirty-year leadership.

**NOTE:**

Source of information was George Maclean, Dr. Ken Maclean's nephew; Nev. Bd. of Med. Exam. records; *Reno Gazette-Journal*; AMA records; *Mayo Clinical Proceedings*; and University of Michigan records.

## DR. GEORGE THOMA
### "RENO STREET NAMED IN HIS HONOR"
## By Dr. Anton Sohn

Dr. George Thoma was a leading physician in nineteenth century Nevada and his importance merited a street in Reno to be named in his honor. Thoma Street is located two blocks north of the VA Medical Center and runs east-west between Virginia and Yori Streets. Thoma was born in Montgomery County, New York, in 1843 to German immigrants, and he graduated from Albany Medical College at the age of twenty-one.

Like many German descendants, he pledged his life to his new country and joined the Union Army as a surgeon in the Second New York Heavy Artillery. He was at the front with Ulysses Grant's Army when Lee surrendered.

Attracted by adventure and reports of wealth in Nevada, he joined a freight wagon train for Salt Lake City. From there, he drove a mule and wagon with two companions across the desert and mountains in 1867 to the Reese River Valley (now Austin, Nevada) to work in the mines. When he arrived in the valley his clothing was in tatters, and he and his companions were exhausted by exposure and deprivation. He supported himself as an ore sorter in a quartz mill, and years later, friends recalled he enjoyed recounting his experiences in the mill. In the evenings, after a hard day in the mill, he pursued his first love—practicing medicine.

Mining discoveries took him to Eureka, Hamilton, and finally in 1872, to Pioche where he was involved in the first attempt to form the Nevada State Medical Association. The doctors formulated a fee schedule, but the association would not be permanent until 1904.

Dr. Thoma was civic minded and was elected to the Nevada State Senate. He served as senator from 1884 to 1888. During this period he went to Sacramento, where he met his future wife. They returned to Nevada where he finished his tenure in the legislature and his new wife taught school.

In 1887, they established a permanent home in Reno where they would reside until his death in 1907. Early in 1891, he was appointed superintendent of the Nevada Mental Hospital (now Northern Nevada Adult Mental Health Hospital) in Sparks, and he served one year in that capacity.

In Reno, he strove to improve the practice of medicine and helped to pass the 1899 state law that regulated the practice of medicine in Nevada. He was also prominent in the formation of the Nevada State Medical Association and served as its second president in 1906. In Reno, Dr. Thoma had extensive real estate holdings, and, with Mr. Bigelow, he built a building at First and Virginia, which became the home of the Woolworth 5¢ and 10¢ Store. He had two daughters, who became Mrs. Roy Hardy and Mrs. George Wingfield, Sr. Dr. Thoma died January 30, 1907.

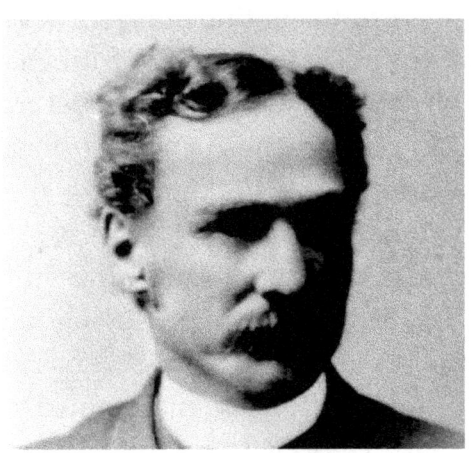

Dr. George Thoma, 1900s

## More on Dr. George Thoma
### By Dr. Owen Bolstad

Dr. George H. Thoma may have been one of the most widely known and highly respected physicians who practiced medicine in Nevada during the second half of the nineteenth century.

He was born on October 14, 1843, in Montgomery County, New York. His father was an emigrant from Germany, who made his living as a clock maker. His mother was born in Montgomery and was of Dutch descent. George received his primary education in Amsterdam, New York, then, enrolled at Albany Medical College where he got his MD degree in 1864. Immediately after graduation from Albany, Dr. Thoma volunteered for the Union Army and was designated as an assistant surgeon in the Second New York Artillery Regiment. He served with the Army of the Potomac until the surrender of the Confederate Army at Appomattox, where he was present to observe the Flag of Truce that signaled the end of the Civil War.

About one year after the cessation of hostilities, attracted by the reports of mineral wealth and driven by a spirit of adventure, Dr. Thoma set out for the western frontier. By the time he reached the Missouri River, he had spent his meager savings and was forced to sign on with a freighting outfit to continue his journey.

After reaching Salt Lake City, he resigned his job with the freight company and set out walking across the Great Salt Desert with two companions and a mule pulling their supplies on a small cart. They arrived at the Reese River Valley during the summer of 1837, almost more dead than alive.

At first, he took employment as an ore sorter in a stamp mill to finance his immediate needs. By 1868, he began practicing his profession of medicine once again in the Austin area. Sometime later he moved his practice to Eureka, where he maintained a successful practice for fourteen years. George Thoma immersed himself in his medical practice and into the affairs of his community as well. It has been said he would answer a call to a miner's hut as readily as he would to the home of a wealthy man. He was well respected by the people of the area, and in 1884, he was elected to the State Senate where he served for four years.

In 1887, Dr. Thoma moved his practice to Reno, where he practiced until his death in 1907 at the age of 64 years. He was well thought of by his colleagues. George Thoma loved his adopted state and often spoke of the peace he felt as he viewed Nevada's rugged mountains and deserts. He lived and worked in Nevada for 40 years and during that time he contributed a great deal to that young and growing western state.

**NOTE:**
This story was adapted from an article in the March 1907 *California State Journal of Medicine*. It was brought to our attention by Mr. Albert R. Paulson of Menlo Park, California.

## ALFRED DOTEN JOURNALS, 1849-1903
### "NUMBING THE SKIN AND ITS CONTENTS ON THE COMSTOCK"

### By Richard G. Pugh

Alfred Doten was a prolific recorder of life in Virginia City for over five decades. His diary not only captured the essence of a colorful era in early Nevada, but it also recorded helping doctors when they needed anesthesia for their patients. In his three-volume diary of 2,300 pages Doten recorded his daily activities, freelance writing for the *Territorial Enterprise* newspaper, assistance in medical procedures, and activities of hard rock miners. His canine companion Keyzer accompanied him in his travels and adventures during the frenetic gold-rush period.

Doten was particularly adept at painting a picture of the daily successes and excesses of flamboyant miners that resulted in violence necessitating a physician and anesthesia. He helped and frequently was called by local physicians to assist in surgical procedures by administering the preferred anesthesia chloroform. Records from Doten's diary indicate he was one of the first "lay anesthesiologists" in Nevada.

He recorded numerous gunfights in Virginia City and related the various ways in which disputes were settled. He wrote about a man who was struck with a miner's pick after a violent argument and nearly died. Virginia City justice was swift in that case as the assaulting man was summarily struck with the same pick for punishment.

Then, there was a case in 1864 where one of the townspeople was seriously injured, not in a gunfight or mine injury, but while exercising in a local gymnasium. Doten assisted Dr. Frederick Hiller, a homeopathic physician, in setting the patient's leg.

On another occasion, Doten was called to assist the doctor in treating a man who was injured when his gun exploded while rabbit shooting. Two middle fingers were amputated while Doten administered the chloroform, and afterwards he wrote, "The gun was over-loaded and had not been shot for three weeks."

Alfred Doten later joined Dr. Hiller in amputating the "preputium" (prepuce) of a miner living in the nearby community of Dutch Flats. Infection of the foreskin was not uncommon in the nineteenth century and was treated by circumcision.

On another day in September 1866, Doten and Keyser traveled to Summit Mill to assist Dr. C.C. Green in treating a head injury patient. The patient was hit by a stone playfully thrown by a friend. Even though he was called to administer the anesthetic, none was given. The man underwent surgery suffering much pain, taking it like a major, but Doten received $5 for being available. Life during the Comstock Lode era was often perilous but never dull.

In addition to his medical duties, Doten participated in many of the cultural activities of Virginia City such as performances at Piper's Opera House. He once attended a lecture by Mark Twain.

Doten: "It was one and a half hours long, but I heard it all and it was mighty good." When not recording the daily temperature and weather swings in Virginia City, assisting physician, recording the ins and outs of daily life, and tending to his mining interests, Doten enjoyed drinking cocktails and cruising about town with his dog, Keyzer, and Dan DeQuille, editor of the *Territorial Enterprise*.

**NOTE:**

The information in this article was taken from the Journals of Alfred Doten, 1849-1903. Also of interest was the fact that alcohol was frequently used for anesthesia. In 1874, Dr. George Kober, who was an U.S. Army surgeon at Fort McDermit on the Oregon and Nevada border, mentioned that he used two ounces of whiskey for anesthesia to amputate a soldier's finger. One and a half ounces is the amount of liquid in a bartender's shot glass.

## DR. JOHN EDWARD WORDEN
## NEVADA'S FIRST STATE HEALTH OFFICER, 1936
### By Dr. Anton Sohn

The following article is the result of an inquiry by Melanie Minarik PhD, and Trudy Larson MD, who were interested in naming an award at the School of Community Health Science at UNR in honor of the first Nevada Health Officer. In such matters, I routinely turn to Guy Rocha.

The law creating the Nevada State Board of Health was enacted in 1893, and several physicians were appointed to the board. They were Nevada's part-time health officers. According to Dr. Don Kwalick, who was appointed State Health Officer in 1997, Dr. John Edward Worden was the first full-time officer. John was born in Canada in February 1875. By 1892 he was living in Milwaukee, and on June 15, 1 889, he graduated from Northwestern Medical School. Dr. Worden studied public health at the University of Michigan and was licensed in 1908 in Fallon.

In 1916, he moved to Elko and was appointed its county health officer. In 1936, Governor Richard Kirman appointed Dr. Worden State Health Officer with the princely salary of $2500. Governor Kirman asked for his resignation two times in 1938 because Worden ran for the U.S. Senate, and Kirman felt this was a conflict of interest. Worden refused both times.

In 1939, he resigned after a severe injury resulting from an auto accident. That year he moved to San Francisco to live with his daughter. He died there in 1959. His obituary is in the December 29, 1959, *Reno Evening Gazette*. It includes this picture of him (photo on page 125) and states he had two children—a son, Lt. Col. J.E. Worden, Jr., and a daughter, Shirley. According to Rocha, "Dr. John Worden, without question, deserves the honor (of an award in his name) for his thirty-one years of public health service to Nevada."

## Dr. Anton Tjader, "1859 Adventures"

"Dr. A.W. Tjader, a Russian gentleman now sojourning here, is the one who took care of the wounded immigrants, survivors of the late Indian massacre on the Sublette Cutoff. He performed this kindness without reward or the hope of reward; and is, in my opinion, justly entitled to public gratitude. I am in hopes he will remain with us and practice his profession." (From September 9, 1859, *San Francisco Herald* written by correspondent 'Tennessee" Richard Allen, writing from Genoa, Carson Valley, Utah Territory.)

There is some question about the birthplace of Dr. Anton W. Tjader. Despite his Swedish name, he described himself as Russian, and the headstone on his grave lists his birthplace as St. Petersburg, Russia, in 1825. His grandson, however, claimed he had verification of Anton's birth and registration in Stockholm, Sweden in 1827.

Anton Tjader received his MD degree from the Royal Scandinavia Institute in Uppsala, Sweden, and served as surgeon in the Russian Army during the Crimean Wars of 1854. After emigrating to the United States in 1855, he entered Harvard Medical School, graduated two years later, and served as a United States Army Contract Surgeon for several years.

In 1859, Dr. Tjader joined the movement west, traveling with the Scroggs wagon train from Missouri. It was during this trek that Dr. Anton Tjader was in the Shepherd Train Massacre on the Sublette Cutoff.

William Shepherd with the Shepherd train was traveling one day ahead of the Scroggs train when he became ill with mountain fever (possibly pneumonia). On July 18, 1859, his brother James and another man backtracked the trail in search of a doctor to attend William.

Dr. Tjader agreed to ride up and attend the sick man. Examining the patient, the doctor determined the man's fever had broken and pronounced him out of danger. The captain of the Shepherd train, Ferguson Shepherd was eager to press on, and by July 26, they had reached Cold Springs camp on the Sublette Cutoff and found the camp in a state of shock, according to statements given when they reached Genoa a month later.

"About 6:00 o'clock PM on 26 July, when some men of a small emigrant train camped at Cold Springs on the Sublette cutoff eighty miles from Salk Lake City, were at supper a small party of eight, Indians arrived with rifles, bows and arrows, came down and asked for something to eat. Having obtained some bread, they started to a hill where the cattle were herded by two men. After saluting the cattle guards and passing them, one of the Indians suddenly turned his pony, lowering his rifle, shot one of the men, Mr. Hall, through the heart, killing him instantly. The other man fled to the camp. The Indians were in the meantime running off nine head of cattle and two horses. At the time of the depredation, there were only a small number of train emigrants present, and sometime afterward, at about 9:00 o'clock, the horse train led by Mr. Ferguson arrived ... in the morning Mr. Shepherd's train left at 7:00 o'clock, at the arrival of the Skroggs train despite the warnings of danger."

At 11:00 o'clock, the train entered a narrow canyon seven miles from the Cold Springs camp. A horse which had been sick stopped and would go no further. The men gathered around the horse to discuss the situation. Distracted by the sick horse, their guard was down. Suddenly gunfire erupted. Captain Shepherd and two other men fell seriously wounded. Next, William

Shepherd was shot in the shoulder, then in the forehead. He was the first to die. Uninjured men from the train began to shoot back.

Some began running from the scene heading back toward Cold Springs camp. Annie Shepherd began to run with her baby daughter in her arms. Encumbered by her long dress and the baby, she soon became exhausted and grew faint.

She asked Smith to carry the baby, but Smith had been shot in the arm above the elbow. The bone was broken, and he was losing blood. Soon he became exhausted and faint. Unable to continue with the baby, he set her down in a grove of poplar trees and covered her with grass and leaves. Near dark he lay down in some sagebrush unable to move on. Another man found him and took him, but not the baby, back into the Cold Springs camp, where Dr. Tjader treated his wounds.

In the end, Captain Ferguson Shepherd, his brother William, and two other men were dead. Five people were wounded. The Wrights, traveling with the Shepherds were both shot and stayed with the wagons in the canyon. Throughout the afternoon and evening people straggled back into Cold Springs. Annie stumbled into camp at sunset 'in a state of insanity.' Placed in a bed, she immediately asked to see her baby. "She's in another wagon as requested by Dr. Tjader, and you are too exhausted to see her," said James Shepherd. Annie pleaded with Dr. Tjader, and he finally relented the truth that the baby, just seven months old, was still out on the trail. Annie raved like a maniac the entire night.

Two more wagons joined the party in Cold Springs camp that afternoon and early the next morning the united trains with 52 wagons and 200 men started through the canyon, led by a group of ten armed men. As they reached the grove of poplar trees the men heard shouting, the baby was found alive! Badly dehydrated and sunburned, the baby was barely alive when she was returned to a joyous Annie, who nursed the baby back to health with the help of Dr. Tjader.

"... the bodies of Ferguson and William Shepherd, William Diggs, and C. Rains were found in the road, covered with blood, dead, and bloated by the heat some 24 hours after the attack."

Upon reaching the wagons, the party found Mrs. James Wright lying under a wagon holding a crippled baby in her arms. Mrs. Wright had a serious wound in her back. Nearby lay mortally wounded James Wright, who died ten days later.

The poor sufferers had been attended by their little five-year-old son who supplied their feverish lips with water. The wagon train continued, reaching Genoa on September 2, 1859.

Dr. Tjader established a medical practice in Genoa, then removed his practice to Carson City in 1860. On May 14, 1860, he volunteered for the Carson City Rangers and was involved in the battle of Pyramid Lake. Although reported to have been killed and scalped, he walked back to Virginia City from the skirmish with three slight arrow wounds and resumed his medical practice, which he continued until his death on July 8, 1870, at the age of 44 years.

**NOTE:**

This story about Dr. Anton Tjader was carefully researched and documented by his great grandson, Mr. Gary Tjader of Los Altos, California. It represents only a small portion of the biographical material being assembled by Gary Tjader, who intends to publish the complete story. Our thanks to Gary Tjader for allowing us to use this interesting look at the practice of medicine and life in the nineteenth century.

## More on Dr. Anton Tjader, "1859 Adventures"

On July 27, 1859, Dr. Anton W. Tjader, a graduate of Harvard Medical College, was traveling west with a wagon train to seek his fortune in California. They were one day behind the small Shepherd/White wagon train on the Sublette cutoff some 80 miles east of Salt Lake City when the Shepherd train was ambushed by hostile Indians. The attack resulted in five dead immigrants and several wounded. Dr. Tjader was called upon to administer medical care to the wounded, and later, prepared a letter to the Indian Agent, Frederick Dodge.

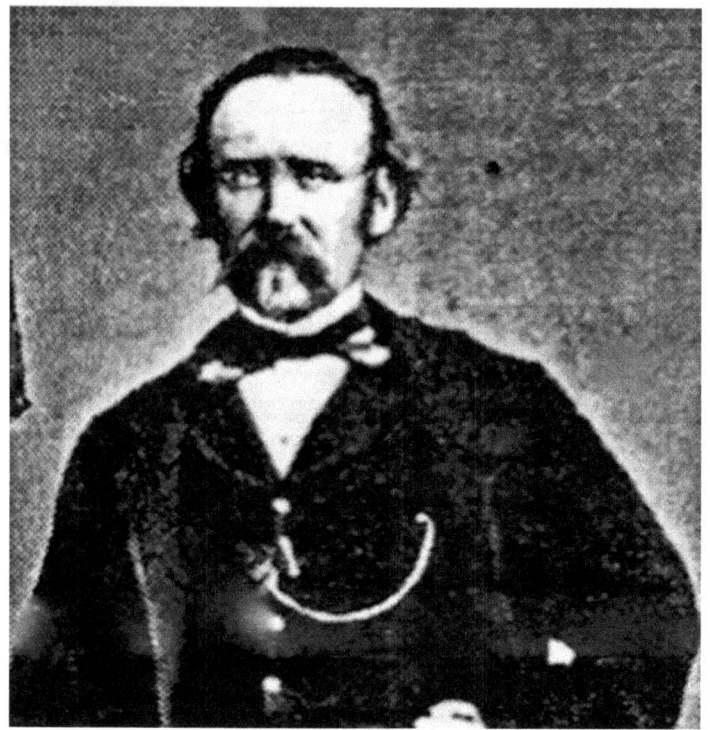

Dr. Anton Tjader, 1860s

Dr. Anton Tjader: "Sir, We have taken into our charge and brought thus far the widows and orphans of the last massacre on the Sublett cutoff at a considerable expense. Mrs. Wright and infant child being seriously wounded and unable to proceed further, and all being totally destitute, we respectfully request that you take charge of them and furnish such aid as may be in your power."

He then prepared a statement of the conditions of the wounded now living; "Mrs. Wright had a rifle ball shot in her back while leaning forward to button up the front part of the wagon. The ball entered half an inch below the right kidney and passed directly downward, grazed the sacral plexus of nerves and pursuing its course downwards and turning inward to lodge somewhere in one of the lower vertebrae. It could not be touched at ten inches from entrance and not seemingly causing any discomfort was allowed to remain. She is now recovering slowly any amount of clothing being partly remised and partly discharged from the wound.

"A little girl daughter of Mrs. Wright aged about 18 months was taken up by the Indians and thrown against the rocks whereby her left thigh was broken in the middle. The poor little thing was partly deranged for some time after. So cruel a treatment. She is now bodily and mentally mending.

"The fracture is united although the bone is slightly bent, the continuous traveling and want of space to apply a proper apparatus (sic) being the cause.

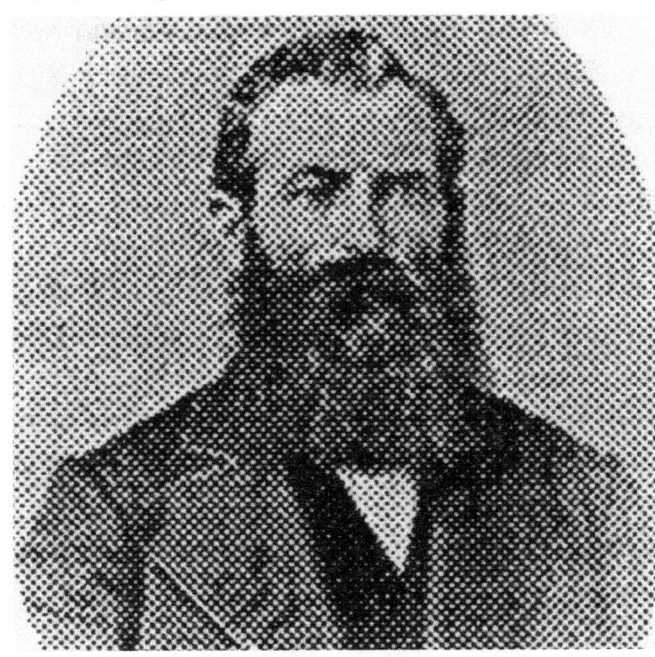

Dr. Frederick Hiller, 1860s

"Another little girl—daughter of Mrs. Wm. Shepherd who was left in the bushes over night was severely blistered all over, neck and legs by the severe sun heat, and her neck injured and remained in pitiable plight for more than a month afterwards. She is recovering, although her neck is still very stiff. The sufferers are now in the hands Maj. F. Dodge, U.S. Indian Agent, who is assiduous in his endeavors to render them all assistance in his power, they are furnished with comfortable quarters, good nursing, clothing, and surgical aid."

## ACCEPTANCE OF FEMALE MDS IN 19TH CENTURY NEVADA
### By Dr. Anton Sohn

The typical medical practitioner in 19th century Nevada was a white Euro-American male. In 1860, Dr. Ada Weed became the first female MD in Nevada. After Dr. Ada Weed, Dr. (Doctress) Helena Jones, practiced in Treasure City, White Pine County, from 1869-'77 making her the third female MD. Women made significant progress in the profession.

Doctress Hoffman, the second female medical practitioner in Nevada, was listed in the Virginia City newspaper, the *Territorial Enterprise* in 1865, and by the end of the century, 22 women doctors were recognized in Nevada. Although the profession would continue to be dominated by men into the 20th century, a steady expansion of the role of women in medicine was occurring. Furthermore, women were making inroads into all the professions.

By the mid-19th century, it became obvious there was a need for women in medical practice. The Victorian ideas of decency and modesty were a barrier to men who wished to practice gynecology and obstetrics. Although there were a few male physicians in the early 18th century who practiced midwifery, many women patients avoided them. Later, in some communities in the West, traditional Chinese doctors were more acceptable to women with "female problems" than American trained physicians who were less sensitive to the needs of women.

Elizabeth Blackwell, the first woman graduate of an American medical school in 1848, was stimulated to study medicine when she observed the sufferings of a friend with a gynecological problem who had been seeing a male physician. However, the medical profession was divided on the education of women who wished to study medicine. Some felt a male student should not study anatomy next to a female student and women should study in all-female classes. Others promoted an all-female medical school on the grounds men should not practice midwifery.

For this reason, in 1848, Samuel Gregory founded the New England Female Medical Education Society which became the New England Female Medical College. His intent was not to create a medical college equal to existing male institutions, but to concentrate on graduating women who would be midwives. He termed his graduates "doctresses." (The term doctress dates back at least to 1800, when a doctress practiced medicine in Bethel, Maine.) Gregory stressed that doctresses should be subservient to male doctors, charge less, and treat only the less difficult cases. Therefore, Doctress Hoffman was probably little more than a midwife.

## Dr. Catherine Post-Van Orden
### Nevada's Third Female Physician

Dr. Post-Van Orden is the first female in Nevada to graduate from a traditional medical college. She graduated in 1879 from Cooper Medical College in San Francisco and practiced in Virginia City, Nevada, from 1879 to 1881.

In 1912, Cooper Medical College became Stanford Medical School. Both Stanford and Toland Medical College (University of California) were exemplary in graduating women MDs.

Cooper Medical College graduated the first woman in 1877, and Toland graduated its first in 1878. From then until 1900, 10.0% of Toland's graduates and 13.4% of Cooper's were women. Records show that at least twenty-three women had practiced medicine in Nevada prior to 1900, about half of them graduated from regular medical schools. However, the battle for equality was not over. There were setbacks in the first part of the 20th century when fewer women attended medical school. Only recently have they begun to enter all sectors of the male dominated world of medicine. There are still obstacles and prejudice that need to be overcome.

## Les Moren, "Outstanding Elko MD"
### By Dr. Owen Bolstad

Dr. Leslie A. Moren of Elko, Nevada. Les first came to Nevada in 1935 and helped to pioneer modern medicine in rural Nevada. Les Moren was one of the founders of the Elko Clinic and was a driving force in the development of that group. A graduate of the University of Minnesota, Dr. Moren practiced medicine for over 50 years. He was active in civic affairs in his hometown and an avid supporter of organized medicine in the state. He served for many years as a delegate to the AMA and was elected president of the Nevada Medical Association in 1973. He served as a member of the State Board of Medical Examiners for over 20 years.

Dr. Moren had been honored as "Nevada Physician of the Year" and as a "Distinguished Nevadan." He died quietly in his home in Elko on December 14, 1994, at the age of 80.In 1992, with the support of the Great Basin History of Medicine Society, I did a series of interviews with Les.

This culminated in the publication of a book entitled *Leslie A. Moren: Fifty Years an Elko County Doctor*. Some excerpts from the book are the best memorial to this outstanding physician.

**1937 (After graduation from medical school)**

"...For a while I considered taking a residency ... but I just didn't have the money. When I started practicing in Elko, I got $200 a month and was surely glad to get that. In that era, none of the medical students that I ever spoke to went into medicine to make money. That was a secondary consideration. We all figured that we would have a comfortable living, but the idea of becoming a millionaire in the practice of medicine never crossed our minds. If you were a good investor and saved money you might, but you're not making it in medicine. I think that was a healthy attitude for us to grow up in. I think that may not be universally true today."

### 1939 (AT THE SITE OF A TRAIN WRECK)

".. Some twenty people had died at the scene of the wreck, and there were survivors and bodies on both sides of the creek. One dead woman was wearing a blue dress with white polka dots, and both her legs had been amputated at the thighs. Her body was just lying there. . . . I sort of had to shudder. I went up in one car that was turned on its side, balanced precariously on top of the bridge. There was a man who had a broken clavicle, and I gave him a shot of morphine, and then he asked me 'How are you going to get me down?' I said 'I'm not going to get you down. I'm not sure that I can get down.'... I came to one man, a Pullman porter, who had a big cut on his scalp and compound fractures of his femur and ankle. I said, 'Well, I'll give you a shot of morphine.' 'Oh Doc', he said, 'take care of somebody who is really hurt.' He was on his second bottle of Scotch whisky by that time."

### 1946 (ON FORMING THE ELKO CLINIC)

".. we started talking partnership, because we thought we could practice better medicine if we pooled our resources ... There were four of us—Dr. Roantree, Dr. George Collett, Dr. Dale Hadfield, and me.

Drs. Secor and A.J. Hood I (Tom Hood's father) were made associates, since they were close to retirement age. We had our offices upstairs in what was the First National Bank building."

## 1992 (ON SOCIALIZED MEDICINE)

"… Complete control of medicine by governmental agencies may occur in our country, as it has in other nations. If it does, I think it will be devastating to many Americans, who will have to wait unconscionable lengths of time to have elective procedures done. You can't expect the physicians in a socialized system to work beyond the usual office hours when they will get their pay checks for just putting in the standard hours. I don't think a government-controlled system is conducive to the practice of high-quality medicine. Somebody said the other day that we would end up with a system that has the efficiency of the U.S. Postal Service and the compassion of the Internal Revenue Service. We may be in danger of developing a dual system, with proscribed government-controlled medicine for the poor people and very expensive, high-quality medical care for the wealthy."

That's the way Les Moren was, honest, open, and a square-shooter. There will never be another doctor quite like him.

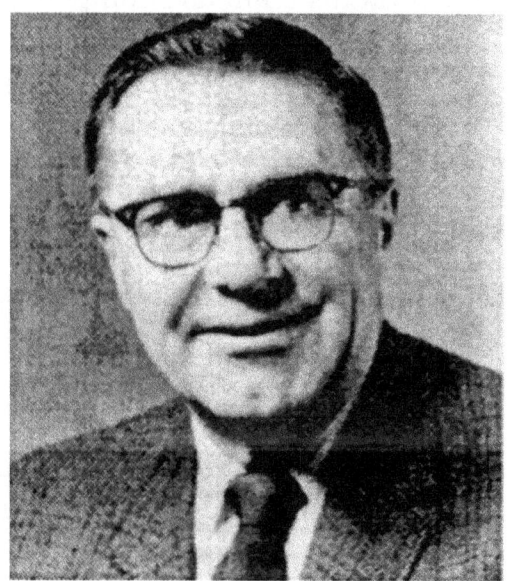 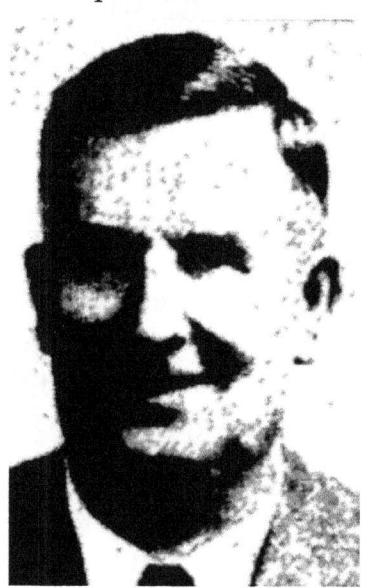

Dr. Leslie Moren, mid-1900s      Dr. John Worden

# Dr. Owen C. Bolstad
## "Stalwart" of the History of Medicine Program
## By Dr. Anton Sohn

Owen died February 20, 2002, in Reno at eighty. I met Owen in 1968 when I interviewed for a position with his pathology group, Western Clinical Laboratory (WCL). It was a Saturday morning, early April 1968, when we met in his office across from Reno High School.

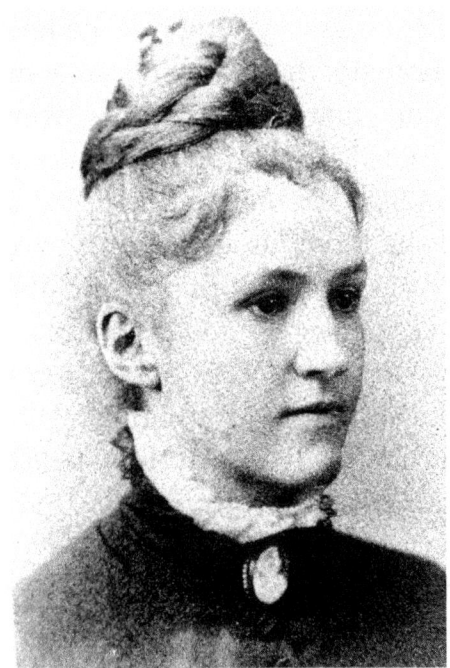

Dr. Catherine Post-Van Orden, 1879

Owen had an appointment with his tax accountant that morning which was a few days before tax filing deadline, but he delayed the meeting, to the chagrin of his accountant, to meet me. Ultimately, I didn't join his group as I was fresh out of my training, and I wanted to practice pathology in a large hospital. Owen's practice involved flying to outlying hospitals.

Four years later, the climate between pathology groups changed from competition to becoming partners when Owen's group, WCL, and my Reno group, Laboratory Medicine Consultants (LMC), merged. The merged group of twelve pathologists became Sierra Nevada Laboratories (SNL) and served fifteen hospitals in Nevada and California.

It is now owned by Laboratory Corporation of America (LabCorp). Shortly thereafter, Owen and I became best friends as we pursued our mutual interests of the outdoors, nature, and history.

Owen was born and raised in Appleton, Minnesota, and was Norwegian to the bone. As a young boy, he knew and loved the lakes around his hometown, and he became an inveterate duck hunter. "OCB" and his school chums were fiercely loyal Americans. They joined the Minnesota National Guard. Shortly thereafter, Owen enlisted in the regular Army, and Pearl Harbor and World War II shattered his age of innocence.

His history of military life during World War II is told in his 1993 book, *Dear Folks: A Dog-faced Infantryman in World War II*. He recounts traveling to Camp Clairborne, Louisiana, for basic training; but before shipping out to England, North Africa, and later Italy. He and an Army buddy traveled the back roads of Louisiana's Bayou Country on a used Indian "Big Twin" motorcycle.

Owen Bolstad and his wartime friends from Appleton were members of the U.S. Army's famed 34th Red Bull Division. For this exemplary military service, he received the Bronze Star, but this was never mentioned to me as his Combat Infantry Man's Badge was more prized. From time-to-time Owen talked about the war years, and with the help of Jack Daniels whiskey, we spent many an evening around the campfire enjoying the bawdy songs and poems of the infantry.

After discharge, Owen attended the University of Minnesota and graduated from medical school in 1951. During the second year of medical school, he met his future wife, Katie, through a roommate, and they were married the following August. His son,

Roger Bolstad, was born during his internship, and Susan Bolstad, Carol Bolstad, and Anne Bolstad came later. Owen tried his hand at family practice in Little Falls, Minnesota, but his real love was pathology. After completing his pathology residency at the VA Hospital in Minneapolis, he moved his family west to settle in Reno, Nevada, in 1965.

He was director of the Carson-Tahoe Hospital laboratory and was its first full-time pathologist. Owen practiced in Reno and Carson City.

Owen also was a pilot and flew to outlying hospitals. He retired in 1985 but was active during his retirement. He was co-founder of the Great Basin History of Medicine program at the University of Nevada School of Medicine with me and was editor of our quarterly bulletin, *Greasewood Tablettes*.

In addition to writing about his wartime experiences, Owen wrote and edited several other books, including *Leslie Moren: Fifty Years an Elko Doctor*. He was an active member of the Navy League, which also utilized his literary talents. Owen was the longtime editor of its monthly bulletin, *From the Sea*, and was awarded the Donald M. Mackie Award, a national honor for best-published Navy League newsletter.

Owen was witty and knowledgeable. His depth of information amazed me. He seemed to have read everything. He had a keen memory. His presence in the history of medicine program was powerful and stimulating. I looked forward to having coffee with him and our friend, Roy Hogan, former WMC laundry manager, in my UNSOM office every Wednesday morning. During these coffee hours, we hammered out future issues of *Greasewood Tablettes* and planned the future course of the history of medicine program.

Owen was an avid outdoorsman and loved the solitude of his duck camp near Fallon. We spent many weeks and weekends on the back roads and mountains of Nevada hunting game, but the most memorable was the week visiting the sites of the nineteenth century forts (Scott, McDermit, Ruby, Halleck, Bidwell, and Churchill) of the Great Basin. Most are now obscure ruins, and it was through Owen's contacts in Elko that we were able to enter private ranches and locate the foundations of the early hospitals. It was on this trip that Owen taught me the secret of his famous lemon pepper chicken.

Every fall, we roamed the mountains of Idaho and Nevada hunting deer and elk together. Some evenings we sat in front of the fireplace reciting poetry. One evening one of the hunting guides came to our cabin and quickly left. He reported back to the other guides, "You won't believe what those guys are doing. They are sitting in front of the fireplace reciting poetry." A favorite poem of Owen's was John Masefield's, *Sea Fever*.

---

### *Sea Fever*

I must go down to the seas again, to the lonely sea and the sky,
And all I ask is a tall ship and a star to steer her by,
And the wheel's kick and the wind's song and the white sail's shaking,
And a gray mist on the sea's face and gray dawn breaking.

I must go down to the seas again, for the call of the running tide
Is a wild call and a clear call that may not be denied;
And all I ask is a windy day with the white clouds flying,
And the flung spray and the blow spume, and the sea-gulls crying.

I must go down to the seas again, to the vagrant gypsy life.
To the gull's way and the whale's way, where the wind's like a whetted knife;
And all I ask is a merry yarn from a laughing fellow-rover
And quiet sleep and a sweet dream when the long trick's over.

---

Before he died, I named the conference room in the new Nevada History of Medicine Museum/Library, The Doctor Bolstad Conference Room.

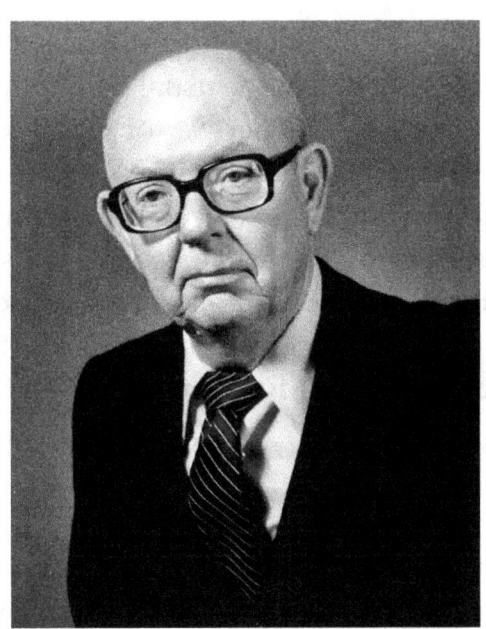

Dr. Owen Bolstad, 1980s

## Fallon Clinic

### By Dr. Anton Sohn

The history of the Fallon Clinic was brought to my attention by Dr. David Klubert, who is married to Barbara Caffaratti Klubert, daughter of Dr. Darius Caffaratti. Dr. Caffaratti's medical legacy includes his daughter Barbara (Ward), who attended our two-year School of Medical Sciences, son John, who went to medical school at the University of Oregon, and a granddaughter, Angela Caffaratti Exline, who graduated from the University of Nevada School of Medicine in 2000. I also have fond memories of the Fallon Clinic. In 1968, as a new pathologist I was assigned to make monthly visits to Fallon Clinic's laboratory.

The annual meeting of the Churchill Hospital staff was the weekend duck hunting season began, and Dr. Dingacci hosted the hospital medical staff at the Greenhead Club.

Memories also linger of Dr. Caffaratti's keen sense of humor. He performed autopsies while the pathologists completed the microscopic evaluation. Each of his autopsies started with the words: "The body is opened in the usual manner with a linoleum knife." This curved knife was perfect for the task and was used by pathologists to open the chest cavity.

I prevailed on Dr. Rod Sage, who knew the Fallon doctors, to provide a description of them. He received assistance on the following article from Joan Elliott, Pat Dingacci, Dr. David Klubert, Dr. Barbara Klubert, Ciligia Littlefair RN, and Bunny Corkill of Churchill County Museum.

## Fallon Clinic, 1949-'90, "Ding, Caffy, Si, and Len"
### By Dr. Roderick Sage

The nicknames Ding, Caffy, Si, and Len rekindle fond memories of the much-loved quartet of physicians who served the Fallon, Nevada, area for upwards of 100 doctor years.

Dr. A.J. Dingacci was universally known as "Ding" to his many patients and friends. Dr. Darius Caffaratti logically went by "Caffy." Dr. Verlyn Elliott was known as "Si," a moniker he acquired in childhood. Dr. Leonard Miller was simply "Len."

These medical practitioners were the sum and substance of the Fallon Clinic from 1949 to the early 1990s.

Dr. Darius Caffaratti, with his friend and colleague, Dr. Leonard Miller, had worked together in Hawthorne, Nevada, before coming to Fallon, where, in due time, they collaborated on organizing and building the Fallon Clinic, which opened its doors in January of 1949.

They left their offices on Auction Road near the old hospital to move into the 4,000 square foot, up-to-date structure at the corner of Taylor Street and Williams Avenue, where it soon became a local landmark.

It remained so until it was demolished in favor of a *Jack in the Box* eating establishment in the mid-1990s, after the four doctors had departed, one way or another.

Ding was born in 1915 in San Mateo, California. After high

school, he attended Santa Clara University graduating in 1937. From there he went through medical school at Creighton University in Omaha, finishing in 1941.

Caffy's life began in Italy in 1916, but at the age of 2 he came to San Jose, California with his family. After prep school at Bellarmire Academy, he too, attended Santa Clara, where he became Ding's roommate and lifelong friend. Caffy graduated from St. Louis University Medical School in 1941, his academic career having been capped by selection for membership in Phi Beta Kappa at Santa Clara and Alpha Omega Alpha at St. Louis University, the well-respected undergraduate and medical scholastic honor societies.

Both young doctors returned to Santa Clara County Hospital for their internships. Ding continued for two more years of surgical training after which he served as an army surgeon in Europe until his discharge in 1946.

Caffy, whose lifelong hearing impairment excluded him from the service, started his career as director of a tuberculosis hospital in Oroville, California. He followed this with two years of work as a resident physician and clinician at the Butte County Hospital in Oroville. Then, in 1946 he launched his own family practice in that Northern California community where he served for 18 years.

Dr. Darius Caffaratti left Oroville in 1962 for a year of European travel with his family.

He used this opportunity to obtain more medical training in Vienna and London, returning to the United States in 1963, Dr. Caffaratti contacted his old friend, Ding, and promptly became an associate in the Fallon Clinic.

Verlyn "Si" Elliott was born in 1924 and grew up in Eastern South Dakota. He served in World War II as a Navy radioman, then returned for premed at Yankton College. He completed the two-year medical curriculum at the University of South Dakota, then obtained his MD from Colorado University in Denver, in

1952. Si interned at the Public Health Service Hospital in San Francisco, then went on to the Walker River Indian Service Hospital in Schurz, Nevada, for three years.

Followed by a stint of general practice and employment with Kennecott Corporation in Ely, Verlyn Elliott in 1958 joined Ding at the Fallon Clinic.

The fourth member of this group, Dr. Leonard Miller, had practiced with Dr. Alphonse Dingacci for two years in the late 1940s, then helped to establish the Fallon Clinic. He stayed until 1953 at which time he entered a three-year psychiatry residency program, variously in Mexico, Hawaii, and New York City.

Dr. Miller, a native of Kansas, was born in 1912, acquired the necessary schooling there, then was awarded the MD degree from Kansas University in 1938. He interned in Detroit, did general practice in Dodge City, Kansas, then worked for the Civilian Conservation Corp. in California, before becoming a navy doctor. He ultimately was the medical officer for a flotilla of mine sweepers in the Pacific Theater.

Dr. Leonard Miller practiced psychiatry in San Francisco for 18 years, where he was associated with the University of California and did research in substance abuse problems and at the California Facility in Vacaville. For two years in the 1960s, Len Miller demonstrated his free and independent spirit by living in (or out of) a van on the side of Mt. Tamalpais in Marin County, sleeping under the stars, then going about his necktie and white coat doctor-role during the day.

In 1975, Dr. Leonard Miller pulled up stakes again, heading 300 miles east, back to the God's Country of Fallon, Nevada, where he rejoined the Fallon Clinic, which he had left 22 years earlier.

Len was a man of medium size, sturdily built, and with a sartorial elegance akin to that of Buffalo Bill Cody.

Between them the four doctors treated well over 100 patients daily in the clinic; in addition to this they made hospital rounds once or twice a day and many house calls.

Their scheduling allowed one doctor to be off for periods of five days, while night calls were rotated amongst the others. This amounted to a work week of 60 to 90 hours per physician. They needed those five free days just to recover.

The doctors enjoyed a variety of hobbies and interests outside of medicine. Alphonse Dingacci was an avid duck hunter and knew the Greenhead Club Marsh intimately. He was also an accomplished musician with special abilities on the accordion, clarinet, and organ. Though his wife, Pat, was an excellent horsewoman, Ding shunned this sport, but was regularly the attending physician at the area rodeos. Ding was a small and wiry man, possessed of a mischievous twinkle in his eye and an enviable sense of humor.

Darius Caffaratti was dark complexioned, compact, and loquacious. His many opinions about life in general, and especially medicine, were expressed with his quite distinctively rasp-like voice. In the 1960 presidential election, while still in Oroville, Caffy managed the regional campaign for Jack Kennedy, but in due time abandoned the Democratic party to become a staunch Republican.

He was an avowed enemy of socialized medicine, worked to legalize prostitution in Churchill county, and served as the County Public Health Officer.

Caffy was an inveterate collector; including old cars, cameras, swords, and firearms. He had his own photographic dark room in addition to a wood working shop. He excelled artistically in both endeavors.

After 18 years with the Fallon Clinic, Darius Caffaratti died quite suddenly in September 1981 leaving his wife, Rose, daughter, Barbara, an internist in Portland, Oregon, and a son, John, a cardiologist in Ohio.

In contrast to his clinic partners, Si Elliott was somewhat angular of build, quiet, and taciturn by nature. A caring and attentive physician, he became active in medical politics, eventually serving as president of the Nevada State Medical Association in 1970-71. He followed this with a term on the Medical Board of Review. Si and Joan raised four children in Fallon, the oldest of whom is currently a physician with the Navy in South Carolina.

They also trained horses at their ranch on the outskirts of Fallon. Si Elliott enjoyed duck and deer hunting, but especially each autumn, he savored a trek to his native south Dakota for pheasant shooting. He was also the team physician for many of the Fallon high school sports activities.

In 1976, Si moved from Fallon to a new practice in Reno. The following year he suffered a severely disabling stroke which forced him to retire from medicine completely. He died in 1990 at the age of 66.

After preparing our history of the Fallon Clinic, we learned only recently of two other physicians who were members of the clinic staff. The two doctors are Conrad Frydenlund MD , now retired, and Gary Ridenour MD , who is still actively practicing in Fallon. Drs. Kurt Carlson and Tim Hockenberry were also valued colleagues, but not clinic members.

Our thanks go to Bunny Corkill of the Churchill County Museum and Archives and Willi Whomes RN, former chief nurse of the Churchill Public Hospital for this added information. Dr. Jack Flanary of Reno was stationed at the Fallon Naval Air Station and knew Dr. Frydenlund in the late 1950s and brought him to our attention.

In mid-May 1981, the city of Fallon sponsored a '"Thank You Doctors Day" in honor of the clinicians and their medical facility. This was expressed with an open house, featuring many speeches and mementoes of affection. The celebration '"Thank You Doctors Day" was in-the-nick-of-time because Dr. Caffaratti died suddenly just four months later.

Drs. Dingacci and Miller continued in the Fallon Clinic for several years with the help of capable temporary associates, including Ding's son, Dr. Mike Dingacci, a 1983 graduate of the University of Nevada medical school. He finished a residency in family practice, then came back to his hometown for three years before relocating in the Seattle area.

During their practices, all the doctors gave generously of their time and clinical expertise as preceptors for the training of UNSOM medical students.

In 1987, Dr. Dingacci retired from his medical practice. At the same time he was named Clinical Emeritus Professor UNSOM.

Pat and Ding found a winter haven in Arizona where they basked in the warm winter sunshine, while learning the intricacies of the game of golf. Summers were spent amongst their many friends back in Fallon.

Ding's later retirement years were tragically disrupted by a severe neurologic injury he suffered in a fall from a pickup truck while helping to prepare a barbecue supper. Though confined to a wheelchair, Ding was cared for with great skill and compassion by Pat. His spirits remained indomitable until the end of his life at the age of 88 in January of 2004.

Dr. Miller maintained a part-time practice until the early '90s, eventually succumbing in 1995 at the age of 82. He was survived by his wife and two children.

After serving as a bombardier in World War II, flying 52 missions, and being a prisoner of war for nine months, Dr. Conrad Frydenlund finished medical school at the University of Minnesota in 1951, followed by a year of internship at San Bernardino County Hospital. After briefly practicing in Minnesota, he returned west to Reno, being employed for three months as a clinic doctor for Washoe Hospital.

At this juncture, he learned Dr. Dingacci needed an associate to replace the departed Dr. Len Miller. Connie's proposed short locum tenens stretched into an eight-year stint with the Fallon Clinic. On his second day in Fallon he was called to attend an elderly sick woman in Hazen, 15 miles to the west.

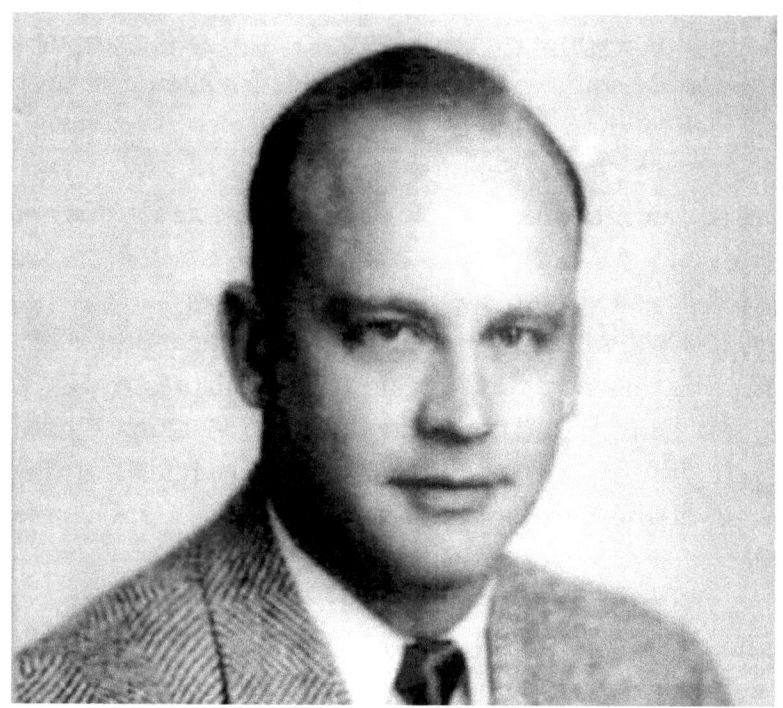

Dr. Leonard Miller, 1979

He found, to his consternation, a badly bloated and decomposed corpse of an old woman lying in a shack, half buried in filthy blankets. Soon after that he delivered six babies in one day and made the first of several house calls to Austin, out east a hundred miles. That's called jumping in with both feet.

Dr. Conrad Frydenlund left Fallon in 1961 to pursue a radiology residency in Santa Monica, then practiced in that city. He is now retired and still living in Saline, Michigan, relatively hale and hearty at 87.

Gary Ridenour MD, the second of the two other Fallon Clinic doctors, grew up in Cleveland, matriculated at Hiram College in Ohio, then earned his MD degree at the University of Guadalajara in Mexico in 1978.

He followed this with an intern year at St. Louis University. He came to Fallon in 1980, practiced solo for a year, then joined the clinic. He submits a telling record of his experience with Dr. Dingacci and a fascinating commentary on his maturing as a young doctor.

As Dr. Ridenour relates, "When I first came to Fallon, I was a 'hot doctor' from the East. Ding took me into his practice. I thought I was doing a good job, but Ding had a very dedicated following. I then began to appreciate that Ding sat down and simply visited with his patients, obtaining more information about their ailments than I ever did."

Once he said, "If you really listen to the patient, they will tell you what is wrong with them. Never be arrogant, never get mad.

"They are paying for a service and expect a little more than you are popping into a room, then popping out. If you want to get rich, go into business. If you want to be happy, do what I do." I chose happy.

On my first day with Dr. Darius Dingacci, he showed me my office. I sat down in the swivel chair at the desk. As I rocked back, I immediately flipped over. Ding chuckled and said, "Watch that chair Gary, Dr. Caffaratti once got a subdural from it!" The next day it was fixed.

I hadn't had on cowboy boots for years, when I noticed Ding's alligator boots and told him I liked them. "They are comfortable," he noted, "and easy to get on in the middle of the night. And you don't have to wear socks." "I have worn them since but usually with socks."

When I first went to the store with Ding, everyone said, "Hello." I frowned and said, "I don't have to be their friend, just their doctor." Ding frowned back and observed, "In a small town, you are a big part of it and not invisible. Get used to it. It's fun." I once complained to Ding that some of his elderly patients were 'crocks' with not much wrong with them. Ding smiled, "They are all alone and scared of dying. They look forward to coming to us. It's our job to help them."

I was once surprised when Ding, with a sly grin, greeted an elderly woman with, "Well, you-old-bat, what's wrong this time?" The old lady smiled and began her story.

He explained later that making fun of getting old was good therapy. "Getting old is something we all have in common, and we should not let it get us down."

Dr. Gary Ridenour concludes by saying, "Of all the doctors I have known and learned from, Ding was head and shoulders above the rest. When he didn't know something, he asked other doctors. He has earned a spot in my heart as a kind, gentle, and caring man. Give 'em hell in Heaven, Ding!"

Lucky was the community of Fallon to have been served so long and so well by this worthy quartet of skilled and dedicated doctors, who just happened to also be men possessed of multiple interests and an unusual depth of character.

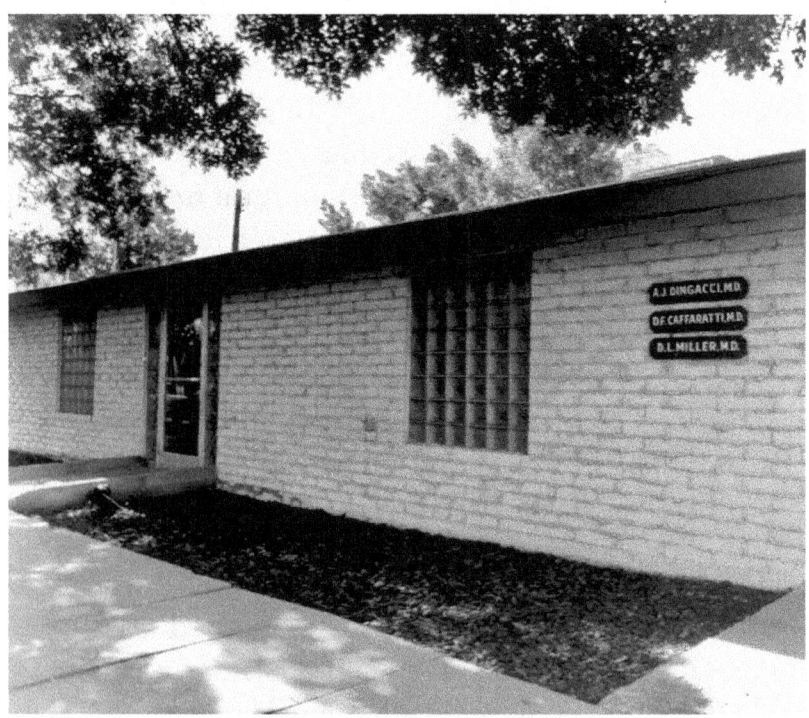

Fallon Clinic, 1979
(Photo, Churchill Co. Museum and Archives)

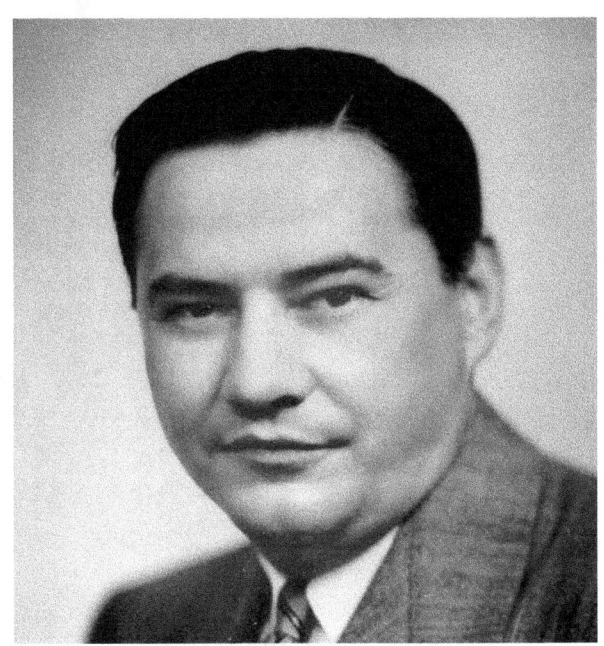

Dr. Darius Caffaratti
(Photo from Dr. David Klubert)

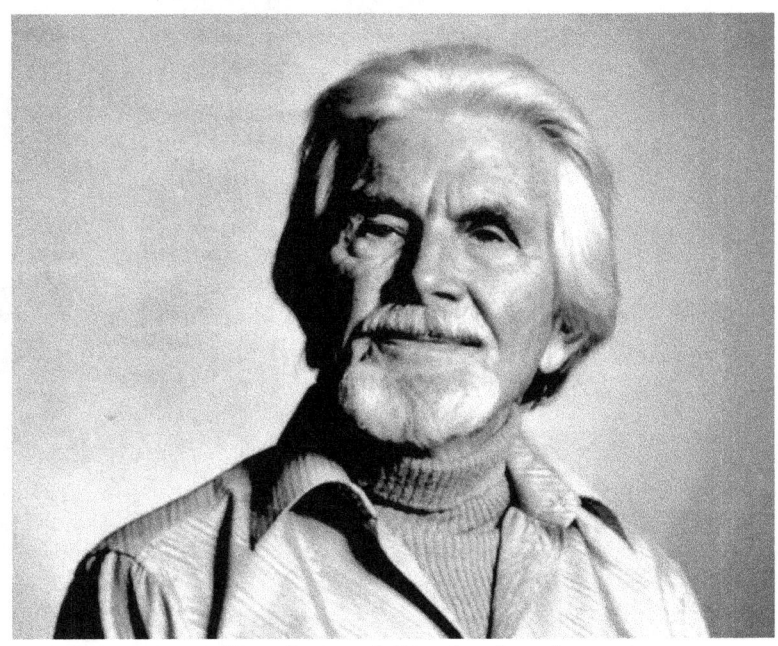

Dr. Conrad Frydenlund

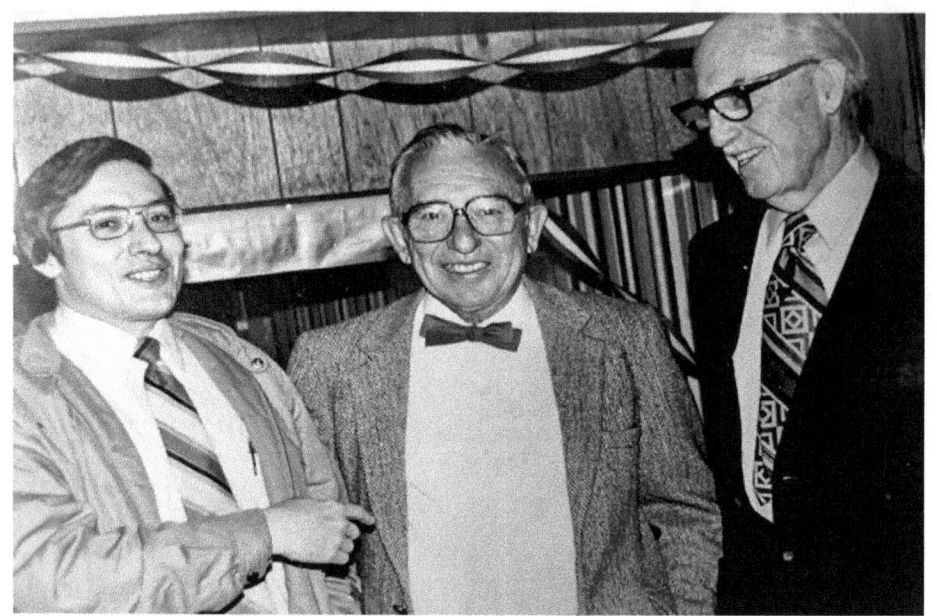

Drs. Michael Dingacci, A.J. Dingacci, F. Anderson, 1985
(Photo, Fallon Eagle-Standard & Lahontan Valley News)

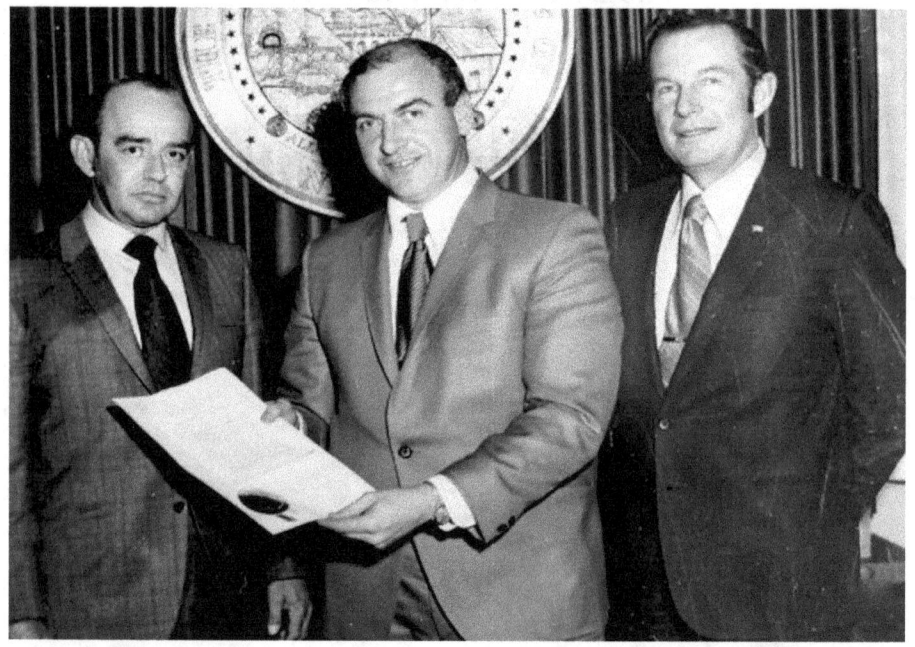

Nev. State Med. Assoc. Rep. Dr. Si Elliott, Nevada Governor
Mike O'Callaghan, and Nev. State Senator Norm Glazer, 1971

## Dr. Alice Thompson, Reno's "Blueblood" Pathologist and American Patriot
## By Dr. Anton Sohn

No physician in Reno's history had more "blue blood" than Alice Lillian Thompson; she is the granddaughter of Myron C. Lake known for Lake's Crossing and founder of Reno. Alice was born January 4, 1876, on the Lake Ranch south of Reno. She attended the Normal School (Teachers College) of the University of Nevada graduating in 1897 and taught school for fourteen years before attending the Oakland School of Medicine. She transferred to the College of Physicians and Surgeons, an eclectic medical school, in San Francisco and graduated in 1914, specializing in pathology and laboratory technology. Dr. Thompson interned at the San Francisco City and County Hospital before leaving the Bay Area to become laboratory chief of Santa Barbara Cottage Hospital.

True to the American patriotic spirit, she joined the war effort during World War I and directed the laboratory at Base Hospital Unit No. 47 in Beaune, France.

After the war, Dr. Thompson returned to Nevada and became its first known female pathologist. She was licensed in Reno in 1920 and became director of Saint Mary's Hospital Laboratory and the State Hygienic Laboratory, now Nevada State Public Health Laboratory. In 1934, Dr. Thompson became the first fulltime pathologist at the Washoe County Hospital (now Renown Regional Medical Center) for $200 a month.

That same year the Board of Trustees authorized the hospital to refer all its laboratory tests to the State Hygienic Laboratory for fifty dollars a month because the hospital did not have funds to start a laboratory.

During World War II, Dr. Thompson was physician for the Reno School System. She also was physician for women at the University of Nevada for over twenty years.

She died December 3, 1960, at the age of 84.

**NOTE:**

Information for this article is from the *Reno Evening Gazette*, December 3, 1960, Dr. Alice Thompson Pioneer Doctor Dies, and Silas E. Ross, *A Directory of Nevada Medical Practitioners Past and Present*, 1957.

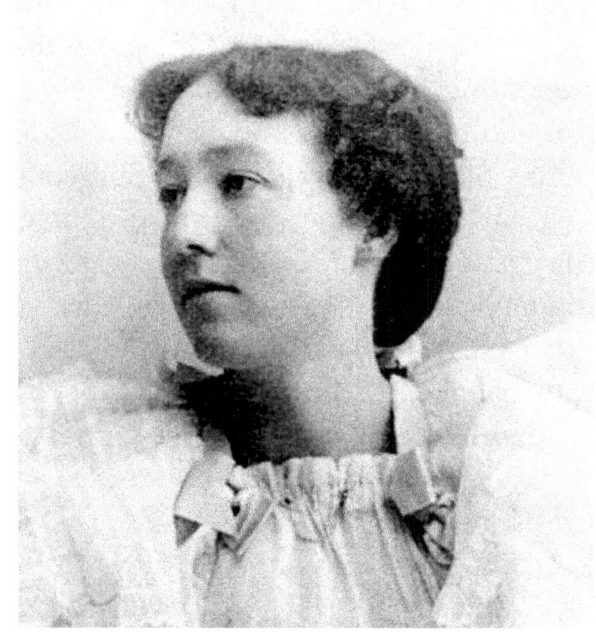

Dr. Alice Thompson, 1920s
(Nevada Historical Society)

## DR. O.P. JOHNSTONE, NEVADA'S FIRST PATHOLOGIST, 1909

### By Dr. Anton Sohn

Oscar Johnstone was born in Iowa in 1871. After graduating in 1905 from Rush Medical College, he instructed at Columbia University, practiced in Pittsburgh, and was an instructor at the Denver College of Medicine. In 1909, Dr. Oscar Percy Johnstone came to Reno to be Nevada's first pathologists and oversaw the State Hygienic Laboratory. He was succeeded by Dr. Mark Boyd.

He resigned after five years to associate with Dr. W.L. Samuels in a clinic.

At 1:00 PM, November 9, 1916, Dr. Johnstone was found dead sitting in his office chair. An office attendant, Miss Ada Hussman, had noticed him two hours earlier sitting in the exact same position and thought him to be asleep. Doctors Sidney K. Morrison, and Mullins did the autopsy and cause of death was atheromatous degeneration of the heart.

Johnstone was one of the leading authorities on the West Coast in bacteriology and pathological diagnosis. (NSJ, Nov. 10, 1916) He was a member of the Nevada State Board of Health and vice president of the Washoe County Medical Society. Two weeks after Dr. Johnstone's death his widow, Bertha Shryock Johnstone, administered chloroform to kill herself and their three children, Eric-six years, Thorwald-four years, and William-less than six months.

**NOTE:**

Dr. Mark F. Boyd graduated from the University of Iowa Medical College in 1911, was licensed in Nevada in 1914 as a pathologist, and became director of the State Hygienic Laboratory.

Dr. Johnstone was the start of pathology in Reno that in 1970 expanded to eleven pathologists, who serviced fifteen hospitals in an area of 120,000 square miles extending from Elko, Nevada, to Roseville, California, and from Hawthorne, Nevada, to Alturas, California.

## Dr. Olga Kipanidze
### Reno's First Fulltime Anesthesiologist, 1935

Sally Zanjani's book, *From Siberia to Reno: A Memoir* by Olga Kipanidze is a great story of survival and success. It is about a Russian doctor who settled in Reno in 1935 and practiced until a few years before her death.

Born in 1897 and growing up during political turmoil, she enjoyed a happy childhood in a well-to-do Russian family that was replaced by a scarcity of food, clothes, and communist brutality. She went to medical school in Moscow where food was a luxury and survival on potatoes and cabbage was the norm.

Her fiancé, Vladimir, an army officer in the Russian Army, fled from the Red Army to Manchuria. Olga gave up a promising career in medical research and joined him.

They married and after six years in Manchuria emigrated in 1930 to America.

She took the California medical licensing examination with about 120 young doctors, including one other woman who didn't return the second day.

Olga passed the exam and began practice in San Francisco. Vladimir enrolled at UC Berkley and died tragically in an automobile accident. Olga struggled with his death. In fact, she never fully recovered or remarried.

A call to the anesthesia department at the San Francisco hospital, where she worked, from a Dr. Hood at Washoe County Hospital (now Renown Medical Center) requesting a full-time anesthesiologist changed her life. She fell in love with Reno and devoted her life to medicine in her new town.

Quotes from her obituary, Nevada State Journal, June 6, 1976.
1. "Her patients became her friends" — office nurse
2. "To know Dr. Kip was to love her" — June Broili
3. "Our family gatherings included Dr. Kip" — Evelyn Scott
4. "She was a perfectionist" — Judge Bill Beemer
5. "Warm, brilliant, wonderful, kind, and a great friend"
6. "She was unpretentious" — Judge Bill Beemer
7. "Even physicians came to her bedside when she was ill"
8. "She was loved" — Evelyn Scott

Dr. Kip gave her 88,000-word memoir to her attorney, Sallie Springmeyer, who was Dr. Zanjani's mother.

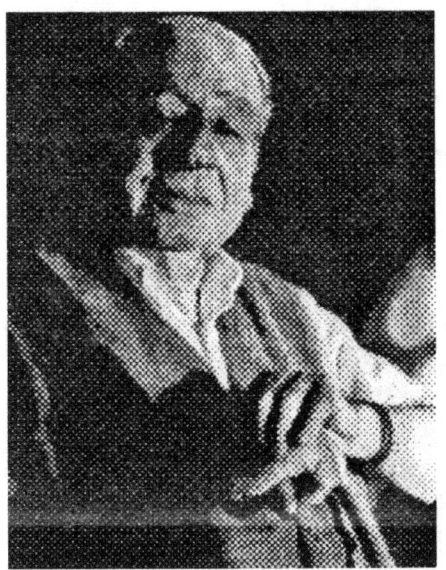
Dr. Kurt Hartoch

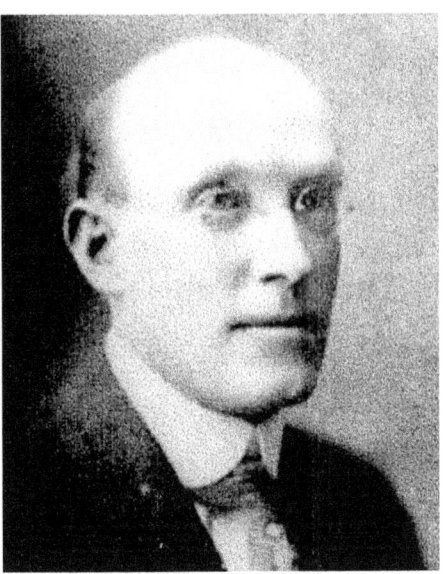
Dr. Sidney Morrison, 1910

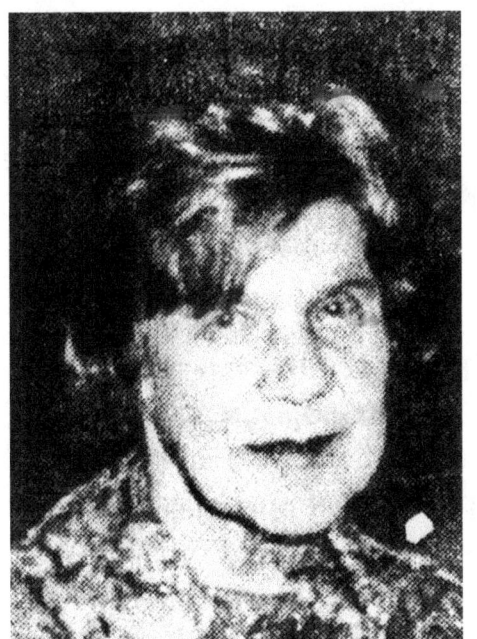
Dr. Olga Kipanidze

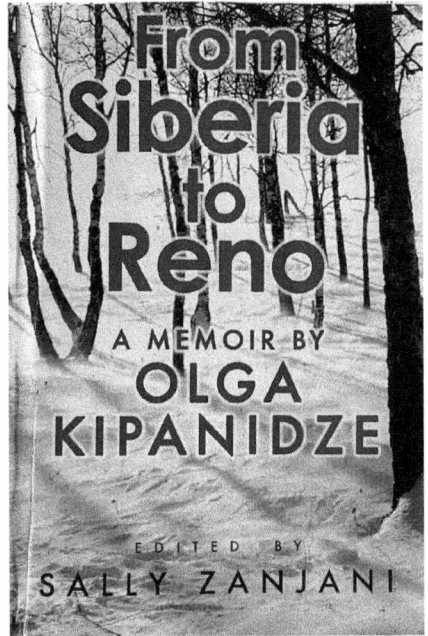

# DR. RAYMOND ST. CLAIR, "SAGA OF MISSING LEGS"
## By Dr. Anton Sohn

David Toll's 1983 book, *Commitment to Caring*, the history of Reno's Saint Mary's Hospital, states that the original hospital had a hand-driven rope lift (elevator) that was used for patients. Toll: "The single exception was Dr. St. Clair... who had lost both legs." Millie Mitchel from the University of Nevada Libraries asked the author to help verify or disprove this fact.

She had an inquiry from St. Clair's granddaughter, Nancy, and grandson who were researching their grandfather and questioned that he had lost his legs.

I researched our medical archives and visited the Nevada Historical Society for information on Dr. Raymond St. Clair, who was one of Saint Mary's founders and found nothing about his missing legs. I remembered Dr. George Gardner had lost both of his legs and practiced in Nevada.

In *Greasewood Tablettes* spring 1998 issue and our book, 150 Years of Nevada Medicine Dr. Rod Sage wrote a brilliant and witty article, A Spunky Kid: Dr. George Gardner. George, born in 1875 in Carson City at the age of 12 fell under a cattle car. Sage: "His legs went one way, and he went the other—in a wheelbarrow..." Gardner with a 'pair of cork legs' entered the first class at Stanford with Herbert Hoover who worked his way through Stanford managing a laundry. Sage: "George often mentioned with some pride that his shirts and underwear were washed and ironed by a future president of the United States."

After graduating from San Francisco's privately owned Cooper Medical School in 1896, Dr. Gardner practiced in Nevada communities: Gold Creek, Rawhide, Elko, and Fallon for 20 years. Dr. Sage: "(Gardner) remained in Fallon until 1917 when he moved his practice to Reno, joining Dr. Raymond St. Clair."

It is highly improbable for two physician partners to walk like the famous French artist, Henri Toulouse-Lautrec, with stub legs in the halls of St. Mary's. For sure, Toll in his book mistakes Gardner for St. Clair. Eureka! We found Dr. St. Clair's missing legs.

St. Clair was born in 1870 in Missouri and graduated from Keokuk, Iowa, College of Physicians and Surgeons. He was licensed by Nevada as an MD in Cripple Creek, Nevada in 1907, and moved to Reno that same year. In addition to being one of Saint Mary's founders, he was honored by the medical profession and elected president of the Nevada State Medical Society (Nevada State Medical Association) in 1917.

His residence in Reno was 1119 Wells Avenue. The St. Clair's moved to Piedmont, California in 1924, where Mrs. St. Clair died 5 May 1925 of a self-inflicted gunshot wound. She had been in poor health for 20 years. Dr. St. Clair remarried, died in Sonoma December 2, 1948, and was interned in Santa Rosa. (Information from Michael Maher of the Nevada Historical Society).

Gardner graduated from Cooper Medical School in San Francisco after two years of required study. In the 1800s, all U.S. medical schools required only two-years for an MD degree. San Francisco's Cooper Medical School, founded by Samuel Cooper in 1858, was bought by Stanford University in 1912, which allows Stanford to boast that its School of Medicine is one of the oldest in California.

Dr. Rodney Sage: "George Gardner finally removed his cork legs for the last time and quietly died at the end of 1970, a month shy of his 96th birthday. He was acclaimed to be one of the last surviving members of the illustrious first class of Stanford."

## NINE DOCTORS OF WASHOE CITY, 1861-1871
### By Eileen Barker

During the ten-year period 1861-1871, and for varying periods of time, nine physicians practiced medicine in Washoe City, Nevada. Those physicians were L. Kords, T.C. Allen, B.B. Bonham, G.A. Weed, J.S. Stackpole, W.P.L. Winiham, A.P.

Mitchell, Simeon Bishop, and Henry Hogan. A short history on the rise of Washoe City in November 1861 provides the *raison d'etre* for the presence of so many physicians in the small city.

Farming and livestock production by white man in Nevada began in the Carson Valley in the Spring of 1851.

Other settlers moved in and extended farming and ranching operations into Washoe Valley where the town of Franktown became settled in 1852. In the nearby mountains the discovery in 1859 of rich gold and silver deposits—the Comstock Lode of Virginia City—had an immediate effect on the small valley. The towns of Ophir, Little Bangor, Mill Station, Galena, and Washoe City soon blazed up. The little settlements took on an importance and growth that lasted for several years.

In 1861, Washoe City became the seat of justice for the County of Washoe, one of nine original counties of the Territory of Nevada. Washoe City's population of 543 tripled within the year. Saloon keepers, lawyers, businessmen, journalists, carpenters, masons, general laborers, schoolteachers, doctors, and one dentist moved into the bustling town. By the mid-1860s, the population of Washoe City and surrounding towns reached as high as 6,000. Washoe City is said to have had the first stock exchange in the West, established prior to the San Francisco exchange.

The absence of food, water, and lumber on the Comstock compelled Virginia City to look to the Washoe Valley to meet the needs of its burgeoning population. Lying between the Virginia Range and the Carson Range, the fertile valley was a natural meadow that provided the agriculture, while the nearby dense growth of pine and fir supplied the lumber. The one lumber mill in Franktown was soon operating to the limit of its capacity. Within a short time, there were 15 sawmills in and around Washoe City, all in full operation. Millwrights, lumberjacks, log wagon bullwhackers, teamsters, and machinists moved in. Great quantities of lath, shingles, and lumber for buildings, and large timber to shore up the many mine excavations were sent by freight wagons up the steep grade to the bustling Comstock Lode. Washoe Valley farmers shipped prodigious amounts of hay, alfalfa, barley, oats, vegetables, fruit, beef, poultry, butter, hops for beer production, and honey from the many beehives in the valley. The wagons returned loaded with ore to be crushed and processed in the valley's mills. Prosperity reigned!

By all accounts, these early settlers were a healthy bunch, but epidemics, accidents in the mills, shootings, fights, and other trauma provided the demand for medical services.

Doctors arrived, some to heal and, since those were days of gold-rush fever, some came because of their own "fever." The state law requiring presentation of a medical diploma to the County Recorder was not enacted until 1875, so little is known of the educational backgrounds of these early physicians. Sam P. Davis in his History of Nevada notes: "Of their ability in the profession no one knew and very few cared. The doctors honored the community with their presence and the people, wishing to be sociable, gave them employment." It is known that Simeon Bishop was born in 1833 in Pennsylvania and was educated at the Physiomedical Institute of Cincinnati. Henry Hogan, a native of Vermont, received his medical education at the Burlington Academy of Vermont Medical College.

Dr. Mitchell was from New York, but nothing is known of his educational background. Dr. Kords lived in Galena, was an active member of the Union political party, practiced medicine as a profession, and operated a successful poultry business. Dr. Winiham ran the drugstore in Washoe City. Dr. G.A. Weed was appointed Superintendent of Schools for Washoe County on November 3, 1963.

When an 1862 smallpox epidemic in the population around Watson's Mill continued unabated, the Washoe County Commissioners in the summer of 1864, purchased the Printing Office Building in Washoe City for $1,000 and converted it into a hospital. A tax of $.20 on each $100 of property value was levied to cover the cost of caring for the sick. Dr. Weed was awarded a contract for $2.50 a day to treat, feed and supply medicine.

Meteoric as its rise, so too followed the end of the towns of the valley. Changes occurred and the economy of Washoe City collapsed. While the smelting and lumber mills were built in Washoe Valley, others were erected at Gold Hill. Seven Mile Canyon, and along the Carson River. The Comstock's dependence on the mills of Washoe Valley lessened.

In 1869, the Virginia and Truckee Railroad was completed from Carson City to Virginia City, and the ore could be carried to the mills on the river much more cheaply than it could be hauled over the mountain by freight wagons, while wood and lumber could be shipped by rail from those mills closer to the Comstock. The milling business in Washoe City rapidly died and the town's twin mainstays were gone.

With the transcontinental completion of the Central Pacific Railroad in May 1869, the city of Reno became the hub of commerce. The final death knell tolled for Washoe City in 1871 when Reno was named the seat of Washoe County and all county business was moved out of Washoe City.

In the manner of the tumbleweeds rolling over the valley, some of the physicians who lived and practiced in Washoe City passed through the area leaving scant trace of their presence there or their activities after leaving. Of others, more information is found. Dr Henry Hogan became the Washoe County Physician in 1874. Dr. Hogan was active in the Populist Party and became a state assemblyman in 1898. He died of pneumonia on March 17, 1902, in Reno, Nevada.

Dr. Simeon Bishop moved to Reno and in 1884, became the Superintendent of the Nevada State Hospital. He died in San Francisco, California on February 8, 1920, of generalized arteriosclerosis. Of interest to Nevada history buffs is the fact that Dr. Bishop's daughter was married to Comstock's Territorial

Enterprise noted editor, Wells Drury. In 1936, Drury authored the book, *An Editor on the Comstock Lode, His Reminiscences of Comstock Society* after his arrival on the Comstock in the early 1870s.

The settlements of Ophir and Galena have long disappeared. Franktown has returned to its pastoral, bucolic setting. Today, in the middle of one of its meadows where cattle once grazed, lies a new golf course surrounded by up-scale building sites. In Washoe City, one crumbling commercial building is left standing. A well-preserved cemetery remains.

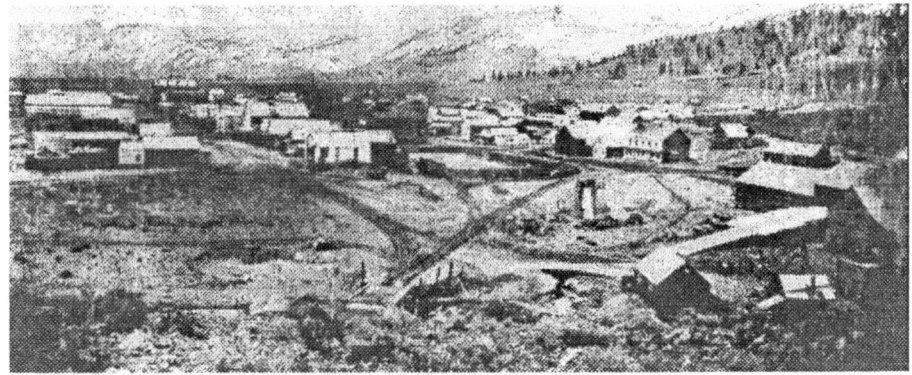

Washoe City, Nevada, 1865

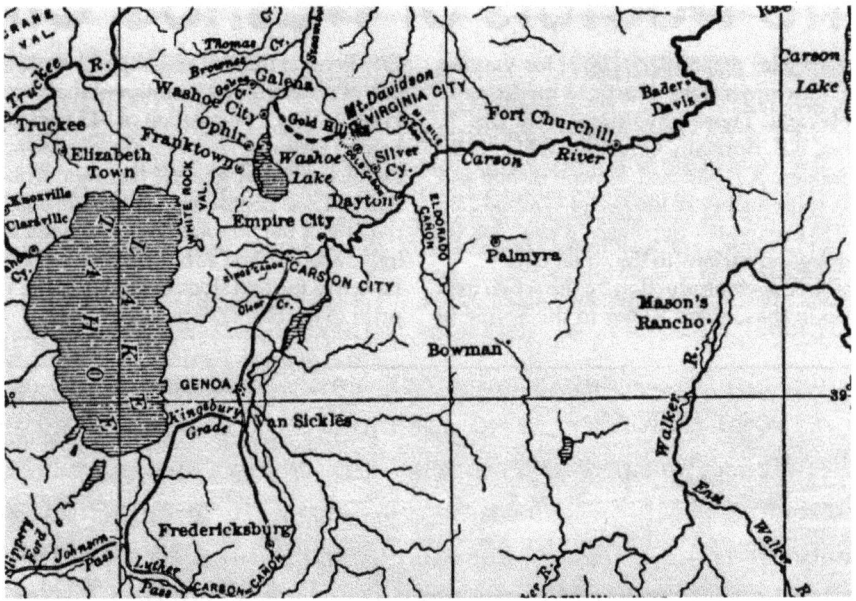

1860 Map of Nevada Territory showing Washoe City

## Dr. Kurt Hartoch's "Proud Dueling Scar"

Kurt Leopold Hartoch MD, was born in Dusseldorf, in the Republic of Germany on June 7, 1908. Son of a middle-class merchant, he suffered during the post-World War I famine and inflationary period. While studying at the university, Hartoch became a member of a dueling society. At German universities dueling societies occupy a niche that may be likened to the modern Greek fraternities on campuses today. Although the stated objectives of the dueling societies were to promote physical exercise, discipline and swordsmanship, the most sought-after goal was a handsome dueling scar upon the graduate's face, preferably on a cheek, as a symbol of one's status. Kurt Hartoch proudly displayed his dueling saber on a wall in his home and proudly demonstrated a dueling scar across his nose until the day he died.

Dr. Hartoch was a unique person with a fine German medical education. He could have practiced anywhere in the world, but circumstances and choice led him to practice in a small rural community in Western Nevada.

He was educated at the University of Koln/Rhine at a time when German medicine was rated among the best in the world. Early in the 20th century many American doctors traveled to Europe for specialty training, and the Germans were leaders in medical research and teaching.

Although Kurt Hartoch became a naturalized American citizen in 1935, he never really lost his rich-guttural way of speaking and his brusque- Teutonic mannerisms. His family wanted him to become an attorney, and he did study law for a period at the University of Koln but found the subject boring and switched to medicine. He was proud of his German medical education, which at that time was quite different from our American system. German students "read" medicine under the guidance of a professor employing a loose curriculum. The success or failure of a student depended entirely upon the diligence of the student and his success was not known until he completed one final comprehensive examination lasting for six months. Kurt scoffed at the tightly controlled American system, feeling that the educators spoon-fed their students.

With the encouragement of his farsighted parents, the new Doctor Hartoch left Germany soon after graduation. He immigrated to Los Angeles, California. There, he obtained an unpaid position as an extern at the Cedars of Lebanon Hospital, working there for about six months. In November 1935, he traveled with a friend to Carson City, Nevada, to appear before the State Board of Medical Examiners to obtain his Nevada medical license. During the journey to Carson City, they encountered ice and snow, skidded off the road, and rolled down a steep embankment. Kurt suffered two broken ribs. Returning to Cedars of Lebanon, he was promoted to the exalted rank of intern, with room and board as well as $10.00 salary per month. During his time as an intern at Cedars Hospital, he had the opportunity to examine and treat several Hollywood notables, including: Al Jolson, Ruby Keeler, Alice Fay, Charlie Ruggles, and Arthur Treacher. This interesting internship ended in July 1937.

After opening his practice in the Cheney Building on South Virginia Street in Reno in 1937, he struggled alone against the established medical groups in the community.

Living in an apartment, he cooked his own meals, washed, and ironed his own clothes, and scrimped to save his money.

Washoe County Physician George Cann, seeing Hartoch's dire straits, appointed him Assistant County Physician, a post that paid a princely $50.00 per month. While serving in this position, Dr. Hartoch achieved a moment of national fame one winter when he traveled with a driver and guide in a homemade snowmobile into the high country near Weber Lake in the Sierra Nevada Mountains to minister to a suffering caretaker at Hobart

Mills. They struggled through snow and ice for fifteen hours, leaving the good Samaritan tired, hungry, and aching all over from the bumpy ride.

As county physician, it was his duty to attend indigent expectant mothers, and since transportation was not available, he was expected to make regular prenatal visits and deliver babies at home. On one occasion he delivered a premature infant weighing just over one pound in a home in Washoe City. The little tyke was put into the proverbial shoe box lined with cotton and got along just fine. While practicing in Reno, Dr. Hartoch was approached by several representatives from Winnemucca, who urged him to move to their community. When the boss of the Getchell Mining Company promised to send their industrial cases to him, Dr. Hartoch decided to check out the town.

The first visit to Winnemucca was not promising (at that time the entire state of Nevada had a population of something over 100,000). A second visit was more encouraging, and after due consideration, the decision was made to move to Winnemucca. His first office consisted of four upstairs rooms accessible only by a steep 'neck-breaking' staircase, with the rooms divided by board partitions. There was no insulation, and the place was heated by a single oil stove. After ten years, Dr. Hartoch moved his office into an old bakery building next to the Post Office on 4th Street and spent about $7,000.00 to convert it into a medical office. It was not until 1962 that he built his own modern, well designed, medical office building on the corner of 5th and Bridge Streets in Winnemucca.

When Hartoch first arrived in town, the hospital was old and inadequate, with long dark corridors. It was run by a single nurse, Wilkie Pinson RN. She was the head nurse, receptionist, bookkeeper, X-ray technician, laboratory technician, and bill collector. She was the medical authority for the city and county and really ruled-the-roost.

After the move to Winnemucca, Dr. Hartoch's wife remained

in Reno until they sold the Reno property. In Winnemucca, they lived in a house on Garrison Street where in January 1942, their daughter Carole was born. In August 1943, Mrs. Julia Hartoch underwent a minor surgical procedure at St. Mary's Hospital in Reno. Something went awry during the operation and within a month she died from complications of surgery. In 1948, Kurt married Wilma Peraldo. They had two children: son Mark, who was killed in a truck accident in 1987, and a daughter, Marlese, who lived in California.

In the 1940s, the cost of medical care was low. Dr. Hartoch's fee for an office visit was $2.00 or $3.00, depending upon the severity of the patient's problem. A hospital visit was more expensive, as was a house call—$5.00. He made house calls until he closed his practice in 1983. Prenatal care, delivery, and postnatal care was $150.00, but during World War II he delivered many babies for a total charge of $45.00 because that was what the government would pay.

From time-to-time, Dr. Hartoch dabbled in business investments, not all of them successful. In 1939, he was offered some mining property for $100.00 (1/2 cent a share.) He refused this offer and was chagrined a few years later when a mining company bought up those shares for $16.40 per share. Then he became involved in mining on Willow Creek, buying several claims and grubstaking a miner to work the claim. When he caught the miner selling off the gold nuggets produced in the mine, that enterprise suddenly folded. He bought stock in Bullion-Monarch Mining Company, selling it when the stock went up. Later the same company asked him to reinvest, which he refused to do. This property developed into one of the largest gold producers in the United States. In 1950, he grubstaked a prospector who wanted to mine the riverbed of the American River, but that enterprise fell apart.

He invested in a mining venture in the Rochester District, but that didn't turn out well either. His practice was a well-balanced mixture of general medicine, surgery, obstetrics, and industrial medicine.

Although no tally was kept, he thought he had delivered more than 2,000 babies during his career. On many occasions, he was asked to make country calls, sometimes as far away as the Oregon border. He made many calls to the scenes of accidents in mines, ranches, and train wrecks. He cared for black families and Mexican families. He cared for prostitutes, itinerants, and Indian families, who had a special place in his heart. With a wide and varied practice, he had many devoted patients and maintained a fine reputation in his chosen community.

In 1983, at the age of 75, Dr. Kurt Hartoch retired from the practice of medicine. Health problems began to take their toll. He became almost blind due to uncontrollable glaucoma. He continued to enjoy life with his beloved wife, Wilma, surrounded by his collection of art, stamps, and coins. He enjoyed visits with his two daughters; Carole, and Marlese.

Dr. Kurt Hartoch died in Winnemucca, Nevada on September 19, 1995, at the age of 87 from the infirmities of age. His passing was memorialized by his wife, Wilma, who endowed a gift of $1,000.00 to the Great Basin History of Medicine Museum in memory of her husband.

**NOTE:**

Material in this article was taken from oral interviews done in 1993 by Linda Dufurrena.

## Nineteenth Century Homeopathic Doctors
### By Dr. Anton Sohn

Anita Watson, a graduate student in the history of medicine at the University of Nevada, Reno, talked to the first and second-year medical students about her research on 19th century homeopathy in Nevada. Ms. Watson emphasized that medicine was unregulated in the state during the 19th century, and anyone could practice medicine and be called a doctor. Furthermore, the cause of most disease was unknown and therefore homeopathy was a viable option for medical treatment. There were several successful physicians who practiced that philosophy during the 19th century in Nevada, but Dr. Frederick Hiller was the most prominent.

Anita Watson: "The philosophy of homeopathy embraces treatment with minute doses producing the same symptom as manifested by the disease process." She elaborated on the medical practice of Dr. Hiller who was a successful homeopathic physician in Virginia City. The German physician Samuel Hahnemann devised homeopathy in the late 18th century. As mentioned, he based his medical system on two laws, similars (*similia similibus curantur*) — use of a drug that produces the same symptoms as the disease — and infintestinals — the smaller the dose, the more effective the treatment. Drugs were diluted to the point where they had no effect.

This system appealed to many Americans who were fed up with harsh treatments, such as bloodletting and treatment with mercuric compounds to the point of poisoning, etc. — by regular doctors. The homeopathic system spread rapidly across America and several medical schools expounding its philosophy were established. The most notable was Hahnemann Medical College, which later became a regular medical school.

In Nevada, the conflict between homeopathic and regular physicians was waged most prominently on the Comstock. The well-known newspaper man, Alfred Doten, sided with Homeopathic Dr. Hiller. They published two pamphlets: *Common Sense vs. Allopathic Humbuggery* and *Medical Truths and Light for the Million*.

Doten was hardly an unbiased, objective observer. He was paid by Hiller; assisted him in surgery, gave anesthesia during his operations, collected his medical bills, and defended him in the *Territorial Enterprise*. Doten pointed out that patients came to Hiller after treatment prescribed by regular doctors had failed. In 1871, Dr. Hiller retired to San Francisco.

Although Hiller and homeopathic medicine was anathematized by regular doctors, very few physicians at that time were homeopaths. Only five percent of practicing doctors in 19th century Nevada had graduated from a homeopathic medical school. Obviously, with the lack of regulation or medical licensing in the state at that time, there could have been more physicians who had not graduated from a homeopathic medical school but adhered to its philosophy. However, it is unlikely they constituted a significant number.

## "Lucky" Bill Thorrington & Dr. Benjamin King, 1850s

### By Dr. Gary Ridenour

"Lucky" Bill Thorrington lived in the Carson Valley in the 1850s. He was a giant of a man, and his friendly nature and generosities were as well-known as his skill at gambling and drinking. He made fast money playing three card monte and thimble rig. Sometimes these winnings included land and personal property, which always led to bad feelings. Two of these losers were John and Enoch Reese, founders of Mormon Station in Genoa. Their debt was an astonishing $23,000 and they were forced to turn over their ranch, all hay and grain from that year, eight yoke of oxen, ten head of horses, sixty head of hogs, seventy chickens, the blacksmithing tools, dry goods, groceries in the store, all furniture, cooking utensils, and the claim to the Eagle Valley Ranch and Old Emigrant Road.

Bill accepted the payment and promptly moved to the ranch with his girlfriend Mary Lamb, a woman from the Sacramento saloons, while his wife and son tried to ignore the situation and live in Genoa near Honey Lake on Barter Creek.

Henri Gordier began to build a herd with some of the finest cattle in the valley. One day in 1858, a neighbor, Sol Perrin, noticed a rider passing by his ranch and recognized him as Lucky Bill Thorrington, a gambler he knew in earlier Placerville days.

Bill, in his usual pleasant demeanor, asked where Henri Gordier could be found, for he was interested in buying some cattle from him. Sol gave him directions to the Gordier place and Bill rode away. Two days later he stopped by Perrin's place and told him he would be sending some men back for the cattle that he had purchased.

A month or so later neighbors of Henri Gordier heard the Frenchman had suddenly sold out and left for parts unknown. A man named Asa Snow was living on the old Gordier ranch. Soon John Mullen and William Combs joined Snow and began working the ranch. This was not the first time someone had given up life in the West and gone home, but Gordier's freeloading alcoholic brother began writing to the neighbors inquiring about Henri's welfare. Mullen and Combs quietly disappeared into the Nevada night.

In late April a group of vigilantes from Honey Lake were out looking for some Indians who were rustling cattle. The campfire talk turned to the missing Frenchman, and one of the men suddenly remembered he had heard a single gunshot about the time of Gordier's disappearance. He was sure it was the one that did in the Frenchman.

A search party turned up ashes, partially burned clothing and blood near Willow Creek, and later they found Gordier's body in a deep spot in the river, weighted down with a rock. A hastily formed jury in Honey Lake found both Mullen and Combs guilty of murder in absentia. Snow and Lucky Bill were found guilty as accomplices. Snow was soon apprehended. He was uncooperative, and while he was being questioned by the posse he died of unknown heart problems. Lucky Bill and Combs were caught and tried in the Sides and Abernathy barn near Genoa. Unfortunately, Bill's appointed lawyer was named Reese, and was probably related to Enoch and John Reese. During the trial gallows were built and both were found guilty and sentenced to death.

The impending hanging interested a Dr. Benjamin King, who was experimenting with galvanic cells. He told the curious that he was interested in reviving the dead by electrical shock, feeling that if electricity could take a life, it might be able to restore it.

Dr. King talked to Bill Thorrington, and he agreed to the plan, providing that he was properly buried after the experiment.

Bill was hung near the Clear Creek Ranch from the back of a wagon. He sang, *The Last Rose of Summer* and was a gentleman until the end. Combs then confessed he and Mullen had killed Gordier, and that he knew nothing of Bill Thorrington. Combs was later hung near Janesville. While Combs confessed, Dr. King quickly retrieved Bill's body and successfully revived him with electrical shock. Ten years later witnesses from Colorado reported Bill Thorrington was living in that state. The vigilantes opened Bill's supposed grave and found only rocks. Lucky Bill Thorrington never returned to Nevada and supposedly died of old age. Dr. King left town soon after the episode, and we hear no more of him or his electrical devices.

# References

1. George and Bliss Hinkle, *Sierra-Nevada Lakes*, University of Nevada Press, 1987.
2. Michael J. Makley, *The Hanging of Lucky Bill*, Eastern Sierra Press, 1993.
3. Norm Nielson, *Tales of Nevada*, Tales of Nevada Publication, 1991.
4. Phillip I. Earl, *Lucky Bill got lucky again...or did he?* Nevada Appeal, 1982.

## SIX DOCTORS HOOD, "NEVADA'S FIRST FAMILY OF MDS"

Over the past century the name Hood has been prominent in Nevada medicine. At the request of the Great Basin History of Medicine Society the most recent member of that distinguished group, Dr. Thomas K. Hood, a retired surgeon from Elko, Nevada, has researched and recorded the history of his family for us.

Following are biographical sketches of the six Doctors Hood. The History of Medicine Library is named after the six Doctors Hood.

## DOCTORS HOOD GENEALOGY

---

Charles J. Hood, William H. Hood, and A.J. Hood I are brothers.
A.J. "Bart" Hood II and Dwight L. "Dutch" Hood are sons of William H. Hood.
Thomas Knight Hood is son of A.J. Hood I.

---

## Dr. William Henry Hood

William Henry Hood was born on a farm near Adrian, Michigan, on January 6, 1862, the son of Andrew Jackson and Mary Knight Hood. Although he was the second born son, he was the first to obtain an MD degree and the first of the Hoods to practice medicine in the State of Nevada. After graduating from church affiliated Adrian College, he earned an MD degree from the University of Michigan and moved to Battle Mountain, Nevada, to begin the practice of medicine.

While establishing himself there he worked for a period at a local ranch until securing his professional status. He married Eunice H. Standerwick of Vallejo, California and fathered two sons, Arthur, and Dwight. The family also included Harry Standerwick, an older son of Mrs. Hood's by a previous marriage.

In 1899, while still practicing in Battle Mountain, William H. Hood was issued license #1 from the Nevada State Board of Medical Examiners. When one of his sons was asked about this, he answered that his father was one of the few doctors in the state who could afford the $2 fee.

He was active in the Nevada State Medical Association and in 1929 was elected president of the Pacific Railway Surgeons, a prestigious professional organization. His wife, Eunice Standerwick Hood, was the first woman to serve on the University of Nevada Board of Regents.

Although he had a rewarding professional career, he became involved in several business ventures prior to the great depression. These investments included ranching interests, a bank, an insurance company, and the Lovelock Mercantile Company. During the depression these businesses lost money, and many became bankrupt. To improve his position, he turned to family members for help and became quite bitter when aid was not forthcoming. There were periods when he refused to communicate with his sons and his brother. In his advanced age he became chronically ill. He died on November 29, 1942.

Dr. William H. Hood developed a reputation as a caring and compassionate physician and was a well-respected member of the medical community. He deserves the title of Nevada's #1 Licensed Physician.

## Dr. Charles John Hood

Charles John Hood was born February 23, 1860, in Adrian, Michigan. He attended public schools and graduated from Adrian College. After spending a year or two in Buffalo, NY, he studied at the Business College of Bryant and Sons.

He returned to Michigan and entered Michigan's School of Medicine, graduating in 1887. Although he was the oldest in his family, his brother William Henry, one year younger, graduated one year before him in 1886.

Traveling west, he set up practice in Spokane, Washington. There he enjoyed a successful period until 1894, when he moved with his new wife Loise to Elko, Nevada, where they would make their home.

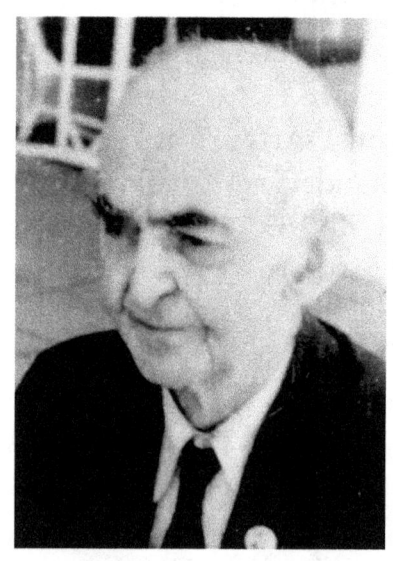

Dr. William. H. Hood

His decision to move may have been influenced by the fact his younger brother had been practicing in Battle Mountain, Nevada. In 1895, he acquired the medical practice of Dr. Joe Henderson, and in 1903 he was joined in his practice by a younger brother, Dr. A.J. Hood I. They shared an office on Railroad Street in Elko. In 1908 he retired from full time work and moved with his wife back to his boyhood home in Adrian, Michigan. He would occasionally return to Nevada to relieve his younger brother, A.J. so he could take further postgraduate training.

As has always been the case, in the 1890s there were many patients who were unable to pay for medical services. To rectify this problem, Charles joined together with two other physicians—Dr. E. McDowell and Dr. G. Gardner—and persuaded the County Commissioners to authorize $125.00 each month for the care of indigents and jail inmates.

Prior to that time, they had been paid nothing for indigent care. This agreement was continued until sometime in the 1940s.

Much of the care Dr. C.J. Hood provided was for railroad workers. Railroad employees required medical care, and accidents were frequent. The contract physician was assured payment, so the position as railroad surgeon was a coveted one. In 1894, Dr. Charles J. Hood was appointed as Surgeon for the Southern Pacific Railroad. This position was handed down to his brother, and later to the physicians of the Elko Clinic.

A typical accident encountered occurred in 1918 when a passenger train carrying several Hollanders bound for Java was wrecked in the Carlin Canyon. Dr. Charles J. was standing-in for his brother A.J. at the time, and a light engine was dispatched from Carlin to pick him up and transport him to the scene of the accident.

In their later years, Charles and his wife spent the cold winter months in Los Angeles. On February 27, 1931, while out for a stroll, Dr. Charles John Hood suddenly became ill. He sat down on a curb and died.

## Dr. Arthur James Hood I

Arthur James Hood was born November 10, 1871. Like his older brothers, he attended Adrian College and in 1903 graduated from the University of Michigan School of Medicine. With his MD degree in hand, he traveled to Elko, Nevada, by train. Arriving in the summer of 1903, he joined his older brother Charles in the practice of medicine.

By this means he could repay the $3,000.00 owed to his brother for his medical education. Their office was a small building facing the Southern Pacific corridor between 4th and 5th streets. When Charles retired and moved from Elko, Arthur continued to practice. He later associated with several partners including Dr. W.W. West, Dr. M.J. Rand, Dr. R.P. Roantree, and Dr. Charles E. Secor.

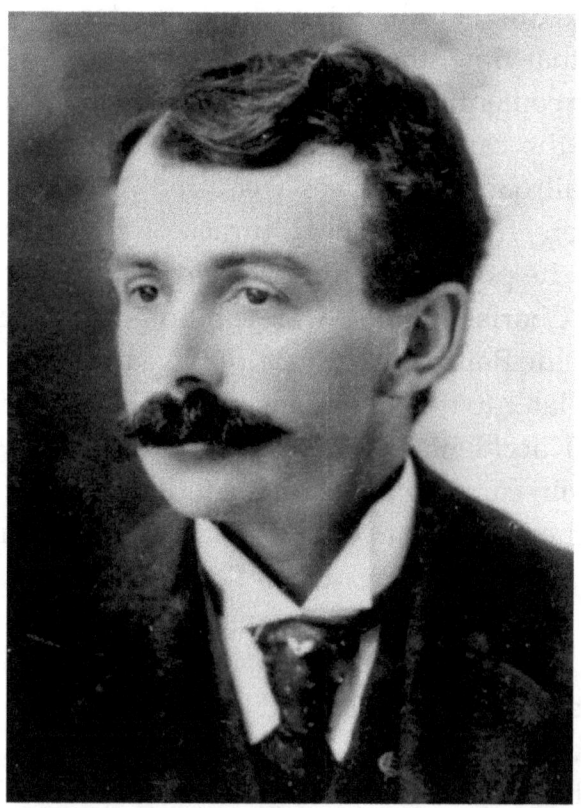

Dr. Charles John Hood (Nev. Hist. Society)

About 1928, a new First National Bank Building was constructed on the corner of 5th and Railroad Streets. Drs. Hood, Roantree, and Secor moved their offices to the second floor of this structure. While practicing there they were associated with several younger physicians, including Dr. L.S. Moren, Dr. Dale Handfield, and Dr. Paul Del Guidice. After the arrival of Dr. George Collett, the Elko Clinic was formed and moved into a building at 946 Idaho Street. Dr. A.J. Hood remained a partner in this group until his retirement.

Dr. A.J. Hood married Irene Hunter, the daughter of a local cattleman, and took up residence at 431 Pine Street. The marriage produced four children, Edith, Charles, Thomas, and Patricia. The first, Edith, died at the age of 6 from pneumonia. Charles graduated from Stanford University and lived in Elko until his death. Patricia also became a physician, graduating and serving a residency in internal medicine at Stanford. Her entire medical career was spent in the Bay area and hence is not included in this history.

The first medical problem Dr. A.J. Hood encountered after arriving in the Great Basin was typhoid fever, which also claimed him as a victim. This disease remained endemic until the water supply for Elko was changed from the Humboldt River to deep wells, along with the Kittridge Canyon Springs.

For the first thirty years of his professional life, considerable time was devoted to caring for the somewhat isolated population scattered from the Bruneau River to Eureka. This required much travel by horse and buggy, train, and later by automobile.

In 1906, Drs. A.J. and C.J. Hood invested in one of the first X-ray machines in the State. As befell many doctors in the early days using fluoroscopy excessively, he received irradiation burns to the fingers of his left hand. The development of skin cancer on his ring finger led to subsequent amputation.

Dr. Arthur Hood felt his most rewarding endeavor was his involvement in securing an adequate hospital for Elko County.

In February 1919, his trip to Carson City to lobby for an enabling act, allowed Elko to build a new hospital.

One of his greatest disappointments occurred later in life, when he did not hear a telephone ring in the middle of the night. The patient, who was seen by another doctor, turned out to be the former President of the United States, Herbert Hoover, who was one of A.J.'s idols. During his last year he became debilitated from repeated episodes of hematuria (blood in the urine). He died on September 18, 1958, from a renal neoplasm.

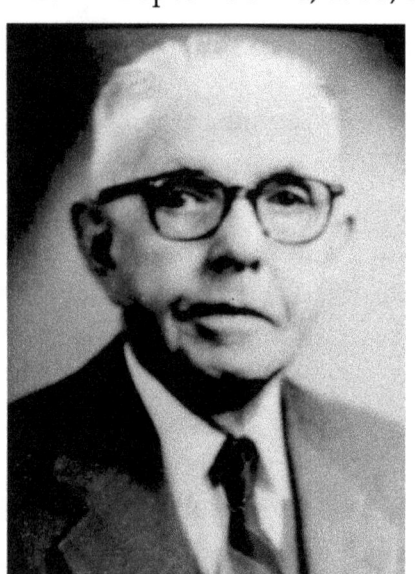
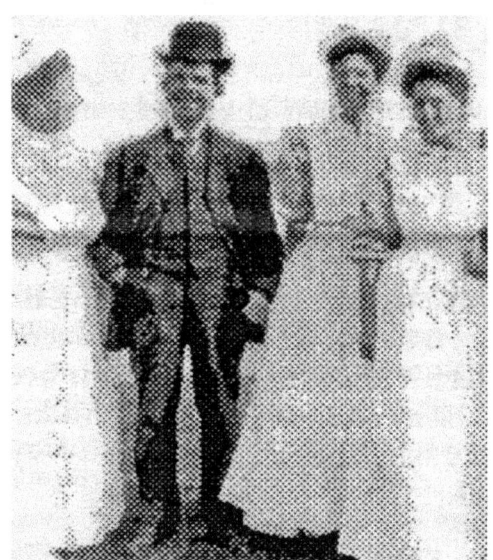

Dr. Arthur James Hood I

## Dr. Arthur J. "Bart" Hood II

Arthur James Hood II was much better known by his friends, family, and associates as "Bart." He was the son of Dr. and Mrs. W.H. Hood of Battle Mountain, Nevada, born April 1, 1895. In 1904, his family moved to Reno. He attended public schools and the University of Nevada. He was a member of the Sigma Alpha fraternity. After graduating from the UNR, he attended Stanford University SOM and in 1921 was awarded an MD degree.

He began medical practice in Reno, Nevada, in 1921. Although he had no formal internship or residency training, he did post graduate work in Vienna, Austria. Much of his professional activity was in the field of surgery during 36 years of practice. He was on the medical staff of St. Mary's Hospital and Washoe Medical Center.

Bart served the State of Nevada as a consultant for the Nevada Industrial Commission, a position that exposed him to a life-threatening experience when a disgruntled claimant brandished a gun at him. He held a commission as a captain in the United States Army and was given an honorary commission as a colonel in the Nevada National Guard.

Bart was a part time inventor. He devised an innovative barbecue that was powered by an electric fan. With a very small amount of fuel the barbecue could even roast a turkey. Some of these barbecue outfits were manufactured and sold. Bart was a rather large and heavy man physically. He was an inveterate cigar smoker and he loved to travel. He got along well with his many friends. He belonged to the Bohemian Club in San Francisco and was a member of the Prospector's Club in Reno. He was also an Elk, a Shriner, and a member of the Sons of the American Revolution.

His first marriage was rather short-lived, producing no children. His second wife was Elizabeth Charleton whose family was among the founders of the Woolworth chain. They had two children, Eunice, and Arthur James III. He also gained two stepchildren, Earle P. Charleton II and Thelma. After the death of Elizabeth (his second wife) Bart married Juliette Toy, the widow of a San Francisco hotel man.

After the surgical removal of a malignant renal tumor, Bart's health slowly deteriorated, and he died in Reno October 23, 1980.

## Dr. Dwight Lincoln "Dutch" Hood

Dwight Lincoln Hood was the second son of Dr. and Mrs. W.H. Hood. He was born in Battle Mountain, Nevada in 1902. He moved to Reno in 1904.

He graduated from the University of Nevada in 1925, earning

a BA degree. Dwight attended the medical school at Washington University in St. Louis, where he was a member of the Phi Rho Sigma fraternity. He received his MD degree in 1929 and returned to Reno where he began a general medical practice, holding Nevada State License #1277. Known by his friends as 'Dutch' he developed an interest in cardiology, and for many years interpreted EKGs at St. Mary's Hospital.

He was granted a commission as captain in the National Guard in 1936 and was inducted into the United States Army early in World War II. Dr. Hood was promoted to rank of colonel during his military career. Active in medical affairs he was a member of the Washoe County Medical Society and the Nevada State Medical Association. Dr. Hood was President of the Nevada State Medical Association and presided over its 51st annual meeting in 1954.

Active in community affairs, Dr. Hood was a member of the American Legion, the Prospectors Club, Elk Lodge, Sons of the American Revolution, and the Retired Officer's Association.

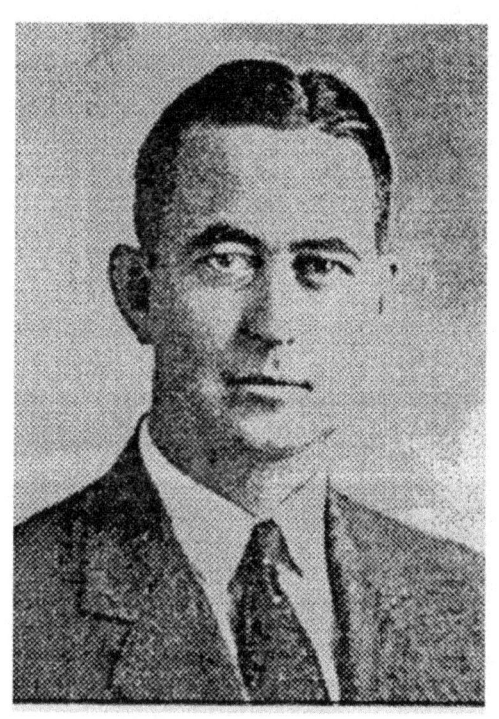

Dr. A.J. Hood II

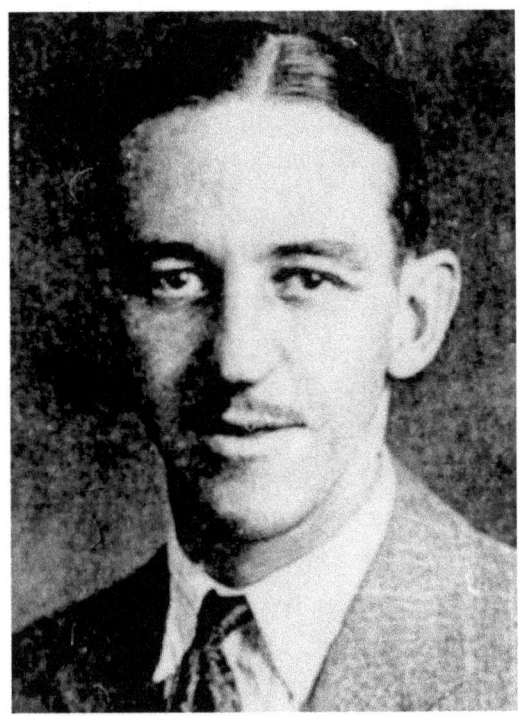

Dr. Dwight L. 'Dutch' Hood

Despite a successful professional life, Dwight's family life was tragic. His first marriage was to Florence, who gave him a healthy son named Henry, whom they nicknamed "Hanky." One evening Dutch returned from delivering a baby to find Florence and her unborn baby had been killed in a fall down the basement stairs. After this tragic accident Dutch devoted much of his time to Hanky's welfare, but sadly he was killed by an accidental gunshot while duck hunting with his father near Fallon, Nevada. A second marriage ended in divorce after only a few months.

His third marriage to Beulah Brown was a happy one and lasted until she died of emphysema near the time of Dwight's retirement. His last marriage was to Keitha. It was a happy marriage, but it was cut short by Dutch's death from emphysema and coronary heart disease on October 15, 1979. Keitha survived, living in Reno until her death.

## Dr. Thomas Knight Hood

Thomas Knight Hood, the third child of Dr. and Mrs. A.J. Hood I, was born in Elko, Nevada, on May 13, 1921. Educated in public schools, he graduated from Elko High School in 1939. He entered Pomona College in Claremont, California. The advent of World War II caused acceleration of his education and after three years at Pomona College he entered Washington University School of Medicine in St. Louis, Missouri. He enrolled in the Navy V-12 program, and with accelerated year-round schooling earned his MD degree in June 1945.

During his senior year at Washington University he married Irene Segelhorst, a nurse. He served a general internship at the Navy Hospital in Shoemaker, California. After serving for two years as a medical officer in the Navy, he entered a three-year surgical residency program at St. Joseph's Hospital in San Francisco.

After completion of his residency program he moved to Elko, Nevada, joined the Elko Clinic, served a preceptor with Dr. George Collett, and was certified by the American Board of Surgery.

Dr. Tom Hood's surgical practice was dominated by trauma, with cases generated by highway accidents, railroad accidents and mishaps from surrounding ranches. His practice at the Elko Clinic was in association with several fine surgeons, including Dr. Hugh Collett, Dr. Matern and Dr. Owens. This arrangement allowed time for continuing post-graduate education. Dr. Tom was a member of the American Medical Association, the American College of Surgeons, the Southwest Surgical Congress, and the Pan Pacific Surgical Association. He served as president of the Nevada State Medical Association in 1973-74.

Dr. and Mrs. Hood had three children, Victoria, Thomas, and Jacqueline. Their son Thomas died at the age of 36 from a amelanotic melanoma. Victoria is married to a psychiatrist, and Jackie is married to a neonatologist. Sadly, there is no other descendant to carry on the Hood medical tradition.

Tom Hood is proud of his small-town background and has been very active in community affairs. He is a Rotarian, a Shriner, member of the Navy League, and member of St. Paul's Episcopal Church.

He had been involved with the development of the Elko Auditorium and Convention Center. He retired from the practice of medicine about ten years ago but continues to be active in civic affairs. Dr. Thomas Knight Hood was honored as a distinguished Nevadan by the University of Nevada and was honored with a *Praeceptor Carissimus* award for teaching med students by the University of Nevada School of Medicine.

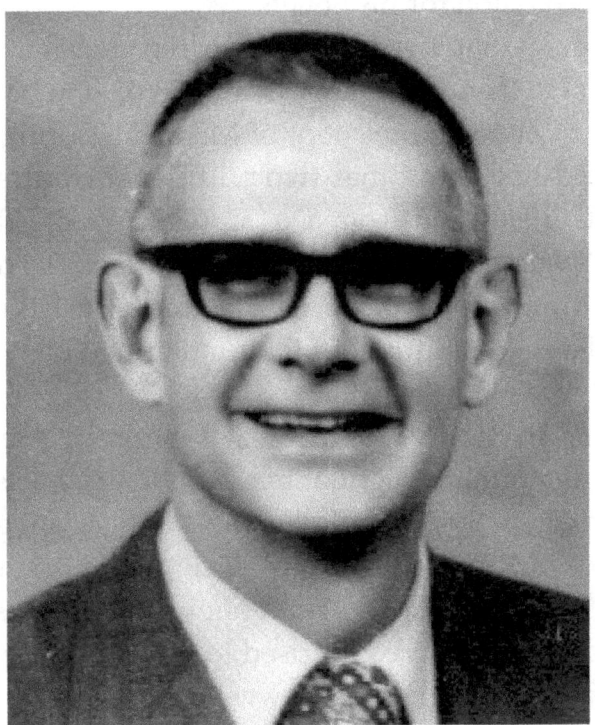

Dr. Tom Hood

# DeTar Family, "Four Medical Legacies"
## By Dr. Robert Daugherty

**John DeTar, 86,** Urologist, Reno (Died November 2011). I knew Dr. John (Jake) DeTar from afar during my twenty years as Dean. For several years, he would write me a very respectful letter strongly suggesting that as Dean of the Medical School I should not be on the Board of Planned Parenthood because he believed they were performing abortions. As I learned over the years, Jake had a fervent belief against abortions.

The more I learned about his activities and beliefs, I realized he and I did not agree; however, I certainly admired and respected his passion for his beliefs.

I also knew that two of his children became physicians, Josephine b (1987) and Michael DeTar (1989), who both attended the University of Nevada School of Medicine during my tenure as dean. I did not know that two additional children, Edward DeTar (MSU 1998) and Tom DeTar (USC 1986), also became physicians. Twelve siblings and four physicians! To have a third of one's children become physicians led me to seek out these four siblings and ask what influence their father had on their choices. Below are their responses.

**Tom DeTar,** Otolaryngologist, Coeur d Alene, Idaho: "Although I am number eight of twelve siblings, I was the first to pursue medicine. Both my father and physician grandfather inspired me, but I also have an uncle and cousins who are physicians. My father kept an extra phone in our house linked to his office, so patients were surprised to hear his voice when they called his office in the evening or weekends.

"His personal attention to his patients served as a wonderful example to me, as I now call my patients at home after their operations.

'I attended UNR with a major in premed studies and a minor in German. Dad encouraged me to keep my education as broad as possible, as professional school tends to narrow a mind's perspective. I thank him to this day for such wonderful advice. Reading Virgil, Goethe, and the classics was possible then, but it would be difficult now.

"I have always felt it was a privilege to take care of patients, enjoying the challenge of diagnosis, and improving my surgical skills. Perhaps, my enthusiasm for medicine is why my son, Will, is a junior at UNR and planning to apply for medical school this coming year. I have never regretted my decision and remain indebted to my father and grandfather for showing me the way."

**JOSEPHINE DETAR,** anesthesiologist, Elmira, New York: "I went to college, intent on teaching physical education as a career. Of course, along the way, I changed my mind and decided to put my love of physical education and sciences together to become a doctor.

"Would I do it again? Most definitely. I have always felt I had been given a great privilege to be accepted into the medical profession and to receive the mantle of a physician. There have been several times when I know my involvement in a patient's care has made the difference between living and dying.

"And I say that those few instances are why I travelled the road I did-just to be there, at that time-and make a difference.

"I am also blessed to be able to say I still love my work. I'm not just working for the weekend. I thank my following mentors, over the years, for making it possible for me to do what I do: My father for teaching me how to ski, sail, ride bicycles, for his foresight in our home-'no TV'-just books from ceiling to floor in every room where a wall was available; for English grammar lessons at the dinner table; for taking us to Mass every Sunday; teaching us about ethics and logic; and handily having a lot of interesting literature lying about the house.

"My teachers: Mr. Riordan, at Bishop Manogue High School; my first-grade teacher, Sister Maryanna, my sixth-grade teacher, Sister Boniface; my chemistry teacher at UNR, Mr. Chuck Rose;

and Mr. Loper in the physical education department. I also must add Dr. Anton Sohn to my list because he let me come to the coroner's office to watch autopsies, which helped me get into medical school. So that's where my path came from and where it led."

**MIKE DETAR,** pathologist, Coeur d Alene, Idaho: "Our family has several physicians, including my father and his father before him, and they certainly played a large role in my decision to pursue medicine.

"I recall as a boy attending a ranch style picnic with my father at the home of a long-time country doctor, Dr. Mary Fulstone, in Yerington, where I met Dr. Salvadorini, a Reno doctor. When I later asked my father what kind of doctor he was, he told me he was a pathologist. I didn't know what a pathologist was and queried about that as well. My father responded by describing a pathologist as a Doctor's doctor who must know everything. That seemed like a daunting area of medicine to me, and I didn't really think about pathology again until my second year of medical school.

"I studied under Doctors Anton Sohn, Roger Ritzlin and Jacob Malin at UNSOM. I have encountered many in medicine who have lost the joy of 'Practicing the Art.' The administrative burden is huge, and the 'compliance' requirements have made the practice of medicine unwieldy and hazardous.

"Despite these challenges, I consider my choice of specialty to have been a wise and personally rewarding one. When people ask me if I would go through medical school, if I had to do it all over again, I tell them, 'Yes, it was a challenge, but when young, fearless, and foolish, and when 'securing the prize' seems attainable, the sacrifices are well worth the effort, and I would do it again."

**EDWARD DETAR,** surgeon, Coeur d Alene, Idaho: "I am the youngest of the twelve John DeTar children and have always felt my family was unique and wonderful. I have been blessed to have such a one-of-a-kind father and have so many great older siblings. In fact, I think the uniqueness of my family is perhaps why I am a doctor today.

"As a child I always felt drawn to medicine and from my earliest days I recall wanting to be a doctor. I admired what my grandfather, father, and older siblings did, and I felt it was the noblest of professions.

"I applied to medical school and was granted two interviews. I did well on one and totally bombed the other. Someone from admissions called me a week later and told me they would like to grant me a third interview since my first two were so polarizing. My third interview started off benign, then the interviewer asked me about my family. This led to a one-plus hour discussion about my family. In the end, she found me, by virtue of my unique family, to be a good candidate and I was accepted. To this day, I am convinced I was accepted to medical school partially because of my achievements, but mostly because of my unique large family with my one-of-a-kind dad. I now practice general surgery and vascular surgery with five partners. I thoroughly enjoy my practice and cannot imagine doing anything else. I am in my 9th year since finishing residency and feel today as I did at age thirteen that medicine is a noble profession, every day is fascinating, and there is nothing I would rather be doing."

## Dr. David "Snowshoe" Thompson, 1970

### By Dr. Roderick Sage

The first mountain man to carry the nickname of "Snowshoe" was John Thompson, who carried the mail to folks living along the Genoa, Nevada, to Placerville, California, corridor in the heart of the High Sierra. He became famous for serving his clients year around from 1856 to 1876. In the wintertime, he delivered the mail travelling on skis, otherwise on-foot or horseback.

Despite his well-known moniker, John Thompson rarely

resorted to snowshoes, which when compared to skis were a cumbersome nuisance. His favorite mode of travel was by heavy, 10 feet long skis supported with a single sturdy spruce staff generally held by both hands.

Our own mountain man, Dr. David Thompson (1923-2013) acquired the name of "Snowshoe" after many years of recreational skiing, both downhill and cross-country in the Sierra, and on occasion in the Rocky Mountain West.

Dr. Dave Thompson, no relation to the original "Snowshoe" Thompson or the later Don Thompson, was an Ohio native who attended medical school at the University of Michigan, followed by residency training in internal medical and hematology.

To pursue his fondness for the Western mountains, Dave chose Reno for his medical career, joining the small enclave of Michigan doctors. Surgeons Ken Maclean and Bill Tappan and internists Stephen Phalen and Peter Rowe in the mid 1950s.)

Dr. David Thompson's epic one-man cross-Sierra adventure occurred in the late winter of 1970. Comparatively, he outdid "Snowshoe" John Thompson by skiing a greater distance, at a loftier altitude, and for five days compared to two. Of course, John Thompson had a job to do, delivering the mail, while Dave Thompson's trip was motivated for esthetic pleasure.

Dave Thompson retired from medical practice in 2006. He died in 2013, the day after his 90th birthday. He exploited his fondness for outdoor Nevada for over 50 years.

Few of his contemporaries have matched this Lincolnesque mountaineer's skill or his exceptional endurance. He was 6 feet 5 inches, spare and fit, a perfect counterpart to the original "Snowshoe" Thompson.

We should mention the third "Snowshoe" Thompson, the well-known local sportsman, writer, and entrepreneur, Don Thompson, who promoted skiing and related activities for many years in the California area.

In Dr. Thompson's words: "My route over the Great Western

Divide was around Triple Divide Peak. It is necessary to start climbing on a long shallow traverse from the river until a point is reached above the small lake. This will put you past the cliffs, which make up the north wall of the canyon at this point.

"Then, one turns due north and climbs steadily over open slopes until the ridge (12,000+ feet) stretching east of Triple Divide Peak can be crossed. At this point, about 200 yards of scrambling puts one in the notch east of Glacier Lake where one has a pleasant short run down around the Lake and into the notch containing the tiny lake at the head of Cloud Canyon At this point, I had intended to proceed westerly, crossing Copper Mine Pass, then along the ridge to Elizabeth Pass and from Elizabeth Pass across the tableland to Pear Lake. However, the weather again worsened abruptly with a strong wind and a double cloud deck to the west. The snow slopes down to Lion Lake were topped by about a half-inch of splendid corn, and I had promised to be back home by April 1 for my granddaughter's birthday, and I headed downhill.

"Unfortunately, below Lion Lake, the visibility deteriorated, and I would have welcomed a couple of bottles of Mummery's Bouvier. (A.F. Mummery was a renowned 1900s alpine mountaineer who preferred Bouvier, an alcoholic drink.)

"It was necessary to follow the streambed carefully and this is not the most suitable route down this canyon on skis. Two sets of cliffs are present; one set above Tamarack Lake and the 2nd set between the 10,000 and 10,400-foot contours higher up.

"The next morning, when visibility improved, it was obvious both sets could be circumvented via open slopes to the south of the stream. However, because of the lack of visibility, I was required to crampon down a narrow but not particularly steep couloir along the creek through the upper cliffs. I spent the 4th night above Tamarack Lake and, after sleeping somewhat later than usual the next morning, I had a pleasant run down to High Sierra Trail Junction at the end of River Valley.

"Although I was able to ski around Bear Paw Meadow into Buck Canyon for about three-quarters of a mile, the ski crossing officially ended at the River Valley Junction and from there to Giant Forest it was a pleasant spring hike.

"I spent one more night on the trail just below Seven Mile Hill, caught a ride from Giant Forest to the Fresno Airport and was home the evening of the 6th day. The route west from Triple Divide Peak to Pear Lake certainly seems feasible and probably would be preferable when traveling west to east. As a matter of fact, the run down from the shoulder of Triple Divide Peak into the Kern-Kaweah River on a west-east crossing would be fantastic.

"As far as equipment is concerned, I would like to put in a good word for Harscheisen. These seem particularly adapted to late winter Sierra snow conditions. They are small metal plates, which fasten vertically on the sides of the ski under the foot. When skis covered with skins, they obviate the need for crampons in climbing steep, hard slopes, a common early morning problem.

"The Kern Basin is a lovely wild place and is twice as beautiful under a mantle of snow. Late winter is the best time, and you won't encounter any snowmobiles."

**NOTE:**

The following account by Dr. Thompson is excerpted from the November 1970 of *Summit* magazine. Sadly, the magazine ceased publication shortly after this issue. Dr. David Thompson practiced in Reno, Nevada, from 1954 until 2006 when he retired. He was born in 1923 and died in 2013.

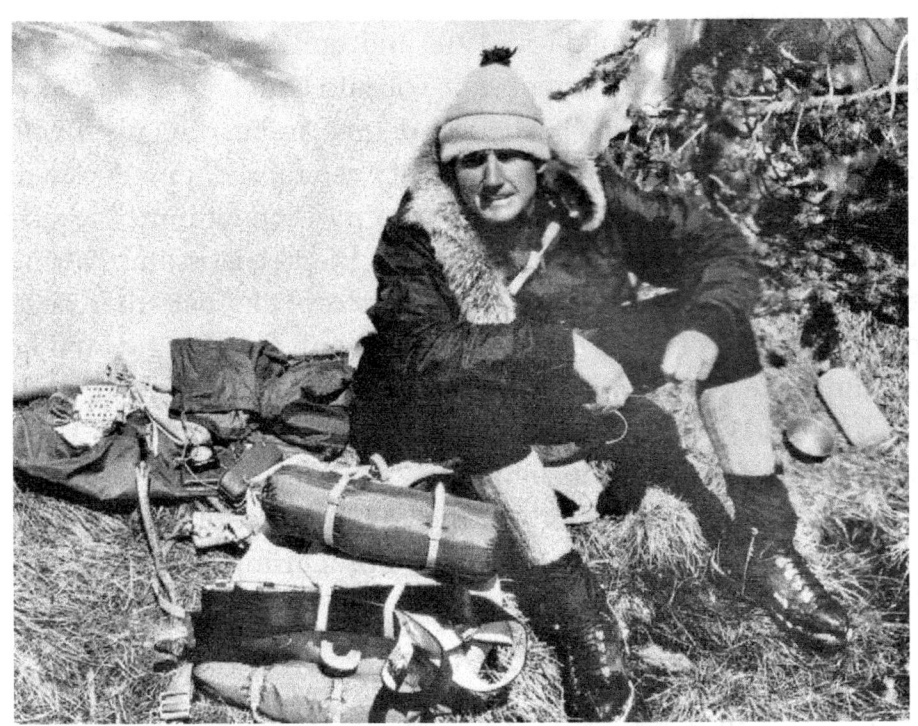

Dr. David "Snowshoe" Thompson, 1970

## DR. WILLIAN RIRIE, ELY, NEVADA, LEADER
### By Lori Romero

Dr. William Bee Ririe was one of the most beloved citizens of Ely, Nevada. He was born in China on Christmas Eve. He was the son of Canadian missionaries who were working deep in Western China. The name William Bee Ririe will be well remembered in Ely, as the local hospital was named after him.

Ririe's first formal schooling was under the instruction of Quakers. He attended the American Quaker School in Chung King and later the China Island Mission School in Chefoo. He studied in 1913 at Oxford University; London, England for a single year. He then entered Toronto University in Canada, where he enlisted in the Canadian Army. During World War I, he was sent to Europe and spent over two years on the Western Front as a medical corpsman. When the armistice was signed, Dr.

Ririe returned to Canada in 1918 and enrolled in a course in biological and medical sciences at Toronto University.

He graduated with a bachelor's degree and earned his MD in 1922. Dr. Ririe served an internship at hospitals in New York and Detroit. In October 1930, he accepted a position with the Nevada Consolidated Copper Company at their Steptoe Hospital. During the Great Depression, Dr. Ririe would accept any patient in need of medical care, even when he knew his only payment would be a handshake.

In 1934, William Bee Ririe was married to Evelyn Dunn and was transferred to Consolidated Copper's hospital at Ruth, Nevada, but his devotion to the Steptoe Hospital kept him involved with the day-to-day operations. During the 15 years he became an American citizen.

In 1949, Dr. Ririe transferred to Kennecott Copper Company's hospital in McGill, Nevada. After 31 years spent mending injuries and treating illness, he retired from the company hospital in 1961. Purchasing a home across the street from Steptoe Valley Hospital, he entered the private practice of medicine. When the copper company deeded the Steptoe Valley Hospital to the county, a new medical group was formed by the younger doctors in town, and Eastern Nevada Medical Center was formed.

In 1968, construction was begun on a new East Ely facility, which opened in June 1969. By almost unanimous consent, the new hospital was named the William Bee Ririe Hospital. He continued to practice medicine, earning the honor of "Physician of the Year" from the Nevada State Medical Association. He was also honored by the Nevada Industrial Commission for his contributions to the working man. In March 1976, Dr. Ririe retired from practice. He died two months later.

**NOTE:**

This article about Dr. William Bee Ririe was researched and written by Ms. Lori Romero, who is library director of the White Pine County Library in Ely, Nevada.

# Dr. George "Spunky Kid" Gardner
## By Dr. Roderick D. Sage

George M. Gardner must have been a spunky kid—bright and plenty spunky. He was born in Carson City January 30, 1875. His father, Matthew Gardner, was a Virginian who came west in 1803. He was a major land holder and lumber baron in the South California area.

Gardner Peak was named in his honor. As a youngster, he played about his father's lumber mill and on the trains. In about 1885, Matthew Gardner sold his lumber empire to E.J. "Lucky" Baldwin, the Nevada entrepreneur, and entered the cattle business in Eagle and Smith Valleys.

George often helped his dad ship cows off to market. One day, he lost his grip on the train coupling and fell under the wheels of a cattle car, crushing both his legs just below the knees. His legs went—one way, and he went the other—in a wheelbarrow to the nearest hospital. George survived, and perhaps it was at that time he decided to become a medical doctor.

Deprived of his lower limbs at age twelve and living in a relatively primitive area with little medical care, George was sent to live with an aunt in Oakland, California. He attended a special school, where he prospered both intellectually and physically. With a working pair of cork legs and the determination to use them, he obtained an excellent high school education.

George Gardner did well enough to gain admission to the first class of Stanford University, graduating four years later in 1895 in what has been described as "that famous first class" featuring among others, Herbert Hoover, who worked his way through Stanford managing a laundry service. George often mentioned with some pride that his shirts and underwear were washed and ironed by a future president of the United States.

Gardner entered Cooper Medical College (Now Stanford) in San Francisco, finishing the two-year curriculum in December

1896. Without the benefit of internship, this brand new 22-year-old doctor signed on as physician and surgeon for a mining camp at Gold Creek, near Elko, Nevada, a move that had to take a lot of spunk. The following summer, in 1897, he opened a medical office in Elko where he stayed until 1904, practicing in partnership with Drs. C.J. Hood and Samuel S. McDowell. In 1904, he moved again this time to Fallon, Nevada.

During his early years in Fallon, Dr. Gardner contracted his services to the Newlands and Lahontan Dam projects, the Fairview mining district southeast of Fallon, and the Tonopah Railroad Company. He also served the mining town of Rawhide, not only as a physician, but also as the town druggist. This arrangement ended when Rawhide burned to the ground, along with his apothecary shop.

For a while Dr. Gardner owned a stage line serving Tonopah, Rawhide, Fallon, and parts in between. The stages were two big Royal Tourist Cars, costing about $4,000 each. They held four passengers, and performed nobly, but service was often hampered by the fragility of their tires. George estimated a tire would survive about 50 miles before a blowout. He spent $600 per year on tires alone.

Dr. Gardner's pride and joy was a Pullman Touring Car which he purchased in 1911 for use in his busy practice in Fallon. Because of his infirmity related to the leg prostheses, he engaged several young lads in Fallon to chauffeur him about on house calls, including this writer's father-in-law, Jack Price. Dr. Gardner practiced widely in northern Nevada. He relates, "Treating a miner in Carlin, Nevada, for a bullet wound in the hip, ultimately making 23 round-trips by train to do so."

Other than his near fatal leg injuries, George's closest call came one Sunday morning when he stopped in a saloon for a glass of beer with a friend. A former patient, Joe Fuller, already in his "cups," wrote him a check for $12 for an overdue fee then, followed it up with a glancing blow to the jaw. This infuriated

George, who immediately flattened the rascal with his cane. Fuller extracted a small pistol from his pocket. Fortunately, it snagged briefly on the lining of his pocket, enabling George to make a fast exit. Fuller fired just as the saloon door slammed shut. In a panic, Fuller turned himself over to the county attorney, thinking he had killed Dr. Gardner. He probably would have, too, but the bullet was deflected skyward by an iron brace on the barroom door. So much for "Sunday Fun" in Fallon.

Dr. Gardner remained in Fallon until 1917 when he moved his practice to Reno, joining Dr. Raymond St. Clair. In 1921, his beloved wife, Louise, died during a major surgical procedure. After this George move to the San Francisco Bay area, opening an office in the Flood Building in San Francisco. He soon remarried, this time to Blanche Miller, a literate and charming former teacher. They made their home in the East Bay Community of Kensington. This necessitated a daily commute by ferry to his office until the Bay Bridge was opened in 1937.

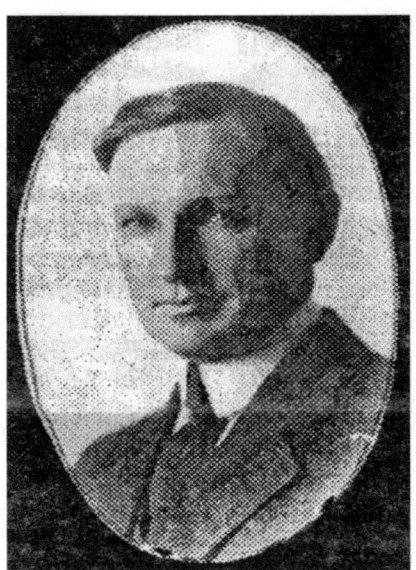 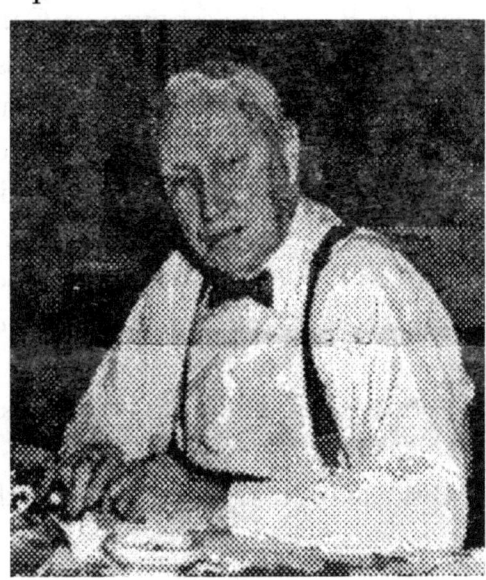

Dr. George Gardner, 1915     Dr. George Gardner, 1975

As he grew older and after a long day at his office, George sometimes removed his prostheses and stumped about on his foreshortened legs, reminding his friends of the famous French artist, Henri Toulouse-Lautrec. He continued in practice until 1946, when he retired, so he and Blanche could enjoy their elegant Lake Tahoe shore front home near Meeks Bay during the summer months and his home in the Berkeley Hills in the winter months. George Gardner finally removed his cork legs for the last time and quietly died at the end of 1970, a month shy of his 96th birthday. He was acclaimed to be one of the last surviving members of the illustrious first class at Stanford University.

## Dr. Anton Tjader
### Nevada's First Autopsy, 1860

The first legal execution occurred in Carson City on November 30, 1860, when Nevada was part of the Utah Territory. Bernard Cherry who lived in Carson City was shot and killed near Dr. B.L. King's house in Carson City by Jonathan Carr, a former rider on the Pony Express and an outlaw who robbed emigrants on their way to California. After the murder, Carr fled to California where he was captured in Tuolumne County.

Carr confessed to the crime and was tried and sentenced to be hanged near the residence of Dr. Benjamin L. King where the crime had been committed. Doctors George Munckton and Charles Daggett pronounced Carr dead and Dr. Anton Tjader did the autopsy. For his efforts, Dr. Tjader was paid fifty dollars which was equivalent to two weeks salary for a doctor.

**NOTE:**
Information is from Guy Rocha, Archivist for the State of Nevada.

# W.H.C. Stephenson, Virginia City Nevada's First Black Doctor, 1863

## By Elmer R. Rusco PhD

Nevada's small Black population during the nineteenth century included a physician who practiced on the Comstock for at least twelve years. Dr. W.H.C. Stephenson was an outstanding and respected leader of his African American community and of the wider community of the preeminent mining and population center during this critical period in Nevada's early history. In addition to his medical contributions, he took the lead in protesting racial discrimination.

We do not know where Dr. Stephenson received his training, although apparently, he was from Rhode Island. In 1867, he wrote; "I am ... a practicing physician and have my diploma and passed a successful examination before entering upon the practice of medicine." In 1868, he wrote that he had been practicing medicine for twenty years; if this is correct, he must have become a physician around 1848, when he would have been 23 years old.

We know he was living in Sacramento and Marysville in 1862 or 1863. He first appears in a Comstock directory in 1863, where his address was given at a laundry on South G Street between Smith and Washington. The same directory lists him as a trustee and clerk of the First Baptist (colored) Church that was organized April 26, 1863. It was the first Baptist Church on the Comstock.

For the next 12 or 13-years, Dr. Stephenson practiced medicine on the Comstock, mostly in Virginia City but also in Gold Hill, Silver City, and Dayton. In addition, he took trips back east for at least two periods.

Various sources list his office in Virginia City, usually on C Street, in 1864-1865, 1867, 1868-1869, 1871-1872, and 1875. In an 1878-79 directory, his wife was listed as living at the 120 South C Street address, which was also used for an office.

In several advertisements, Dr. Stephenson described himself as an Eclectic Physician. Eclectics had their own medical schools, journals, and a National Eclectic Medical Society before the Civil War. Besides the obvious factor of favoring treatment procedures from a variety of different sources, Eclectic physicians at this time were noted for their avoidance of a wide variety of harsh medicines or methods of treatment, such as purgation, lancing, the promotion of fevers, and the prescription of mercury compounds, which were then common among physicians. In some respects, eclectics often provided better care because less harmful techniques were used than those used by many other physicians.

The statements made by him about a diploma and passage of an examination suggest the Dr. Stephenson graduated from an eclectic medical school, but further research is needed. As Dr. Anton Sohn has pointed out, "Not all those who called themselves physicians were educated in the healing arts. Licensing laws were virtually non-existent and educational requirements had not yet been established to ensure that all physicians were trained."

In 1868, Comstock's pioneer black physician wrote a column on smallpox which was printed in the *Territorial Enterprise*. In it, he reported this disease had been spreading in San Francisco and several other California cities, had reached Gold Hill and Virginia City, and had become a matter about which Nevada citizens ought to be alarmed. He offered several suggestions for prevention and mitigation of smallpox on the Comstock, starting with vaccination but also including total abstinence from all intoxicating liquors, the destruction of all bedding used by persons who have been afflicted with the disease and disinfecting houses where there had been patients ill with the disease. Dr. Stephenson ended by advising physicians to change their clothing after treating smallpox patients. He offered the opinion that not all physicians would agree.

Nevada's first black physician was obviously well educated and quite intelligent as several letters to the editor and his leadership in various community matters attest. In 1870, when Black men were allowed to vote for the first time after the 15th Amendment became part of the U.S. Constitution, Dr. Stephenson and other Black Nevadans registered to vote.

The *Territorial Enterprise* reported that a person of lighter skin, but darker heart refused to register because he would not place his name under the doctor's. The newspaper offered the opinion that Dr. Stephenson would not have objected to placing his name after that of this man because Dr. Stephenson has intelligence enough to see that it would not detract from him to have his name follow that of an inferior.

His important role in the first Baptist Church on the Comstock has been noted. The first pastor of the church, Rev. Charles Satchell, left after about one year and was succeeded as minister by Dr. Stephenson. However, the church ran into debt and the building was sold at auction in 1866. Some members of the congregation criticized Dr. Stephenson when he purchased the building and kept the proceeds.

When Nevada became a separate territory in 1861, and a state in 1864, there were various relics of the barbarism of slavery imprinted in the statute books of Nevada, as an 1865 address to Nevada citizens from a black organization headed by Dr. Stephenson put it. For example, suffrage was restricted to white females, negroes, Mongolians, and Indians. They could not be educated in the public schools unless a separate school was set up for them. Members of the same groups could not marry whites and these three groups were forbidden to testify against white persons in either civil or criminal cases (with the curious exception that Chinese were allowed to testify against whites). In the latter case, Dr. Stephenson was specifically affected to a substantial extent. In 1867, he protested: "I have three thousand dollars due to me, in the State from Anglo-Saxons, for professional services, which I can only collect through sufferance; and this, in sums of ten to forty dollars, is a dead loss, from the fact that the parties have shielded themselves through an Act of the State which leaves me no redress."

In supporting his call for repeal of the testimony law in civil cases, the *Territorial Enterprise* asserted that Dr. Stephenson no doubt paid more tax than…both-of-the-two legislators who had killed the bill to repeal this law during the 1867 session. Dr. Stephenson asserted in 1870: "My Country and State taxes for the year 1869, in gold coin, were $40, city tax $16, government (federal occupational) tax $50."

Dr. Stephenson was one of the leaders of the African American community who protested these discriminatory laws and sought their repeal. During the 1865 legislative session, a petition requesting African Americans be allowed to testify against whites in criminal cases was sent to the legislature and a bill allowing this, although ambiguously worded, was adopted. During the same year "Black Comstockers" led by Dr. Stephenson, organized to seek an end to exclusion from voting, testimony, and schools.

In a vigorous attack on the school law in 1870, the physician reported the taxes he had paid during 1869 and protested that the exclusion of black taxpayers from the public schools was grossly unfair and a violation of the right to an equal protection of the laws…and equal school rights with the Anglo-Saxon. He suggested that the question was whether "people of color" were as human beings, entitled to any school privileges whatever. The 1870 census of population reported Dr. Stephenson and his wife, Jane, had a daughter who was 13 that year. No doubt his own child was one of the children not allowed to attend public schools.

The efforts led by Dr. Stephenson were rebuffed in both the 1866 and 1867 legislative sessions. Equal access to public schools was not achieved until 1872, when the state supreme court declared the school law barring non-white children to be unconstitutional. The 1869 legislature repealed the law forbidding blacks to testify against whites in civil cases, while retaining it for other non-whites.

When black men secured the right to vote in 1870, a Lincoln Union Club was organized in Virginia City with Dr. Stephenson as president. This organization held an elaborate celebration of the passage of the 15th amendment on February 3, 1870. This included a parade and a reading of the 1866 federal Civil Rights Act.

While he did not give the main address at this event, Dr. Stephenson made a few remarks, which a newspaper called *sensible and appropriate*.

African American leaders after the Civil War were strongly Republican, because nationally this party had secured enactment of the 13th, 14th, and 15th amendments and several civil rights laws. When a Liberal Republican party was organized in 1872 and put forward Horace Greeley as its presidential candidate, Dr. Stephenson, even though he was at the time in New Rochelle, New York, wrote a vigorous statement addressed to *"Colored voters of Storey County and Nevada."* This document asserted that the Liberal Republicans and the Democrats were involved in a league against Emancipation ... (and) against the Civil Rights bill and the 14th and 15th amendments. He urged black voters in Nevada to vote for the reelection of President Grant and for the "Old Republican Party" which was still devoted to freedom and equal rights.

In short, W.H.C. Stephensen was not only a physician on the Comstock for a decade and half but was also an early advocate of human rights in the state. He deserves to be remembered for these achievements.

**NOTE:**

Elmer R. Rusco PhD, was Professor Emeritus in Political Science at the University of Nevada Reno. The advertisement is from Charles Collins Company *Mercantile Guide and Directory for Virginia City, Gold Hill, Silver City, and American City 1864-67.*

**W. H. STEPHENSON, M. D.,**
MAIN STREET, SILVER CITY,

Gives special attention to the treatment of all

## DISEASES OF THE HUMAN SYSTEM

And from an experience of twelve years of general practice, can
Guarantee Greatest Satisfaction to all who may place themselves under his care.

Special attention given to the treatment of
RHEUMATISM, NEURALGIA, DIPTHERIA AND PARALYZED LIMBS.

## An Advertisement from 1864

Dr. Stephenson Ad. 1864

## DR. ROYCE W. MARTIN, LAS VEGAS' FIRST MD
### By Curator Phillip I. Earl, Nevada Historical Society

Born at Table Rock, Nebraska, on November 16, 1878, Dr. Royce W. Martin was later to become Las Vegas' first physician and the community's foremost booster. The son of a livestock buyer and dry goods merchant, he attended Wesleyan University for a year and received a business degree from Omaha Business College in 1898. For a time, he taught school in rural Nebraska before entering upon medical studies at University Medical College, Kansas City, Missouri, where he got his degree in 1903.

Known to his friends as Roy, he once told an interviewer he had taken up medicine because of a boyhood experience: "I was born on a farm, and every time the doctor came, I got a dime for holding his horse. I decided then and there, doctors must have a lot of money and that was what I wanted to be."

Shortly after he graduated as a fledgling physician, he

accepted a position with a mining company in Tampico, Mexico. Upon his arrival, he found himself in a yellow fever epidemic. Sent to a jungle district where one of the company's operations was located, he did his best to care for those down with the disease and himself came-down with the disease.

Following the subsiding of the siege, he returned to the United States. For a time, he practiced medicine in the northern section of the Oklahoma Territory on the so called "Oklahoma Strip," a section 28 miles wide and 100 miles long that had become America's premier "outlaw country" by the turn of the century.

In July 1905, he heard of the boom in Goldfield, Nevada, and decided to try his luck. Arriving in Las Vegas by rail in August 1905, he learned the community had neither a doctor nor a hospital, so he decided to stay and set up a practice. He established an office in an 8-by-10-foot frame shack near Fremont Street and was soon doing a booming business. Four months after his arrival, he was appointed chief surgeon for the Las Vegas & Tonopah Railroad, serving in that capacity until the line ceased operations in 1918. Mining was one of Dr. Martin's diversions over the years, and he became a friend of every miner and mine promoter in southern Nevada. He often accepted mining stock in exchange for his services.

Among the promotions, he was involved in was the Three Kids Manganese Mine some 15 miles southeast of Las Vegas, which boomed during World War I and became one of the nation's premier producers of strategic metal during World War II.

On June 27, 1910, Dr. Martin married Nellie Cotton at Seward, Nebraska. Not long after they arrived in Las Vegas, they moved into a new home on the corner of Fifth and Fremont Streets. By that time, he had moved his offices to the upper floor of the Thomas Building. He subsequently converted the other rooms to a hospital, Las Vegas' first such facility. In July 1918, he purchased the Palace Hotel on North Second Street and was redoing the building for a hospital when the Spanish Flu epidemic hit later in the fall. Dr. Martin was also Las Vegas' health officer at that time and not only treated patients, but enforced measures to close schools, theaters, churches, and saloons to check the spread of the disease.

On December 25, 1932, a new hospital opened in the 200 block of North Eighth Street. Las Vegas had several physicians by that time and Dr. Martin had moved on. He had long been active in community affairs and had served as president of the Las Vegas Chamber of Commerce for ten years. He was also active with the Las Vegas Rotary Club, the Elks Lodge, the Masonic Order, and the Eagles. He also served on the Colorado River Commission for many years, working on plans for the construction of Boulder Dam. In 1922, he was elected to the Nevada Assembly. In addition to sponsoring legislation dealing with medical and dental practice in Nevada, he concerned himself with highway legislation, taxation and matters bearing upon the welfare of his constituents in his home community. Dr. Martin was also a talented amateur thespian.

At the outbreak of World War II, Dr. Martin was retired, no longer practicing medicine, but the shortage of doctors at that time forced him to practice. In April 1943, officials at Basic Magnesium, Inc. hired him to do physical examinations for prospective employees. He and his wife moved to the Basic Town site, now Henderson. In November 1943, he suffered

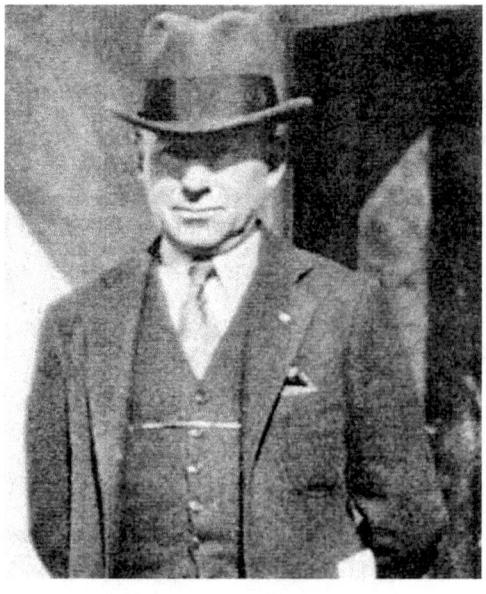

Dr. Royce W. Martin, 1930s

a heart attack and died at Basic Hospital on December 22.

He was survived by his wife and two daughters. Although largely forgotten in Las Vegas today, Dr. Martin's imprint is on every aspect of the history of early Las Vegas. One of the city's middle schools was later named in his honor, but he deserves more recognition.

## Dr. Kirk Cammack, "Frontier Desert Justice, 1960s"

"When I came to Las Vegas in 1960, just out of my surgical residency, the town was still a frontier gambling town. Five or six years later, with the arrival of Howard Hughes, it began to develop into a cosmopolitan city of over a million people—as it is today. Besides the "mob element gamblers" in the valley, there was a group from the western states and gambling ships off the coast of California that had migrated to Nevada where what they were doing was legal. It wasn't very long after coming to Nevada that I operated on one of the Texas gamblers who had been shot in the abdomen. The man survived. This Texas gambling contingent had come to Nevada to escape a dangerous war going on in the Dallas area between their competition. This is when I met Golddollar. He stood six-feet six-inches and had all gold teeth.

"He had been the first black man to be admitted to the Professional Rodeo Cowboys Association. He was the bodyguard of a leading Texas gambler in Las Vegas. He was very quiet, but at the same time a very intimidating man.

One day, Golddollar was in my office waiting to be seen, when this agitated family came in yelling and very upset over the death of their daughter. She had come into the trauma area after having been beaten up and overdosed. It had been difficult to make a diagnosis of her situation, and eventually she died. The family was irate, and threatened to sue me, screaming, hollering, and disrupting my office. I took them into my private office to try to talk with them, but to no avail. They left the office, saying they were going to see an attorney that day and file a lawsuit against me for malpractice.

"Golddollar asked my receptionist, 'Who were those people? and what was the problem?' She briefly explained it to him. He asked for their address, and she gave it to him (It was hard to deny Golddollar anything.) Several days later, I received a call from the family, saying they wanted to talk to me. I told my office staff I didn't want to hear any more of their vituperation, and to do what they had to do. One of the office staff said, 'They are nice now, and they want to talk to you." When I got on the telephone with them, they were very calm and apologetic for their behavior and said, "We are not going to sue, and you should not be concerned with that at all." At the end of the conversation they said, "Thank you very much for your help, and would you please tell Mr. Perry Rose (Golddollar's real name) we are not going to sue, and there will not be any problem." This conversation was followed by their attorney, calling to reassure me there would be no lawsuit and to inform Golddollar.

"The next time Golddollar came into the office, I asked him what he said to those people to get them to decide not to follow up with a lawsuit. He rolled his eyes sideways and shrugged his shoulders and said, "Doc, I don't know what you're talking about." I never mentioned the subject again. It was a malpractice suit avoided by "Frontier Desert Justice, Texas style."

## DR. JACK C. CHERRY, "ONE-OF-A-KIND," 1924

Dr. Jack C. Cherry was most assuredly a "Nevada State Treasure." He came to Nevada in 1924 after practicing in Montana for four years as physician for the Northern Pacific Railroad. That position gave "Doc" many personal and professional awards, but the most prized was marrying his wife, Phyl.

Dr. Cherry: "The mines were going strong in Goldfield, and I had done as much as I could do at Northern Pacific, so I wanted to find a place of my own and get started." When he learned Dr. Blake in Goldfield wanted to retire, Doc arranged to buy his practice and move to Nevada. Goldfield was lacking many niceties like streets, sidewalks, trees, and grass. Many of their friends and relatives couldn't understand why they wanted to go there. "Doctors were a dime a dozen then. After they graduated, they were all out looking for jobs as there was a depression."

Thus, began a career that spanned more than fifty years administering to Nevada's citizens and helping to build our state's health care community. Even though the big companies were ending their mining operations when Dr. Cherry arrived in September 1924, the practice was extensive, and he began making a name for himself. Dr. Cherry: "The big Goldfield Consolidated Mill was closed. Mark Bradshaw and Albert Silvers leased the tailings, which they washed down with hydraulic hose and treated with a cyanide process. They did so well that they refined the process and ran the tailing through again."

Dr. Cherry: "I had contracts with the three railroads, a mill, the mines, and Esmeralda County. My territory ran into Death Valley and as far south as Beatty." In addition, he ran the Goldfield Hospital for nine years. Goldfield's closest call with an epidemic was a case of typhoid traced to the water supply. The water came from springs at Lida. It was pumped to redwood tanks, open on top, in a two-step process and then gravity-fed into the town's wooden mains. The tanks were death traps for birds. "The tanks had to be drained and scrubbed down, but the privately-owned water company didn't want the expense. It took a court order and the sheriff to get the job done. In those days most doctors didn't have a pot-to-sit-on."

Dr. Cherry: "My office in the Goldfield Hotel (two rooms on the second floor) cost me $30 a month. There were quite a few bootleggers out in the hills at that time." Dr. Cherry recalls some of them made real good corn liquor. The only other source was by prescription. He said, "The government allowed us 100 one-pint-prescriptions every three months. They were drawn on drug stores, and the empty prescription had to be returned to the Internal Revenue Service in San Francisco."

One of his regular customers was Walter Scott, better known as "Death Valley Scotty." He came to town regularly for his pint of bottled-in-bond whiskey. "He would arrive in a Model T Ford driven by an Indian. He always wore a white cowboy hat, a white shirt, and a red necktie. For some reason he always rode facing backwards. Scotty constantly talked about building a castle. He was a big "bullshitter." His house was a 14 x 16 ft. cabin in Grapevine Canyon."

Dr. Cherry: "Scotty did get a castle, but in a roundabout way. He never had a dime to his name. It came about through an invitation from A.M. Johnson of Chicago to pay him a visit. Johnson had money, but not very good health. After a couple of months in Death Valley he felt so much better that he decided to build a house. It became Scotty's Castle. Johnson kept more than 100 men on the job, except during the scorching months of July and August. Dr. Cherry was the construction physician: I'd drive the 37 miles through Bonnie Claire and the Grapevine Mountains on Sunday, have dinner and then, conduct sick call."

"Johnson wanted no shoddy monument. He built the castle to endure. Cast iron sewer pipe was coated with tar and wrapped with tar paper." I told him, "The pipe would last for 50 years in this dry climate, even without tar and paper." He replied, "I want it to last for 250 years." The castle's music room with its big organ reflects a special interest of Johnson. He controlled the Wurlitzer business in Chicago. The wrought iron fence and gate in the room were imported from a church in Spain.

Dr. Cherry moved to Tonopah in 1933 when Dr. Percy McCloud of that city died in a flaming car wreck while returning from Ely. On long trips across country the doctors carried extra gas, from five to fifteen gallons. They made a potential funeral pyre.

Dr. Cherry brought in Dr. Gerald Sylvain from Butte, Montana, to take over his Goldfield practice. Dr. Sylvain later moved to Las Vegas. Tonopah greatly expanded the territory Dr. Cherry covered, first in a Dodge, then later in LaSalle Coupe. He usually had a shovel strapped to the rear bumper. He administered to Round Mountain, Manhattan, Silver Peak, and Beatty. In Tonopah he took care of the "Soiled Doves." Every Monday the girls from the cribs arrived for their physicals. That night the police chief checked each for their certificate.

When World War II arrived, Dr. Cherry was offered a commission and went to the Presidio in San Francisco to talk with a general: "I cut myself when shaving, I used a styptic pencil to stop the bleeding. It didn't burn. Puzzled, I took my blood pressure, and it was high as hell." The result was a complete change of plans and a move from Tonopah (elevation 6,000 feet) to Las Vegas (elevation 2,200 feet.) Dr. Paul Jones, a hospital board member, invited him down to look over the town. His first check point was the National Hotel on Carson and 4th.

Dr. Cherry settled into his new home fast. He took over the handling of county indigent cases, a responsibility that paid all of $400 a month. In the summer of 1942, he accepted the job of county hospital administrator when Paul O'Malley quit to run for justice of peace that paid $650 a month.

The hospital was a small, struggling, overcrowded, somewhat makeshift institution-40 beds, patients often overflowing into the halls, a surgery lighted by spotlights strung along two pipes, a well for water and its own sanitation system-a septic tank. The city sewer didn't run that far out on West Charleston. It had two units, an old frame building with 20 beds used mainly for ambulatory patients and old folks, and a newer stucco structure with 20 beds. Dr. Cherry said, "When it rained, we had to set out pans to catch the water in the old building, We either had to have a new roof or a new hospital."

Since dependents of Nellis AFB servicemen were treated

there further compounding the inadequacy of the facility, Dr. Cherry decided to use that as leverage to get federal funds to build a major addition.

He went to Los Angeles to talk to officials of the Federal Works Agency. The initial sympathy of the Feds dissolved into silence. Apparently local opponents of the county hospital had got to them and blocked action. Dr. Cherry said, "For nine months nothing was accomplished. I couldn't even get a letter out of them. Finally, I called Pat McCarran." McCarran, then Nevada's senior senator, was surprised the county was still awaiting word. "If that Los Angeles man doesn't call you in fifteen minutes, let me know," he told the doctor.

The official's call was prompt, and typically mendacious. "We've been waiting for you to come down," he said. "The plans are ready." So, the county got a $456,000 hospital addition by agreeing to come up with the $60,000 needed to equip it. That spawned a new problem. The linen demands for the additional 140 beds swamped the local laundries, so Dr. Cherry went through Los Angeles junkyards buying washers, dryers, a boiler, and a mangle (a large machine for ironing sheets, etc.).

There was a headache with the railroad because ambulances carrying the sick and injured were frequently held up at the Charleston Avenue crossing. Dr. Cherry went after state and county funds to build an underpass. The new hospital was leased from the federal government for $1 a year, until such time as a bond issue could be floated to buy it. Through some tough bargaining, Dr. Cherry negotiated the Feds into accepting $182,000, and that is how Las Vegas got Southern Nevada Memorial Hospital. The hospital is located on what was the county poor farm.

In 1931, county patients were moved in, and it became the Clark County Indigent Hospital. Ten years later, a board was formed, private paying patients were accepted, and the name was changed to Clark County General Hospital with Dr. Cherry hired as administrator. During the early years in Las Vegas, Cherry was also physician for five of the hotels there (Flamingo, Sands, Riviera, Last Frontier, and El Rancho Vegas).

Jack Cherry has been state president of the Elks, Exalted Ruler twice, and was honored with a life membership in the Elks. His loyalty and love for Nevada strengthened through the years, and he was responsible for much of the growth and improvement in Las Vegas. During those years Dr. Cherry has known Nevada's people from grassroots miners to ranchers.

He knew the mountains, deserts, sagebrush, and cities. He gave Nevada the best that he had, and Nevada will remember him well. He died in 1986 at the age of 88.

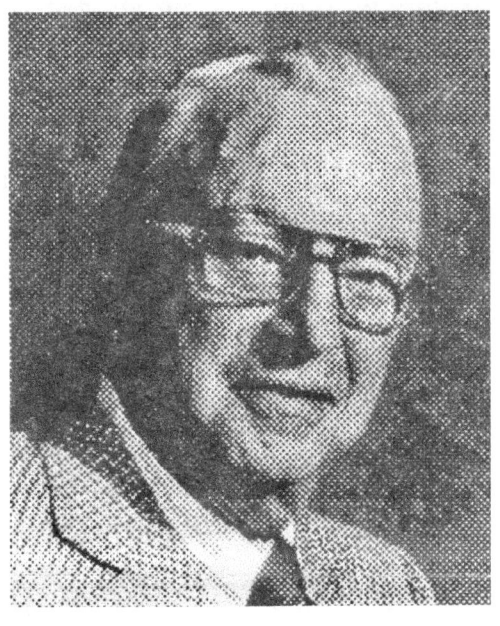

Dr. Jack C. Cherry, 1960s

**NOTE:**

Information is from *Nevada Health Review*, July 1981, *Profiles in Medicine*. Photograph of Dr. Cherry, courtesy of his son, Jack Cherry.

### DR. WILLIAM PATTERSON, "SOLDIER, RANCHER, ETC."
### 1899

William H. Patterson MD played many roles during his lifetime; as a soldier, a husband, a father, a rancher, a horseman, a physician, a statesman, and an administrator. He fought for and represented his country, saved lives, lost a few, made fortunes, lost fortunes, enjoyed good health, and suffered from blindness. He experienced much love and suffered much loss.

He was a risk taker as described by Dr. Frank Farwell, a consulting psychologist to the U.S. Congress, who developed a theory that the U.S. population is largely a nation of risk-takers made up of the descendants of immigrants who took the supreme risk of uprooting themselves to come to the New World-thrill seekers who need a higher degree of stimulation than others to be fulfilled.

Both Dr. Patterson's parents had separately immigrated to Canada in the 1830's, most likely to seek a better life.

His mother, Elizabeth Smith was born in Johnston, Renreshire, Scotland, in 1817, and arrived in Canada in 1836. Soon after her arrival she met John Patterson, also a Scottish immigrant and they were married in 1839. John Patterson was a magistrate. They had five children, including William H. Patterson, who was born in 1843.

The family settled in Almonte, Ontario, Canada, in a stable and secure environment. Elizabeth was widely known for her good works and kindness in the community. Her obituary in the local newspaper spoke of "her quiet and unassuming manner and Christian integrity [that] won the admiration of all with whom she came in contact." Upward mobility appeared to thrive in the Patterson children; both William and his brother James graduated from McGill Medical School, sister Jessie became head of the Art Department at the University, brother Robert became Chief of the Canadian Supreme Court, and sister Mary married a businessman.

Most of his siblings made a good life for themselves, never living far from the family home in Almonte, but William H. Patterson had wanderlust. Soon after his graduation from McGill University with honors he made plans to leave for the United States. The reason for his departure is unknown. Eastern Canada was peaceful at that time, there was no family discord, and his future seemed assured. William was a risk-taker, and the appeal of the wild west may have stirred his adventurous spirit-at any rate he moved to Arizona in 1867 and applied for United States citizenship.

He spent four years as an assistant surgeon (contract physician) in Arizona with the United States Army, then moved to San Francisco. With a new contract with the Army, he served at Fort Bidwell, Modoc County in Northern California as assistant surgeon from March 20, 1872, until October 1, 1873. In this time, Dr. Patterson served in the "Lava Beds" during the Modoc Indian Wars made famous by Indian Warrior "Captain Jack."

When his military career ended, he set up medical practice near Fort Bidwell in Cedarville, Modoc County, California. There, he met and married the town's first schoolteacher, Mary Drouillard in 1874. Miss Drouillard graduated from one of the first classes at San Jose Teacher's College, which later became San Jose State University.

They had four children. His medical practice grew rapidly, and Dr. Patterson was most welcome in the community. According to the local newspaper, "There was no doctor nearer on the south than Reno, on the west than Susanville, and the east than Omaha, and on the north, there was nobody at all."

He set all the broken bones, cured all the fevers, and brought in all the babies in Modoc County, California, Roop County, Nevada, and Lake and Grant Counties in Oregon. He covered an area at least 150 miles square. To cover these long distances, he kept several fine saddle horses, and on a long ride he would change horses once or twice, leaving his horse on the road and hiring one to ride out and back. It was said that he had the largest surgical practice in the United States.

As a successful businessman he began to buy land. He bought the Cottonwood Ranch in Surprise Valley near Cedarville. He bought the Duck Lake Ranch in addition to their home in Cedarville. He invested in property near Tonopah, Nevada. Patterson Lake in Surprise Valley was named after him. It is of interest to note Chief Winnemucca, his wife, and youngest son all died at the southern end of Surprise Valley.

Dr. Patterson was a member of Surprise Valley Lodge No. 235, Free and Accepted Masons, and served as Worthy Master of that Lodge. He was elected as California State Senator representing Modoc, Lassen, Sierra, and Plumas Counties from 1887 to 1888. While in the senate he introduced numerous bills involving Napa State Hospital, the Chinese immigrants, and the mining industry.

In 1899, he accepted an appointment from Governor Sadler of Nevada to serve as Superintendent of the Nevada State Hospital, so he moved his family to Sparks. Two years later in 1902, his wife Mary died at the age of 46 years. Dr. Patterson established the first scholarship at the University of Nevada with a gift of $100. He later married another schoolteacher from Cedarville whose name was Annie Stevens. Within about ten years he separated from his second wife and moved back to Cedarville.

Like many professional men in that time, Dr. Patterson invested in gold mining operations, and apparently made a great deal of money. His last investment in gold mining and milling was not successful.

In his retirement Dr. Patterson was an avid reader with a love of poetry. He is remembered as a real gentleman, impeccably dressed, with an erect posture. He insisted upon proper English and disliked nicknames. In the later years of his life he lost his vision. No longer able to care for himself, he moved in with one of his daughters in Berkeley, California. On March 29, 1925, he died in the Alta Bates Hospital in Berkeley at the age of 82 years.

**NOTE:**

This story was abstracted from a biography by Dr. Patterson's granddaughter, Mrs. Beatrice Rey. Additional information and pictures have been furnished by Granddaughter Mabel P. Baker and great granddaughter Margaret Rey Duensing. The photos are from the family collection and the Riverside Gallery Reno, Nevada.

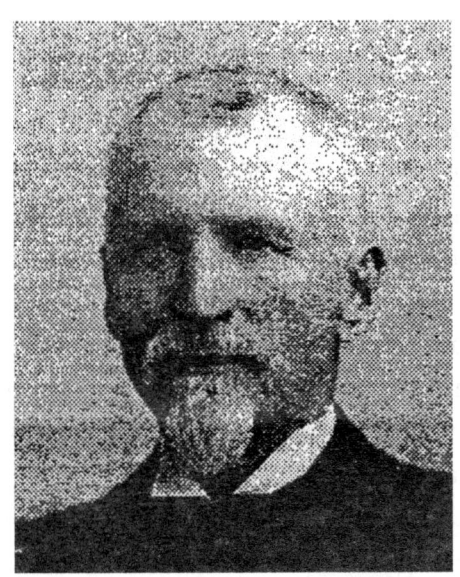

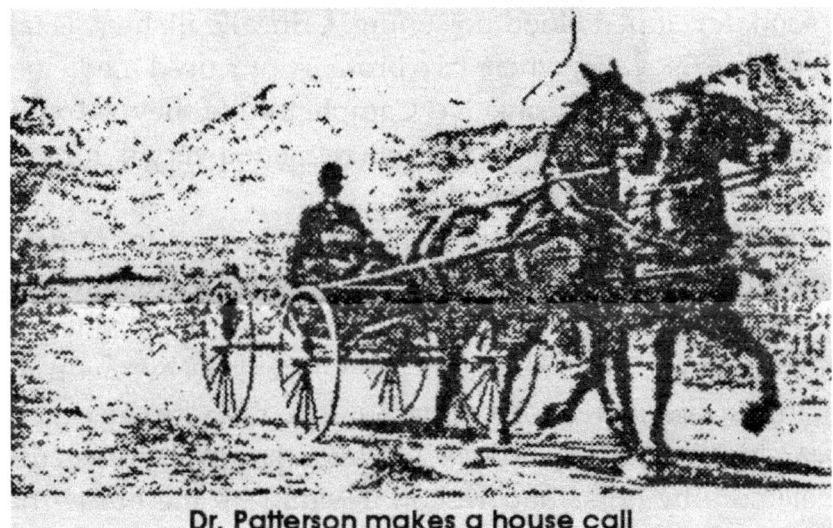

**Dr. Patterson makes a house call**
Dr. William H. Patterson, ca. 1900

## Dr. John D. Campbell, "Tale of the Phantom Hand"

Dr. John D. Campbell of Pioche, Nevada could have easily been the role model for Doc Baker of *Little House on the Prairie*, or the famous 'Doc' of *Gun Smoke*. Like the roles that they portray, Dr. Campbell was a real-life country doctor. Traveling by horse and wagon, regardless of weather conditions, to minister to humble homes or miner's cabin, Dr. John Dalgleish Campbell gave many years of professional care to the residents of Lincoln County.

Born in Hartland, Michigan on 9 July 1853, he graduated with honors from the University of Michigan Medical School. While in Michigan, he married Bertha Haford and fathered one son, Wilkes James Campbell. After the death of his wife Dr. Campbell moved west. He spent some time in White Pine County where he practiced medicine. He married Maggie Leahigh, and soon after moved to Pioche. While in Pioche they had three more children, two sons-Ainslie and Floyd, and a daughter Edith. The early death of Edith was a family tragedy.

In 1902, Dr. Campbell operated on an Indian lady with cancer of the breast. During the operation he inadvertently cut himself and soon developed blood poisoning. Critically ill, he was taken to Delamore, Nevada, where two brothers practiced medicine. In a desperate attempt to save Dr. Campbell's life they amputated his left arm just above the elbow. He remained very ill for a long time, but eventually recovered.

During his convalescence he began to suffer a lot of pain in his amputated hand, which had been buried in Delamore. He said it felt like the fingers of his left hand were clenched together and cramping. The "phantom pain," caused by neuromata growing in the stump of the amputated limb, became almost unbearable. Finally, his oldest son, Wilkes James Campbell drove to Delamore by horse and wagon. He dug up the buried hand and straightened out the fingers. Almost simultaneously Dr. Campbell's pain ceased, and he was much relieved. His wife, Maggie, became his new left hand, assisting in bandaging and other treatments.

During the great influenza epidemic of 1917-18, Dr. Campbell and his son, Wilkes, would travel from house to house with a bucket of soup, giving soup to the ill and quarantined victims of the epidemic. He helped a lot of people, and he developed a reputation as "guardian of the sick."

On many a cold winter night, the good doctor answered calls for assistance across the county. He and his son, Wilkes, bundled up in heavy bearskin coats and hats, would drive many miles in a wagon or cutter. Before they left on a call, they would heat up rocks to help keep their feet warm, but that didn't do very much good as the rocks soon cooled. The cold was sometimes unbearable, but Dr. Campbell never refused a call.

In addition to his medical practice, the good doctor was active in community affairs. He was elected assemblyman from White Pine County in 1889 and 1906 and served two terms as a state senator. He presided over the Senate for one full session in the absence of the Lieutenant Governor. He was a 32nd degree Mason, an Elk, and an Odd fellow.

Dr. J.D. Campbell died at his home in Pioche on January 8, 1928, at the age of 75 years, much respected as the "Country Doctor" of Lincoln County.

**NOTE:**

This story is from Kimberly Campbell, great granddaughter of Dr. Campbell. The information is from a tape recording by Linwood Wilkes Campbell, grandson of Dr. J.D. Campbell in 1998. We appreciate his contribution to the medical history of Nevada. The following portrait was given to the Great Basin History of Medicine by Linwood W. Campbell.

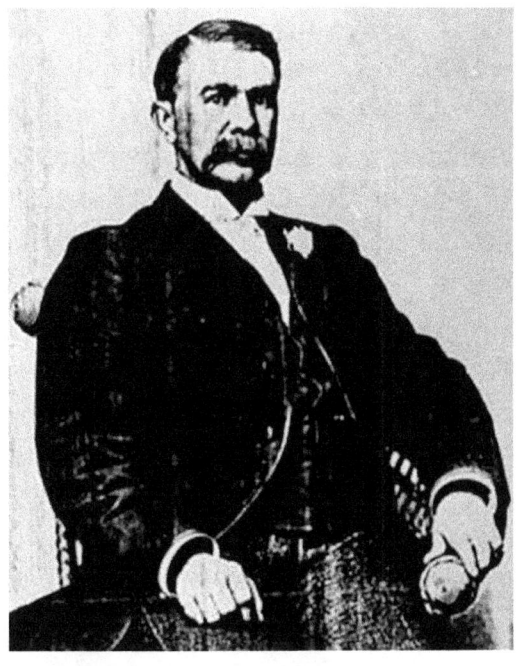

Dr. John D. Campbell, ca. 1910

# Dr. James Barger
## American College of Pathologists President
# By Lisa Puleo

Dr. Barger: "I was born in Bismark, North Dakota, at St. Alexis Hospital. My father was a country banker and my mother, a native of Wisconsin, was a homemaker. I had an older brother whose name was Thomas. Our parents, who were good Irish-Catholics, wanted one of us to become a Priest. I went to school in Linton, North Dakota, graduating from high school in 1934. After spending two years at St. Mary's College (now St. Mary's University) in northern Minnesota, I transferred to the University of North Dakota. My brother was supposed to enroll in pre-med, but after he had been there for a week, he transferred to mining engineering. He also joined the Kappa Sigma Fraternity, although our parents did not approve. I wanted to become a chemical engineer, but mother asked me, 'Why don't you try pre-med?' Well, one cannot 'just try it'; as once I was in pre-med, I was caught.

"After graduating from medical school, World War II came along. I was sent to Fitzsimmons Army Hospital in Denver, Colorado. This was during the early days of blood transfusion. I gave a paper on alkaline phosphatase in Portugal, and while there I met Phillip Levine, a pioneer in blood banking. He stimulated my interest in the Rh system, so when I returned to Fitzsimmons, I began to do some research. Phil Levine and others were making anti-Rh serum by injecting rhesus monkey blood into Guinea pigs. When I tried to do that, I ran into the problem of obtaining rhesus monkey blood. The tuberculosis hospital in Denver was run by a church group which had a monkey colony. I went over and looked at their monkeys, and they were almost as big as me—boy, were they tough! I decided I couldn't handle that job, so I went over to the zoo and asked for help. The zookeeper very nicely got me the rhesus monkey blood.

"When I got back to Fitzsimmons I ran into the chief of service, a Colonel, who asked me, 'Where have you been?' I replied, 'To the zoo, Sir,' and he said, 'What for?'. I told him 'To get some rhesus monkey blood, Sir,' and he asked, What for? I told him I was trying to make some Rh anti-serum. He looked at me, smiled and just walked away.

"I didn't get the Guinea pigs to make the antiserum, and soon received orders to leave Denver.

"I was transferred to the General Dispensary in Washington, D.C. The Dispensary opened in January 1943. It was great; at the dispensary, we wouldn't look twice at anybody in the Clinic unless they had at least three stars. I stayed there until 1944, when I was transferred to the Office of American Affairs. They sent me to a hospital in a jungle town in Eastern Bolivia. At the hospital I met Sister Mercy, who was a real fine person. I spent fourteen months there, traveling to nearly every place in eastern Bolivia. I was looking for beriberi, that had been reported in that region in 1915 or 1920. By the time I got there, beriberi had been practically eradicated. When I searched for patients with beriberi, I was always told they were a little bit further into the interior. I finally got to a place that was in the middle of the Amazon jungle, when I decided beriberi could just stay there.

"I married Susie right after I came back from Bolivia. We married in Douglas, Arizona. I was sent to Colorado Springs, Colorado, but by that time I was on my way out of the service. Susie and I had two children, James Jr. (who will be fifty this year) and daughter Susan Mary. My wife, Susie, died in 1951. I later married my second wife, Josephine. She developed carcinoma of the lower esophagus and stomach. She died from disseminated intravascular coagulation. My third wife, Janie, died from emphysema secondary to smoking. She was always trying to quit, but finally just didn't have any lungs left. After she died, I would find packs of cigarettes hidden here and there in the house. She was a typical addict and was always trying to hide her habit.

"I came to Las Vegas in 1964. I got a job at Sunrise Hospital with a pathologist that I knew when I was in Phoenix. It was a nice place to work because I could do what I wanted. The administrator, Nate Adelson, was one of the toughest negotiators I have ever known. When you reached an agreement and shook hands on it, that was it. If he made a mistake he ate it, and if you made a mistake, you ate it. He was fair, but tough, and he was a great guy.

"He was the one who built Sunrise Hospital. There were other pathologists in Las Vegas when I arrived. Drs. Bob Belliveau and Grayson were at the County Hospital. There was enough work to keep busy, and so it was nice.

"About that time, I started getting involved in the national politics of medicine and pathology. When I first arrived in Las Vegas it was a small, growing town, with not a very big medical group. I knew everyone. We had frequent medical meetings and it was very congenial—a thing I now miss. We would get together and got to know each other. I think that kind of comradeship leads to consultations and exchanges of ideas.

"I have always been a member of the medical society, no matter where I was. If you are going to be a physician, you should be a member of the American Medical Association. Most of the doctors in town were members of the AMA. Everybody seemed more relaxed in those days. I think we should go back to having county society meetings where we could just get together and become better acquainted. We used to have a pathology society too. We would meet about once every three months and have dinner. I was selected as a delegate to the AMA. by the county medical society. We had great times at the AMA and the county meetings. It was fun in those days, and I wish we could bring those days back. I think people are too busy these days. As the saying goes, take a real interest as though it all really mattered!"

**NOTE:**
This story is from an Oral History by Lisa Puleo, Executive Director of the Clark County Medical Society. Dr. Barger was president of the of American College of Pathologists, 1981-83.

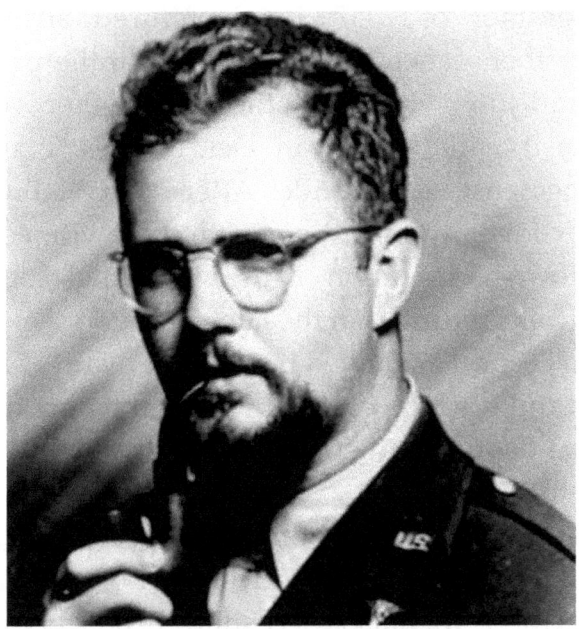

Dr. James Barger, 1940s

## DR. ROLAND STAHR MAKES A HOUSE CALL, 1937
### By Dr. Roderick Sage

Dr. Roland Stahr was a revered pediatrician in Reno from 1939 until his untimely death in 1969, and before that in Fort Dodge, Iowa, where he had practiced for the previous dozen years. He was a hero, not only to his young patients and their parents but to his colleagues as well, serving as president of the Washoe County and Nevada State Medical Societies. He was named Nevada's Outstanding Physician in 1965.

In 1937, Roland Stahr still practiced in Fort Dodge, a city of 20,000 inhabitants in northern Iowa. He was a consultant to family doctors all over that part of the state for general childcare and for pediatric allergies.

My father was such a general practitioner in the nearby town of Eagle Grove, 25 miles to the northeast. He often referred his difficult pediatric problems to Dr. Stahr. The onset of such a request would begin with a terse phone call, "Stahr? This is Sage."

In the summer of 1937, Iowa endured an epidemic of poliomyelitis, then generally known as infantile paralysis. One morning in mid-July, when my father and mother were enjoying a two-day visit with friends in Des Moines, I awoke to an overwhelming sense of lassitude. After nearly falling asleep in my morning cereal, I tumbled back into bed with covers drawn up and window shades down. Thus, I remained, cocoon-like, all day until the folks returned in the late afternoon. They wondered if we shouldn't cancel a planned trip to visit relatives in Waterloo- one hundred miles to the east. However, the next day, I awoke bright-eyed and bushy-tailed, rarin-to-go. We had a splendid two-day-get-together.

The day after we returned home, whatever it was, hit the fan! In addition to a return of that overwhelming weariness and photophobia, there was also a crushing headache, fever, and a steamroller overall aching. I wasn't just under the weather, I was SICK. Then the fun began.

"Stahr? This is Sage." After a few hours of observation and a downhill course, another call and Roland Stahr was on the scene- the first of three house visits he made from Fort Dodge that night.

The physical exam was an ordeal. A few days before I had been a lively, nimble eleven-year-old swimming in the town pool and playing softball.

Now sitting up in the bed was a chore. Groaning with misery, I braced myself with my arms. It hurt to extend my legs more than 60 degrees. The flashlight hurt my eyes and my neck was sore and inflexible. Would that examination ever end?

After a while (after it was dark) Roland returned, armed with PARAPHERNALIA. "OK Roddy, we're going to have to get a little blood out of your arm." Ouch! But it was over in a hurry.

Then the big surprise. "OK Roddy, lie over on your side. We're going to put a needle in your back so that we can draw out some fluid."

Over on the left side, knees drawn up, and back convex. This effort hurt, and I grunted and perspired. The stick in the back was accompanied by an odd, deep nerve aching. In a bit this ordeal ended lights went out and I was able to get some sleep. But believe it or not—it must have been 2:00 am—here was this gadfly and his companion, my father, back to torment me some more.

This time they arrived with an enormous vial of watery-looking fluid, a giant syringe, and a long, skinny needle. The neurological exam was repeated. I was aware of more pain and increasing weakness. This had become a true pediatric emergency. Into the arm vein went the contents of the vial by way of the big syringe-and long needle. This seemed to continue for an eon, until the needle finally came out. Tape and cotton were applied to the arm and at last I was in dreamland again.

The remainder of the night was one of blissful slumber. On 'coming to' at 8:30 AM, the whole world was bright and rosy. Fever down, stiffness and aching nearly gone, my spirits were hearty. To recapitulate a bit: As I lay there in my misery, I heard those two men (Dr. Roland Stahr and my dad, Dr. Erwin Sage) talking about me. The word "polio" was bandied about. That didn't sound too ominous. Dr. Stahr said something about a positive Babinski sign, which sounded like gibberish, so it couldn't be anything bad. Then he told dad he had had two patients with this unknown malady (polio) who received the same sort of serum; one did very well, but the other didn't.

That July afternoon and evening when it became obvious, I was one "sick-cookie," the big wheels started to turn.

Roland Stahr arrived on the scene and checked me out. He went out and returned later with his diagnostic kit to draw blood and do a spinal tap. The disease was moving fast!

When the diagnosis of polio became evident, father called the state health department in Des Moines, 80 miles away and ordered a batch of poliomyelitis convalescent serum. This was how the disease was treated in its early phase in 1937. Venous blood drawn from recovered polio victims was spun down, leaving clear serum loaded with anti-polio antibodies. This serum was injected into the patient's vein. Later, it was found most people had these antibodies, probably from subclinical infection and the serum was more widely obtained.

At midnight, father was on his way to Ames, Iowa, to rendezvous with a State Trooper who had transported the precious supply of serum from Des Moines. By 2:00 AM, he was back home, and Dr. Stahr was again on hand.

The first batch worked for five days, giving way to a relapse with more fever, headache, muscle pain and weakness, but this time a new supply of serum was obtained under less hectic conditions. After this injection I was home free.

Later, when I asked my dad the name of my illness he replied, "anterior poliomyelitis." Big deal! Then I asked him what that meant in ordinary language. He answered, "infantile paralysis." In 1937, those two words engendered terror in the beholder. For a moment, I was scared out of my wits and asked him if I was going to be paralyzed. He assured me I wasn't but let me know I had luckily missed that fate.

Roland Stahr came west to Reno in 1939, after suffering a debilitating problem with arthritis, which persisted for years until he was serendipitously tested for Bang's Disease (Brucellosis). He reported the ensuing orchitis clinched the diagnosis and he was then successfully treated for Chronic Brucellosis.

When I started my dermatology practice in Reno in 1958, Dr. Stahr was on hand to welcome me and introduce my wife Jackie and me to the community. He was a superb consultant for a fledgling dermatologist and is still a hero to the four young Sage brothers.

# Reno's First Pulmonary Doctor Robert Locke, Iwo Jima and Back

Dr. Robert Locke was a quiet, modest man, who did not brag about or mention his bravery during World War II. Although it was known he had been awarded the Navy Cross, his account of privation with honor on Iwo Jima was found after his death, and his involvement in the tuberculosis treatment is described in *People Make the Hospital: The History of Washoe Medical Center*. He never forgot the University of Nevada and served as a full-time physician at the student health facilities.

Bob was born in Mt. Pleasant, Utah, in 1920. The family moved to Reno ten years later. When he attended the University of Nevada, he came under the influence of famed Professor Peter Frandsen, who was responsible for many Nevada students pursuing careers in medicine and dentistry. While Bob was attending the University of McGill Medical School in Montreal, Japan bombed Pearl Harbor. The following year, Bob enlisted in the U.S. Navy, and in 1943 after graduation, Ensign Locke reported for active duty at Treasure Island in the San Francisco Bay. He volunteered for Marine Corps duty, but further training was interrupted by the desperate situation in the Pacific.

Hurry-up exercises on Maui's beaches did not prepare Battalion Surgeon Locke for the horror that was to follow on Iwo Jima. He wrote, "Intensive education as to the exact landing location occupied the last two weeks prior to landing, along with DDT dusting and wax impregnation of all combat clothing to prevent typhus and other pest-borne disease." Then, what history would record as one of the bloodiest battles of the Pacific ensued. The Japanese deliberately ignored the first wave of U.S. troops on the beach of Iwo Jima to trap them and the second wave on the narrow strip of sand.

Senior Officer Locke was placed in charge of the second wave of vehicles on the right flank, but as his lead vehicle reached its goal, "The radio fairly screamed us back to sea in that we were definitely in Japanese territory." As they regrouped, intense mortar fire erupted destroying all landing craft and pinning them down on 30 feet of beach.

During the intense enemy fire, Robert Locke remembered: "I made a flying leap off the front of the vehicle and landed in neck high water and waded on into my unit. A few seconds later my vehicle and the remaining occupants were annihilated. For the next 72 hours, we were totally confined to the narrow beach strip." Locke's Navy Cross citations read, An adjacent unit was in the center of the heaviest concentration of artillery and mortar fire and was suffering extreme casualties beyond the abilities of its depleted medical sections. With total disregard for his own safety, Lt. Locke voluntarily left his covered position and entered the shelled area four times and helped carry wounded to the evacuation station.

During the following 21 days, the Japanese continually killed Americans by creeping out of the tunnels at night and infiltrating their positions. Locke: "It was discovered that the Japanese were infiltrating in American uniforms during the night in small groups and were swimming to sea and coming back in on the beach. Almost every foxhole I visited blew up within seconds of my leaving."

The second part of Locke's citation notes that under enemy fire Lt. J.G. Locke waded out to a small boat evacuating the wounded and forced the crew that refused to leave because of the intense fire to take the wounded off the island. At the end of the Iwo battle Dr. Locke wrote, "Actually, the flag raising on Iwo was very premature to those of us there and was far from the climax. Probably the true climax was our cemetery trips, the last few days before final securing of the island, through the thousands of dead lined beside rows of crosses, attempting to identify and locate lost friends."

After Dr. Robert Locke returned to Reno, he was appointed as the first pulmonary doctor on Washoe Medical Center's medical staff on July 2, 1947. In 1951, the Washoe Trustees agreed with the medical staff's recommendation that he manage all patients on the TB ward. He practiced internal medicine for three decades before retiring. He died at age 82.

### DR. JAMES L. SWANK, "GEM OF DISCOVERY"
## By Dr. Anton Sohn

School of Medicine Assistant Professor Megan Swank was alerted by one of her students that we were displaying a Doctor's Swank medical bag.

Megan approached Pathology Manger Lynda McLellan, who opened the bag with her to find a letter linking the bag to her great-grandfather, Dr. James Levey Swank. We were unaware of the letter that was addressed to Medical Librarian Joan Zenan May 20, 1989. The letter states Dr. Swank came to Las Vegas in 1943 after a divorce in Michigan and practiced until his death in 1961.

Following is the 1989 letter with Dr. Swank's Las Vegas history from Mrs. Dorothy George: Ms. Joan Zenan, "Thank you for coming to our home and picking up the medical equipment, once the property of Dr. James L. Swank. As I mentioned to you, Dr. and Mrs. Swank were long-time friends as well as occupying an office near Dr. George's in the late 40's and early 50's in downtown Las Vegas. Dr. Swank was on 4th street and Dr. George on Carson Avenue (where the Nevada State Bank now stands), just around the comer from each other.

"It is difficult to get accurate information on the medical equipment since Mrs. Swank is also deceased. I talked with her sister who lives here, and she gave me the following information.

"Dr. Swank graduated from the University of Maryland School of Medicine in 1927. He came to Las Vegas around 1943 and was a family physician until his death in 1961.

"His father, James Levy Swank, was a family physician in Shanksville, Pennsylvania. The stethoscope and sphygmomanometer were given to Dr. Swank as a gift from his father and as near as I can pinpoint the date of the age of the equipment is circa 1890. The medical bag was used by Dr. Swank here in Las Vegas far house calls for many years and the blood pressure equipment sat on his office desk for all the years of his medical practice.

"Of interest, when talking with Mrs. Swank's sister, I learned that the late Dr. Pearlman had received many pieces of old medical equipment of Dr. Swank's stored in their garage and discovered after Dr. Swank's death when Ms. Swank was moving to a different home. It included old orthopedic saws, surgical instruments, etc. of the same vintage as the blood pressure equipment. Dr. Pearlman made a huge collage of his 'find' and it hung in his office until his death.

"His wife has since died also and the whereabouts of the collage is unknown.

"I hope the above information is helpful to you for your display of Dr. Swank's medical equipment. We were happy to give it to a new home where others might enjoy it. Thank you again for your visit and acceptance of the equipment. Also, June sends greetings to you. Sincerely, Mrs. Dorothy George."

Jarrett DeCorte: "I'm writing to you today in reference to the most recent 'Gem of Discovery' mentioned in the UNR School of Medicine Greasewood Tablettes.

"Upon reading this article about Dr. Swank, it came as quite a surprise to realize the person who wrote that letter in Dr. Swanks bag was my late grandmother, Dorothy George, spouse of my late grandfather, Doctor Joseph George in Las Vegas. I had to reread it several times as I felt like it was a mistake seeing her name there at the bottom of the letter. Very fascinating, true gems from the past!

"At the time this letter was written, I was 8 years old. Today, I currently live in the George family home in Las Vegas that my grandparents moved into in the 1950s.

"My grandparents were indeed good friends of the Swank family. It was a delight to read this and see both mentioned in history."

**NOTE:**

Dr. Anton Sohn gave Dr. Swank's doctor bag to Megan Swank.

## Dr. John H. Pasek, Sixty Years Minden's Doctor
### By Dr. Richard Newbold

"Doc" John Pasek was born on November 23, 1913, in Huron, South Dakota. His mother was a homemaker, and his father was the CFO for Huron College. He had three brothers (two became engineers and the third became an FAA controller). He received a BA in chemistry from Huron College, then graduated from University of California at Irvine in 1939. U.C. Irvine was established in 1896 as a school of osteopathic medicine. The school in 1962 became the California College of Medicine and granted MD degrees. Prior graduates had their certificates of osteopathic medicine converted to MD degrees.

Pasek was hired by Mono County to practice general medicine in Bridgeport, CA, in 1939. He was there for two years, then went back for anesthesia training in Long Beach, CA. He remained in Bridgeport until 1943, when he moved to Minden, NV. He was the Mono and Alpine County Health Officer for decades.

In 1943, he opened a hospital in in the basement of the Minden Inn and had patient rooms on the 3rd floor of the hospital. This lasted for three years, but he continued to maintain an office across the street on the 2nd floor of the old historic Farmer's Bank. John moved his office to the Stratton Center in 1971 and remained until 1998 when he retired.

He maintained an office practice, delivered many babies, did minor surgical procedures, and set fractures. He remained on the staff of Mono General Hospital in Bridgeport, California, filling in on weekends and holidays for resident doctors. He retired from Mono County in 1986.

Dr. Pasek was also on the Douglas County School Board from 1954-1960. He was an avid hunter and fisherman in his younger, and even in his later, years. In the early 1970s, he bought a 10-acre plot of land in Ruhenstroth and raised alfalfa and sheep.

He was known for "house-calls" and his "gentle-caring" nature. He held a DO Medical License #106 even though he could have had converted to an MD. He practiced medicine for over 60 years and died at home on June 14, 2005, at the age of 91.

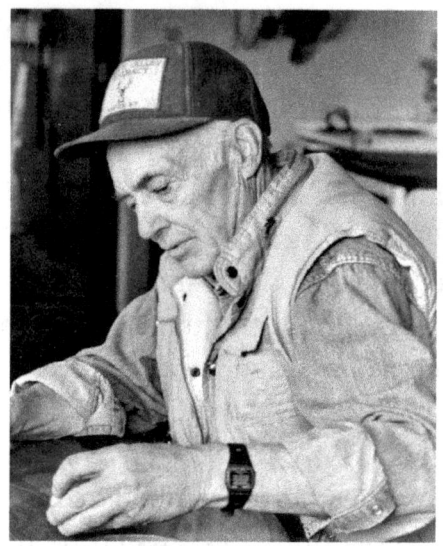

Dr. John Pasek, 1980s

## "WW I Hero" Dr. Delos Ashley Turner
### By Peter Aylworth

Delos Ashley Turner's father, Ephram Turner, followed the goldrush to California in 1849 and later moved to Nevada where he was involved in law enforcement. He was county sheriff and U.S. Marshal before moving to Delamar, Nevada in 1893 where he was captain of the guard for a bullion coach that moved gold 163 miles from mines to the railroad.

Delos Ashley Turner was born in Pioche, Nevada, in 1877,

went to its elementary school, moved to Salt Lake City for high school, and graduated from the Medical Department of the University of Illinois in 1901. He practiced medicine in Salt Lake City for the Salt Lake Railroad before he moved to Goldfield, where he remained until 1911. He served as county physician, health officer, and the first president of Esmeralda County Medical Society.

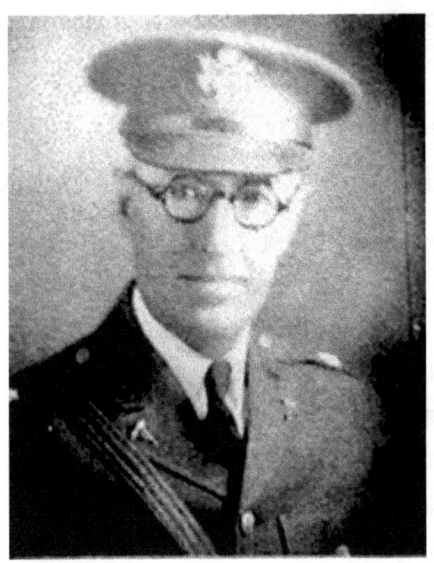

Dr. Delos Ashley Turner, 1907-08

In 1909, Dr. Turner was the president of the Nevada State Medical Association. He served as the Chief Surgeon of the Goldfield mining operations until 1917. During the First World War Turner joined U.S. efforts to liberate Europe. He received medical officer training in Fort Riley, Kansas and served as 1st Lieutenant in the 7th Engineers. In November 1917, he was promoted to Captain and assigned to the 349th Infantry. The fighting ended in November 1918, and he was shipped to France to help with post-war health efforts. Medical officers not only helped those who were wounded but others who had non-combat health issues. He was promoted to major and remained in France until June 1919. The Paris Peace Conference was finalized July 1923 with signing of the Treaty of Lausanne.

Dr. Turner continued his military career in Reno, serving as lieutenant-colonel and executive officer for the U.S. Army Reserves 116th Medical Regiment. He dedicated his career to helping veterans get proper medical treatment. In 1924, he was chief medical officer of the U.S. Veterans Bureau and coordinated Reno and San Francisco healthcare. In 1937, he moved to Hines, Illinois, where he served with the Veterans Bureau from 1938 to 1944. He died in January 1945 at the age of 68.

## Dr. Louis Lombardi
## Nevada Board of Regents, 1950-1980

# Unrecognized Founder of Nevada's School of Medicine

1. Born November 17, 1902, Reno, Nevada, Graduated, Reno High School
2. University Nevada, Reno, AB, 1929
3. St. Louis School of Medicine, MD, 1933
4. Opened General Medical Practice in Reno, 1934
5. Delivered more than 4,000 babies
6. Voted to establish Nevada's School of Medicine in 1969 while a member of Nevada Board of Regents. He was a member from 1950 to 1980
7. Honorary Degree Nevada's School of Medicine, 1981
8. WW II, U.S. Navy Commendation and Bronze Star at Iwo Jima
9. U.S. Selective Service Board for twenty-five years after WW II
10. Past President, Washoe County Medical Society
11. Past Chief of Staff, St. Mary's Regional Medical Center
12. UNR Athletic Department's physician for twenty years
13. UNR Lombardi Recreational Center named in his honor, 1974
14. Died in August 1990, Reno, Nevada

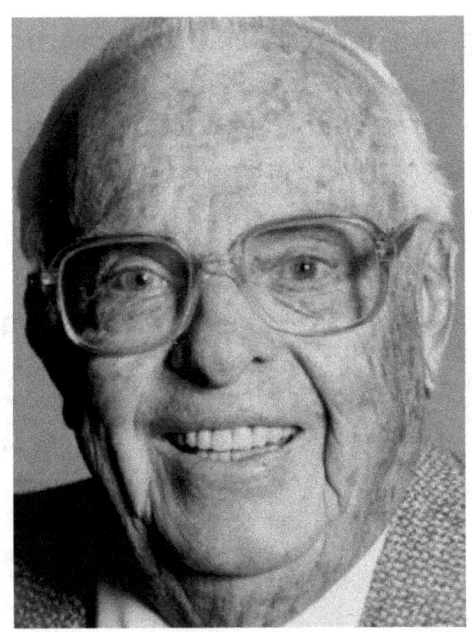
Dr. Louis Lombardi, ca. 1970

## Dr. Donald Pickering's "Monkey Fetus Experiment"

In 1966, Dr. Donald Pickering built a stainless-steel womb for a monkey fetus. He removed a living monkey fetus from the womb of a mulatta macaque monkey and grew it in the artificial womb for thirty-three hours until it died. This was the first time an artificial womb was used, and even though it was a short time, it was a success.

The purpose of this experiment was to develop an environment for studying disease before birth. The mulatta macaque was chosen because it has similar reproduction features to humans. The experiment was initiated because thalidomide in the 1950s caused multiple abnormalities in the human fetus. The drug was banned during pregnancy in the 1960s.

Abnormalities in the embryo has undergone much research, but Pickering's research was the first time an artificial womb was developed. The experiment was published 29 July 1966, in local newspapers and *Time* magazine.

Dr. Pickering was born in 1923 and practiced pediatrics in Reno from 1964 to 1982. He was involved in founding the first neonatal intensive care unit (NICU) in Nevada at WMC in 1973. He moved to Alaska in 1982 and died in Seattle in 2006.

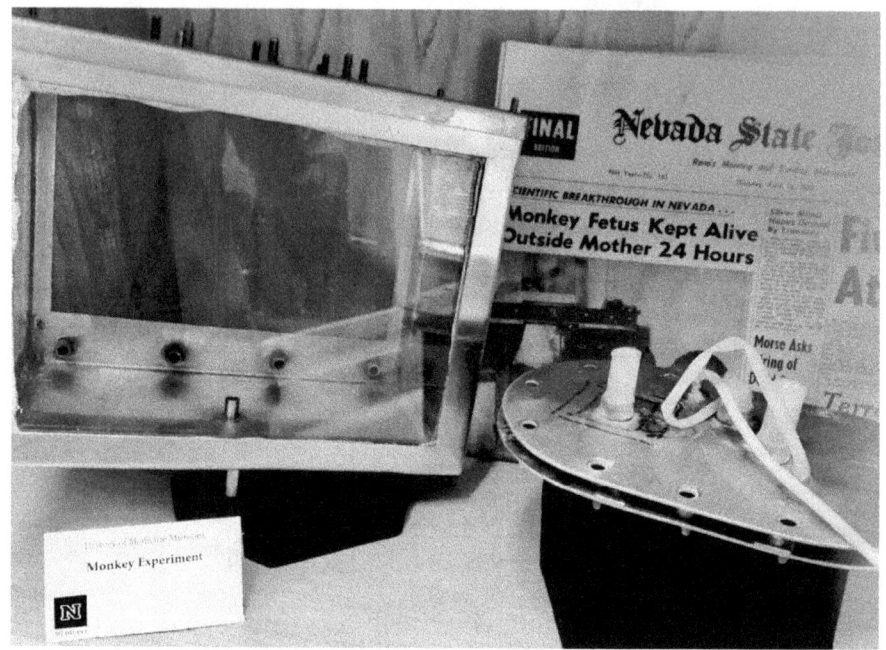

Pickering's Artificial Monkey Womb
(donated by James K Ohl)

## Dr. Charles West, Nevada's First Licensed Black MD

Hank Greenspun in the *Las Vegas Sun* on October 10, 1984, stated that Dr. West's death meant the fight for freedom has lost a true champion.

Greenspun called Dr. West, "a healer of bodies, minds and souls," who led the attempt to reverse "the ugly political and spiritual environment of Southern Nevada in the early 1950s."

In 1954, Dr. Charles West moved to Las Vegas at the suggestion of Bandleader Count Basie. Dr. West became the first black doctor to pass the Nevada State Board of Medicine Examination since it was first given some fifty years earlier.

During his lifetime, Dr. West was recognized for his achievements. President Lyndon Johnson appointed him to UNICEF. He was appointed to Nevada's Governor's Medical Advisory Board of the Aging, and the National Conference of Christians and Jews honored him.

He established the Charles I. West Las Vegas Medical Society for blacks. In 1964, Dr. West received a Nevada Centennial Year Certificate of Appreciation and Gratitude for Outstanding Community Service.

**NOTE:**

Dr. Charles I. West was not the first black MD in Nevada. Dr. W.H.C. Stephensen was the first black MD when he moved to Virginia City in 1863. The MD license act was passed in 1899, and Dr. Charles West was the first black doctor after the licensing law was passed.

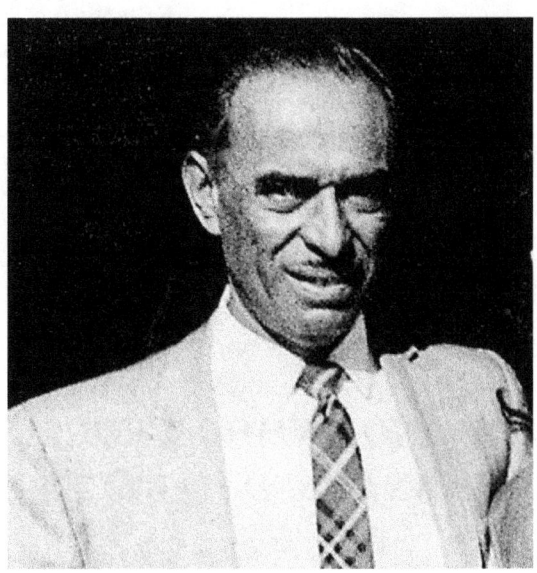

Dr. Charles I. West, ca. 1970

# III

# CHINESE MEDICINE

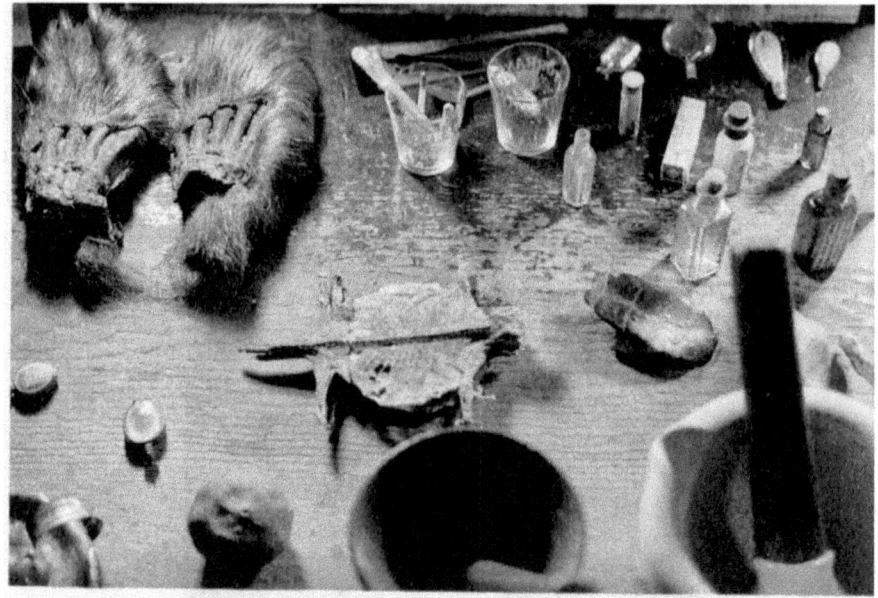

Kam Wah Chung Pharmacy, John Day, Oregon (Great Basin History of Medicine)

## HERBS AND ANIMAL PRODUCTS (BEAR CLAWS) USED FOR TREATMENT

# DOC ING HAY OF JOHN DAY, OREGON, 1887
## By Dr. Owen Bolstad

During the second half of the nineteenth century, American business imported thousands of Chinese laborers to help develop the Western Frontier. Most of these poorly paid workers were employed to build the transcontinental railroads, but many others found employment as cooks, laundry workers, and various other menial jobs. There were truly remarkable men among these migrants, and some made indelible marks upon the American West.

As the railroads were completed and the labor market became more competitive, many of the Chinese laborers returned to their homeland, happy to leave this strange and foreign land where they had been treated with so little respect. Not so was Doctor Ing Hay and his partner in business, Mr. Lung On. Although they retained close ties with their Chinese roots, they had no intention of leaving their new country.

Born in the Kwangtung Province of China in 1862, Ing Hay arose from a peasant background. In the middle of the nineteenth century the ruling Manchu Dynasty had been forced to open China's doors to foreign trade and there followed a series of wars and rebellions that caused great poverty and famine. Members of Ing Hay's family sought relief of their suffering by migration to America. Finding employment here, they wrote to relatives remaining in the old country encouraging them to come to America. In 1883, Ing Hay and his father arrived in the United States, settling in Walla Walla, Washington, near their relatives.

It is not known just when Ing Hay received his training in classical Chinese herbal medicine, but when he moved to John Day, Oregon, in 1887, he intended to open a practice there. Meeting Lung On after his arrival, they became fast friends and soon became partners in-business. They leased the Kam Wah Chung & Company building, a fortress-like stone structure in

John Day's Chinatown and opened for business. The company sold general merchandise, both to the dwindling Chinese population of John Day and to the general population as well. In addition to the store, Ing Hay began the practice of herbal medicine, dispensing his potions and nostrums to the public-at-large.

Doc Hay, as he soon became known in the area, practiced pulsology, making his diagnoses by carefully feeling the strength, rhythm, and rate of his patient's pulse. He would then compound an individual potion designed for the person's ailment and give explicit directions as to its use. Within the apothecary shop in the Kam Wah Chung store there were literally hundreds of herbs and remedies, many imported from China. It is believed there was liberal use of opium and alcohol when making these remedies, perhaps one reason why Doc Hay's ministrations were so popular.

Doc Hay became well known and well respected over much of central and eastern Oregon. Apparently, Ing Hay never resorted to surgery in his practice, and his gentle homeopathic approach to medicine did little direct damage to his patients-something that most of the poorly trained conventional doctors could not claim.

Doc Hay remained in John Day, continuing to do business even after the death of his partner Lung On. In 1948, at the advanced age of 89 years, Ing Hay suffered a fractured hip and died of complications, despite the efforts of modern medicine. The Kam Wah Chung establishment was locked up and left undisturbed. Mr. Bob Wah, owner of the store, deeded the structure to the city of John Day with the stipulation that it become a museum to honor the Chinese community, but it was not until 1967 that the city realized they were the legal owners of the building and began the task of converting the old building into a museum.

Workers' cleaning and organizing the store found a bundle of uncashed checks from Lin Hay's patients totaling over $23,000 ($265,261 in 2022) hidden under his bed. This may demonstrate the nature of Doc Hay's medical practice better than any testimonial. He felt the patients needed that money more than he did. With a grant from the National Trust for Historic Preservation, and with volunteer help and support from the community, the store has been restored to its original appearance.

Today, the Kam Wah Chung & Co. Museum contains literally thousands of interesting artifacts from the early days. The original building is filled with hand-crafted furniture and furnishings. The storeroom is filled with cases of goods, both domestic and imported from China.

Many of the cases are unopened. Doc Hay's pharmacy is intact, with mortar & pestle, scales and implements on the counter. There are bear paws, elk antlers, dried lizards, and pickled rattlesnake on display. The collection of medicinal herbs includes over 500 varieties, undoubtedly one of the most-complete collections in the world. A small religious shrine is present in every room, while calendars and "pin-up" pictures of Chinese ladies hang on the wall. Adjacent to the completely stocked kitchen are four bunk beds, where guests of Ing Hay and Lung On rested while they took a short trip back to China with the aid of an opium pipe. The walls and ceiling of the old building are blackened from smoke, perhaps from the opium smokers. Doc Hay's tiny bedroom remains intact, with his shoes neatly aligned beneath his bed and his clothing hanging on the wall.

The museum is a most remarkable place and a wonderful look back into another time and another culture. Anyone traveling in Central Oregon would do well to visit John Day and Doc Hay's house, even if it might seem out of the way. A visit to this fascinating place will be a rewarding experience and an authentic look into western America's past. Mrs. Carolyn Mienhimer, gave us a guided tour when we visited John Day.

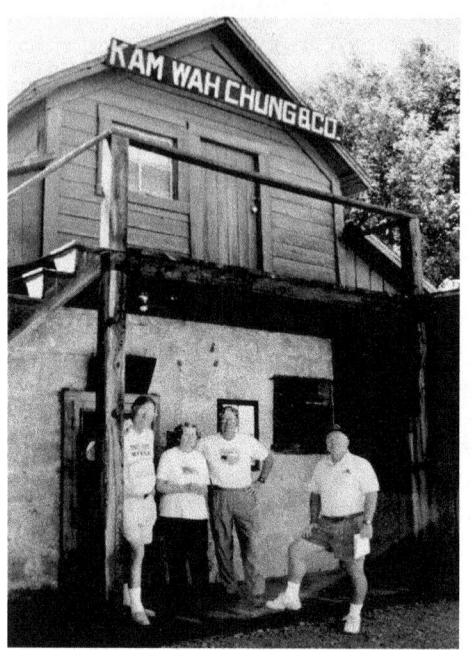

Wm. Thompson, Guide Carolyn L.E. Toole, and Wm. Payne

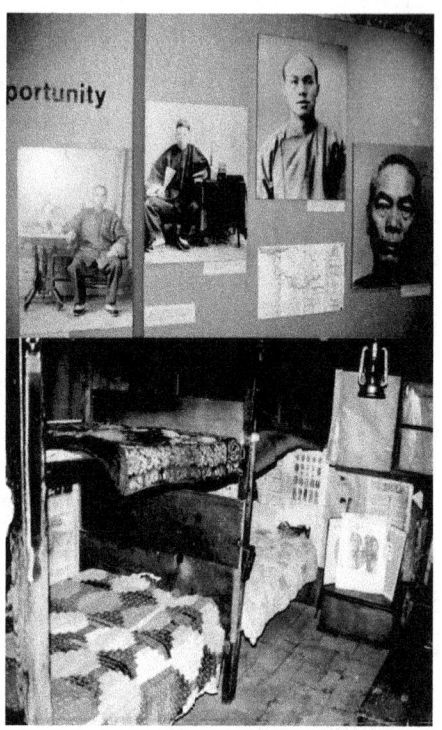

Kam Wah Chung Store, 1999

## MORE ON DOC ING HAY
### By Myra W. Uband, Las Vegas

Such a surprise on opening my *Greasewood Tablettes* last week to discover an article on Doc Hay and his career in John Day, Oregon. I had just returned from my Aunt's 85th birthday in John Day, and my second "official" visit to the Kam Wah Chung Museum. I say "official" because as a child growing up in John Day our journey home from school was directly in front of Doc Hay's building. He was usually standing out front watching the kids "be brave" and walk past his place. He would smile, but we had a real fear of the unknown building's interior. We would race on up the hill.

I did go to school with his great nephews, Eddie Wah who is a dentist in Portland ... Kam Wah Chung is a most fascinating

"Medical" house. Doc Hay made visiting trips for many, many miles around John Day. He had many patients in John Day who would not go to conventional doctors.

**NOTE:**

The steel plates over downstairs doors and windows are for protection from bullets fired by drinking miners from downtown John Day.

## Chinese Doctors in Nevada
### By Dr. Anton Sohn

Chinese merchants and laborers came to the Great Basin through the port of San Francisco in the mid-nineteenth century. In 1860, there were only 23 Chinese in Nevada, compared to 7,000-8,500 Native American Indians and 6,857 white immigrants. Twenty years later there were 5,416 Chinese, mostly males, in the state, accounting for 8.7 percent of the population. These new immigrants worked in the mines and on the railroads.

Afterwards, national opposition and local movements of opposition forced a marked reduction of Chinese. Even though they supplied needed services necessary for western expansion, the Chinese suffered from discrimination and were forced to provide their own medical care and hospitals. Fortunately, traditional herbal Chinese Doctors also came to America and brought a well-organized body of medical knowledge based upon thousands of years of clinical trials, experiments, and careful observations. Unlike American folk herbalists, they were well schooled in their craft and had an organized pharmacopoeia.

The professional Chinese physician was a mid-level practitioner and the backbone of medical practice in the traditional social triangle. At the top was the scholar-physician, usually a member of the royal court, while at the lower end was the folk practitioner.

In addition to herbal medicine, Chinese medicine has a long tradition of surgery. The famous surgeon Hua T'o lived in the second century AD and performed operations, including amputations.

Today the best-known Chinese practice is acupuncture, a practice that was reserved for the royal court in the nineteenth century.

In the New World, Chinese physicians became prominent and influential in both the Chinese and American communities. There were several reasons for their prominence. In many mining districts there was a shortage of medical practitioners, and the Chinese physician fulfilled a need. In addition, for many illnesses, Chinese medicine was superior to medicine practiced in the West. For example, it was more effective in dealing with female complaints, sexual disorders, and psychological symptoms. Furthermore, the Chinese doctor was usually highly literate and well-educated.

Dating from the first century BC, the earliest pharmacopoeia of the professional physician, *Pen-ts ao ching*, attributed to *Shen-nung*, contained 365 drugs classified either non-toxic and 'superior' or 'inferior and toxic'. The toxic drugs were reserved for serious illness. By the sixteenth century 8,160 prescriptions, made from 1,892 ingredients, were listed, and by the twentieth century there were approximately 2,000 described ingredients. On the American frontier, probably no more than 600 of these ingredients were available. Doc Ing Hay had a little over 500 herbs in the Kam Wah Chung Pharmacy in John Day, Oregon, a gold-mining town 70 miles north of the Great Basin.

Although herbs, minerals, and animal parts were important to traditional Chinese medicine, pulse diagnosis based on careful observation was the basis for diagnosis and treatment for nineteenth century patients. Using this method, diagnosis is made by taking the pulse at three sites on each radial artery. Each site corresponds to a body organ and is further divided into a deep and superficial pulse.

Thus, there is a superficial and light pulse, known as *Fu*, and a deep and bounding pulse, *Ch'en*. The third and fourth principal pulses are *Ch'ih*, a slow pulse at the rate of three beats per respiration, and *Shu*, a fast beat at six per respiration. It was said that using pulsology a Chinese practitioner could describe the symptoms and history of a patient without even seeing the patient.

The number of Chinese practitioners in the Great Basin or in Nevada is difficult to evaluate. Many did register their diploma with the county recorder as required by law, but many did not. Some even had their names printed in business directories. When the long arm of the law tried to prosecute them for failure to register, many juries were reluctant to convict the offender. In Battle Mountain, a jury refused to convict a Chinese Doctor who failed to register. It was obvious Chinese doctors provided a service that was appreciated by white settlers. In a community in southern Idaho, most of the white women went to Chinese doctors with whom they had better rapport than with white doctors.

Not all practices brought by the Chinese to the Great Basin were good. They brought opium smoking and opium dens to the fast-living mining and railroad communities. In John Day, Oregon, an opium den was in Dr. Ing Hay's home. A Chinese laborer made $1 a day and spent 50¢ on opium. It has been calculated that 15-30 percent of the Chinese laborers in Nevada were addicted. Initially the habit became prevalent among gamblers and prostitutes, but it eventually spread to the general population. To cope with the growing problem, Virginia City in 1876, enacted a law against opium smoking. Unfortunately, this was not enough to curtail its use. Hypodermics and parenteral use of opiates spread during the 1870s. Opium was even an ingredient in some patent medicines.

An overdose of opium by use of the Black Pill was used by the Chinese to commit suicide. A severely injured laborer without support of family and invalids unable to return to China because of the expense saw suicide as the only option-often with the assistance of friends.

Many Chinese prescriptions were more effective than some nineteenth century drugs used by regular physicians. Western medicine could profit from closer scrutiny of some of the ancient healing practices of the Chinese.

**NOTE:**

Information was taken from book entitled *The Healers of 19th Century Nevada* by Anton P. Sohn MD.

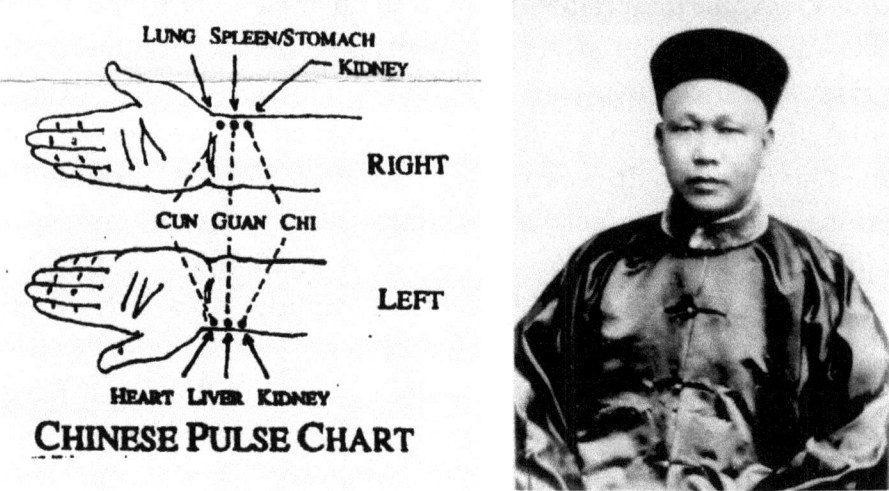

Herbalist Wai Tong, Carson City, 1899

# IV

# MEDICINE AT NINETEENTH CENTURY GREAT BASIN FORTS
## "KEEPING NEVADA SAFE"

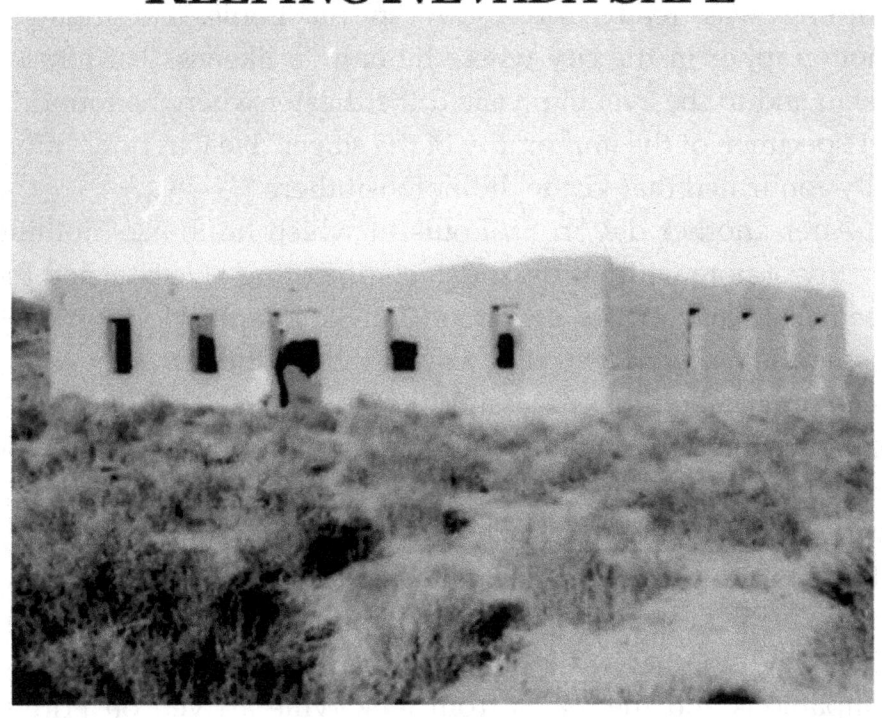

*1993 FORT CHURCHILL HOSPITAL RUINS*

## Fort Churchill and Fort Ruby, 1861

Charles Alexander Kirkpatrick was nearly 26 years old and had just begun his practice of medicine in Grafton, Illinois, when he decided to join a party from nearby Jersey County heading for the California Gold Rush. He arrived at Mason's Landing at 8:00 AM on Monday, April 9, 1849, where he waited until 4:00 PM for a boat to ferry him across the Mississippi River to St. Louis. The long wait gave him opportunity to ponder his decision. He wrote in his diary: "... I will leave it to those who have left home with the intention or with- out the hope of returning, to describe the feelings with which I left my home and bid a final adieu to the friends that I loved."

When the boat docked, he spent the night aboard and in the morning was ready for a day in St. Louis. He found a photographer in the city where he had "a likeness" of himself taken, and in the evening, visited the theater where he found "a fair specimen of the immorality of the stage." He was now "more fully confirmed that virtue did not visit there."

After another day in St. Louis in which he found 'nothing worthy of note without too much commenting'. He boarded the steamer *Timour* in late afternoon for St. Joseph. He took deck passage so to begin a "rough way of living," but he enjoyed the week of travel on the Mississippi River so much that he wished he had farther to go. Ashore, he found himself in a town of 2,000 inhabitants and a crowd of emigrants which included men of every description of character, from the honest, enterprising citizen to the lowest, meanest blackguard. He summed up the latter as "thieves, murderers, liars, Indians, devils, etc."

He had another week of waiting until his California-bound companions and the teams from Jerseyville arrived on Friday, April 28. It gave him time to call on the four ladies he had met on the boat, and they greeted him "as an old acquaintance, and seemed almost as much interested in my welfare as if I had been a relative." He spent two hours with them and bade them 'an affectionate final farewell and returned to camp feeling I had enjoyed perhaps my last hours of pleasure in female society," he wrote, adding, "But so let it be!"

Kirkpatrick was born July 23, 1823, in a log cabin in Pike County, Missouri. In a log house, an Irish schoolmaster gave him his first lessons. When he was ten, his father, a veteran of the War of 1812, moved to Illinois when the offer of military tract lands to veterans offered him a good farm.

After a few years on the farm, young Charles became converted to Christianity and followed a missionary, Dr. David Nelson, for one year, became disenchanted and returned home. In 1841, he enrolled in the first class of the Knox Manual Labor College, working his way through school until he earned a teaching certificate. In 1844, he began a three-year study of medicine with a Dr. Vance in the town of Vermont in Fulton County. In 1847, he attended medical lectures at the Ohio Medical College, and in 1848, commenced the practice of medicine in Grafton, where the Illinois River joins the Mississippi River, not far from St. Louis, Missouri

It was the first week in May before the Jerseyville Company assembled at St. Joseph and started on the road. The rains began to fall almost immediately, producing mud through which the men had to struggle. As they came to the "unbounded plain," their emigrant train of seven wagons was joined by another ten teams. Dr. A.R. Knapp of Jerseyville was elected head of the Jerseyville Company.

As he settled into the daily routines of travel, Kirkpatrick wrote of the contrast of goodness and wickedness of mankind and of his own quest for gold. His diary echoes his concerns about the unfairness of deaths he witnessed in accidents and illness. He wrote of his own ills and of the torture of riding in a wagon for ten days when he was too sick to walk. He did not write of medicating himself or of doctoring others. Instead, he wrote of music and dances.

Monday, July 23, 1849, was Kirkpatrick's 26th birthday, and a day later "some boys" from Pike County, traveling in a nearby company, arrived in the Jerseyville camp with a violin and tambourine to provide a "hoedown" until 11:00 PM.

We may assume this was a birthday celebration for the Pike County native and an exception for a weeknight party, because the rigors of trail travel called for early hours, both bedtime and rising.

Five days later, after a good day's rest on the Sabbath, the Monday morning start on the trail was accompanied by singing. The songs are not mentioned in the diary, but the Pike Company is given credit for producing the first versions of the famous *Sweet Betsey from Pike,* and *Joe Bowers.*

On the Humboldt River, while getting ready to cross the desert, the Pike County boys again visited on August 22. "We had a violin so with this music we had quite a concert." For the next fortnight driving was hard across the sandy desert and up the rocky canyon of the Truckee River, which they were forced to cross numerous times.

On September 3, they were at the "Cannibal Camp" of the Donner Party, where Kirkpatrick took a souvenir tooth from a skull that he found. "The view from the summit was worth all the trouble it cost to gain it," he wrote. The roads were unmercifully steep and rocky, and there had been no feed for the cattle, but the travelers admired the huge trees and scenery as they pushed along on their arduous journey.

On September 8, the wagons did not get underway until noon, and that night, Doctor Kirkpatrick watched some "negro dancing," provided by five men being taken to California by a Missourian who was also taking a lot of "little fellows," meaning Afro-American lads.

Within a week, Kirkpatrick got his first view of California gold miners at work. Some of the men in the party couldn't wait and grabbed wash basins to try their luck, with poor results. After a stop at Johnson's Ranch, the company pushed on toward Sacramento. Kirkpatrick and four other Jerseyville men became sick and did not reach Sacramento until October 5. For the next two months he was too ill to keep his diary. On January 1, 1850, he left to rejoin his partners. He had a sign on his tent pole announcing he was a practicing physician.

He recorded he sought the usual physician's fee for his services which ranged from one half ounce (of gold) or all that his patient had. In November 1850, he was counted in the U.S. Census in Sacramento County.

He moved to Mariposa in March 1850, spending the next winter there, practicing with Dr. Bigelow of Boston and others. In 1859, Dr. Kirkpatrick was in Benicia, where he became the U.S. Postmaster.

Benicia was a U.S. Army post, an important river port, and for a time the Capitol of California. In June 1860, Hutching's California Magazine published an article by Kirkpatrick entitled *Salmon Fishing on the Sacramento River*. It was an account of the decline of the salmon fishery because of placer mining, and the article is still quoted today in environmental studies.

When the Pony Express delivered the call to California in 1861 for volunteers to fight the Civil War, enlistments began immediately. The first troops were dispatched to the Southwest to fend off an anticipated Confederate invasion. The Third Regiment was recruited in the Gold Country, organized at Stockton, and assigned to guard the Overland Route through Utah. The regiment, commanded by Colonel Connor, listed Dr. Kirkpatrick as assistant surgeon. The regiment marched from Stockton with a train of 55 wagons and 3 ambulances. Accompanying them were the carriages of officers' wives and their dependents. The column reached Fort Churchill in the Nevada Territory on August 1.

In route, there had been 30 desertions and other problems.

While at Ft. Churchill the troops made repairs and reprovisioned. Col. Connor wanted to delay garrisoning at Fort Ruby until spring because Ruby Valley is a bleak, inhospitable place, but he was ordered to resume the march.

When Connor's column arrived in Ruby Valley on September 1, snow had begun to fall in the mountains. The soldiers were ordered to extra duty, building cantonments under the direction of the quartermaster. The men gathered stone and timber from the nearby mountains for the first buildings at this former campsite, which had served cavalry patrols for the stage and Pony Express.

In civilian clothes, he rode in the Overland Stage to reconnoiter a site closer to Salt Lake City than Camp Floyd. In October, Connor moved his main body of troops to a new site, which was to become Fort Douglas. Meanwhile Assistant Surgeon Kirkpatrick remained in Fort Ruby with 3 officers and 161 men. Kirkpatrick's wife, Mary, remained with him at Ruby. The Kirkpatrick's had four children and while at Fort Ruby a daughter died in infancy.

In March 1866, Kirkpatrick was mustered out of the army as a lieutenant colonel and moved to Redwood City, California, which had been his wife's home before her marriage. From time-to-time, Dr. Kirkpatrick's medical practice received newspaper attention. In November 1868, a George Rice was injured by a falling tree. Dr. Kirkpatrick treated his fractured skull and amputated his broken arm. Rice recovered to become County Clerk and founded a successful title company.

After another accident, Kirkpatrick set the broken leg of a carpenter, James Crowe. Crowe later became an undertaker. To keep up with modern developments in medicine, Kirkpatrick returned to medical school and graduated from Dr. Hugh Huger Toland's Medical School in San Francisco. Toland's school later become the University of California Medical School.

When Gussie Finger accidently shot Willie McGarvey in the

leg with a shotgun, Dr. Kirkpatrick treated him successfully. Later, when Gussie was hunting alone, he fatally shot himself while crossing a fence. The doctor treated Ned Connors when his arm was broken but could not save George Rice's 13-month-old son when he choked on a screw.

Dr. Kirkpatrick was active in community affairs in Redwood City. He headed a committee to collect money for the victims of the Chicago Fire. He installed the first sidewalk in Redwood City in front of his home. His wife, Mary, was the president of the county's first Suffrage Society.

Dr. Charles Kirkpatrick became ill early in the 1890's and later suffered a stroke. He died at St. Luke's Hospital in San Francisco on April 27, 1892. His former patient, James Crowe, handled the funeral arrangements.

**NOTE:**

This story was abstracted from an article by Nita R. Sprangler, who lives in Redwood City, California. Ms. Sprangler did extensive research concerning the life of Dr. Kirkpatrick, who was a resident of that community for many years.

## DR. WILLIAM P. KENDALL, 1886 FORENSIC EXAMINATION
## By Dr. Anton Sohn

In August 1886, word was brought into Winnemucca by stagecoach that Andy Kinnegar had been shot and killed in his ranch and store. Kinnegar was known as a quiet man who lived by himself in the canyon.

Justice W.H. Minor, acting in the capacity of Coroner, held an inquest concerning this death. The body had been discovered by Mr. J.F. Burgan, who had arrived at the Kinnegar place about one-half hour before sundown on August 12. Burgan, together with a man named Miller, found the front door locked, and entered the place by way of an unlocked kitchen door. Upon entering the house the two men noted a strong odor and found the bloated remains of Andrew Kinnegar seated in a chair. Since the man was obviously long dead, they departed and went out to report the crime.

Mrs. H.H. McColley, wife of the owner of the Willow Creek Station and ranch, testified that on the morning of August 11, an Indian woman named Susie appeared at the kitchen door with a pistol and told her that her husband, One-Armed Jim had killed Kinnegar. Mrs. McColley, under the impression Susie had brought the gun in so Jim would not kill Kinnegar, kept the pistol.

Dr. William P. Kendall, the surgeon at Fort McDermit, examined the body of the deceased and testified that there was "the track of a ball, either rifle or pistol, extending from the right nasal fauces inwardly, downward and to the left, to a point over the seventh cervical vertebra, producing injury sufficient to cause death."

Immediately, Sheriff Fellows began the search for one-armed Jim. Jim had lost his left hand when a gun exploded while he was shooting. The other Indians stated he had become resentful, quarrelsome, and dangerous after his accident. He was captured while hiding in the willows along the Quinn River, about five miles south of Fort McDermit. After his capture he was found to have several items identified as having come from the Kinnegar place.

The murder trial began on November 19, 1886. Jim pleaded not guilty to the charge of murder. His defense was that he had been promised money by a white man if he killed Kinnegar but was not able to name the man who promised him the money. After fifteen hours deliberation, the jury found Jim guilty and sentenced him to be hanged, but prior to the date of execution, ten of the jurors petitioned the Board of Pardons to commute the sentence.

After several petitions and appeals, Jim's sentence was finally commuted to life in prison. Twenty-nine years later, on February 15, 1915, old one-armed Jim died in prison. He was thought to be 109 years of age when he died.

This preceding tale is the result of extensive research by historian J.P. Marden, of Winnemucca, Nevada. The original story appeared in Marden's weekly column in the *Humboldt Sun*. He has kindly given us permission to reprint parts of the article.

William Pratt Kendal was born September 10, 1858, in Pittsfield, Massachusetts. He graduated from Columbia Medical College in New York City in 1882. He was commissioned as a First Lieutenant in the United States Army in 1885 and served four years at Fort McDermit. He became the last military doctor to serve in Nevada during the frontier days when he closed the hospital at Fort McDermit with the following entry in his daily log: "No patients admitted, no births, marriages, or death... No meteorological observations made from [the] 1st. Weather had been very dry and warm: water already becoming scarce in the Quin [Quinn] Rover and adjacent valleys."

Dr. Kendall continued to serve in the United States Army for another twenty-seven years. He retired in 1916 having achieved the rank of Colonel.

**NOTE:**

Meteorological observations taken by Army doctors date from 1814, when Surgeon General James Tilton required all army doctors to keep meteorological, climatic and wind data. The theory was that miasmas from foul air, pollution, and vapors due to decomposition of vegetable and animal matter from marshes and along rivers caused disease.

Surgeon General Joseph Lovell in 1818 wrote: "Every physician who makes a science of his profession or arrives at eminence in it will keep a journal of this nature, as the influence of weather and climate upon diseases, especially epidemics, is well known.

"From the circumstances of the soldier, their effects upon diseases of the army are peculiarly interesting, as by proper management they may in a great measure be obviated.

"To this end every surgeon should be furnished with a good

[weather] thermometer, and, in addition to a diary of the weather should note everything relative to the topography of his station, the climate, complaints prevalent in the vicinity, etc., that may tend to discover the causes of diseases, to the promotion of health, and the improvement of medical science."

Their main concern was to understand the weather and climate as related to the cause of disease and epidemics. If one could control environmental factors such as 'complaints prevalent in the vicinity' and foul vapors, the transmission of disease would be better controlled. Modifications of this theory persisted until the discovery of bacteria in the late 1880s.

Little did Tilton know, his military order was the birth of the United States Meteorological Service, Department of the U.S. Army Corp of Engineers. In 1891, this service was transferred to the U.S. Department of Agriculture. The U.S. Weather Bureau later continued as a part of the Department of Commerce. In 1970 the name was changed to the National Weather Service, where it continues today under the Department of Commerce. The weather statistics kept by the military surgeons thus became the earliest meteorological records in many parts of the country.

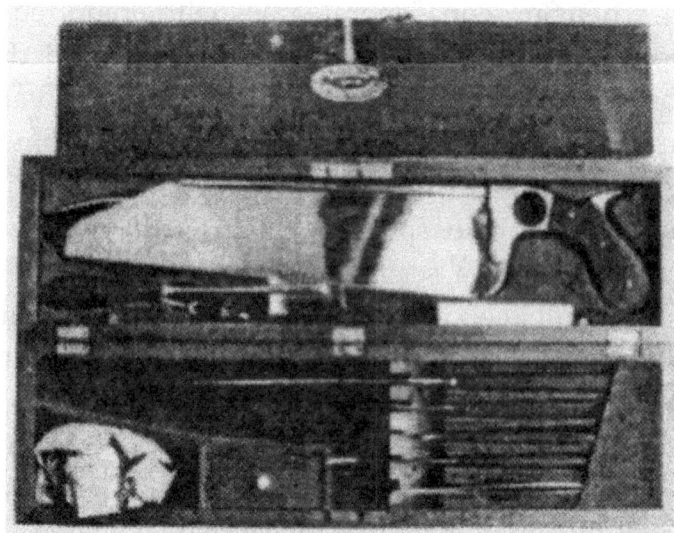

Civil War Amputation Kit (History of Medicine Museum)

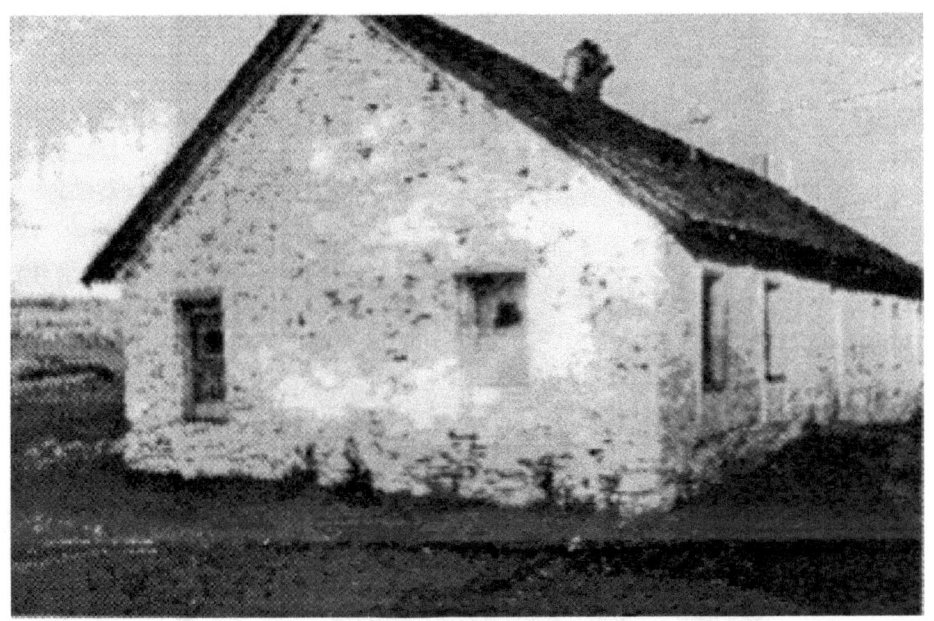

Ft. McDermitt Officers' Quarters, Senior Center, 1993

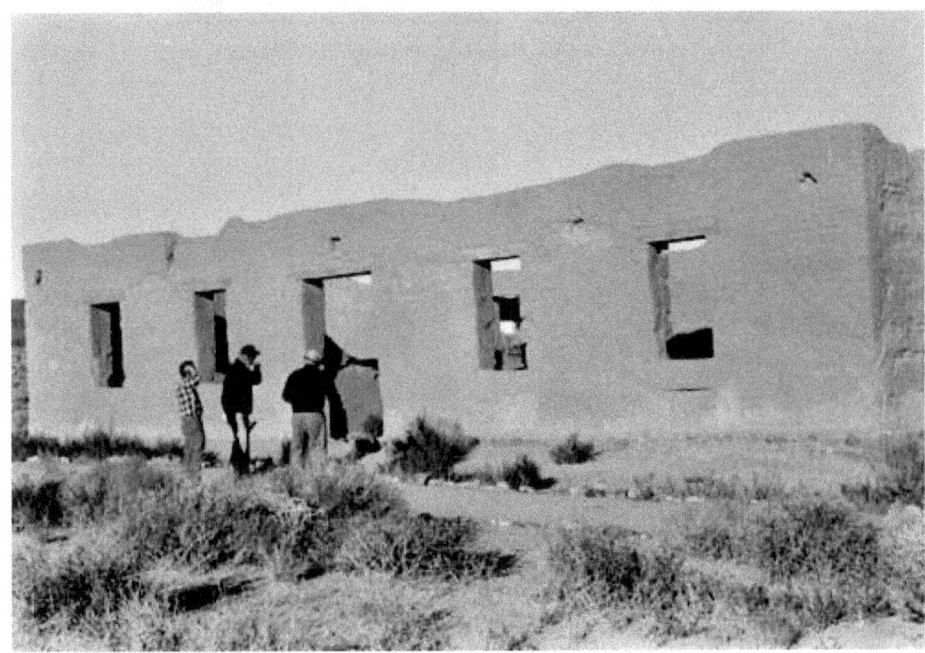

Fort Churchill's Hospital Ruins, 1993
Guide James Prida, Dr. Owen Bolstad, and Roy Hogan

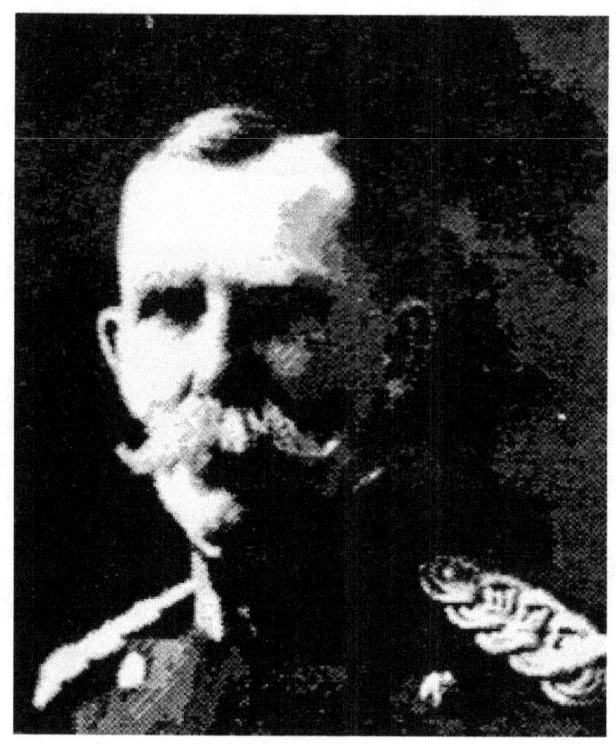
Colonel William P. Kendall MD

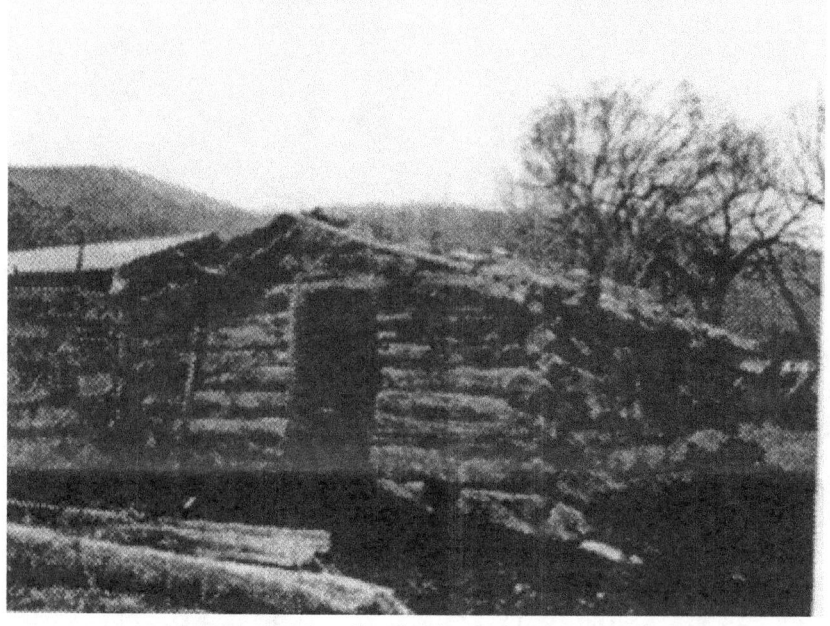
Fort Ruby Sutler's Cabin, 1993

# "Saga of Nevada's Nineteenth Century Forts"
## By Dr. Owen Bolstad

When Dr. Anton Sohn (Andy) returned from his sabbatical study of the history of medicine at Johns Hopkins University, he was filled with enthusiasm about military medicine in the state of Nevada during the period from 1860 to 1890. Armed with a myriad of facts concerning the forts that had been established in the state, and details of the doctors who provided medical care for the troops, he wanted to inspect the remaining ruins of the seven more or less permanent forts in the northern part of our state. After we had discussed this project at some length, Andy invited me, and our hunting and fishing buddy, Roy Hogan, to accompany him on a journey of inspection and research across the state.

We left Reno on October 30, 1993, driving in a rented twenty-six-foot motorhome with Elko as our first destination. Upon arrival, we rendezvoused with Dr. Tom Hood and Mr. Bob Pearce at the Northwestern Nevada Museum. Both Tom and Bob, natives of the Elko area, had expressed prior interest in our project and had volunteered to help us find the locations of both Fort Halleck and Fort Ruby's hospitals.

On October 31, we drove out to Fort Halleck by way of Lamoille on dusty and narrow gravel roads. We easily located the monument marking the location of Fort Halleck, which is by the roadside some 500 feet from the fort. Since the remains of the fort lie on private property, it was necessary to obtain permission from the ranch owners before we began our inspection. The presence of Tom and Bob greatly facilitated this, since they were both well known to the owners of the land where the fort was located.

The best-preserved part of the fort is in an old cottonwood grove, with lengths of stone foundations up to 30 inches wide and 40 feet long. According to maps of the old fort, these ruins represented outbuildings. A search for remnants of barracks and officers' quarters led us to a pasture west of the trees, and after looking around for some time we were able to find foundations of a number of these buildings.

Dr. Sohn was most interested in locating the garrison hospital. There had been two hospitals built at Halleck. The first was condemned.

Both the old and the new hospitals were located by us across the fence on the east side of Route #71 near ranch property. There were even a few medical artifacts-broken bottles and vials-lying about.

Bob Pearce left our party at Fort Halleck. Dick Immenschuh and Paul Sawyer, who had come along to assist us, also returned to Elko. We continued over Secret Pass into Ruby Valley. We drove almost the length of the valley before coming to the site of Fort Ruby. There was no one around to give us permission, so our inspection was brief. Most of the buildings of the original fort have been burned, rebuilt, and burned again so little remained that we could identify. We did find one ancient stone building by a spring which probably represents one of the original structures, possibly the guardhouse or laundry. Not far from there was another structure built of cottonwood logs that probably dates to the time of the fort, but may have been a civilian dwelling, possibly the cabin of a trader or sutler. We took a few photographs then returned to Elko by way of Harrison Pass, arriving in time to receive Halloween trick-or-treaters.

The next morning, we met and visited with Edna Patterson, a well-known Nevada historian and writer, for a delightful hour or so of conversation. Returning to the Northwestern Nevada Museum, a most interesting place now under the supervision of Shawn Hall, several hours were spent examining old newspapers and records of the post-civil war era. Late in the afternoon, we drove to the rest stop at Button Point near Winnemucca where we ate supper and camped for the night.

On to Winnemucca, on November 2 we met Linda Dufurrena, a well-known professional photographer, at the Humboldt County Library. It is a great library! Sheri Allen, the librarian, was interested in our project and did a great deal to assist us with our research. In the afternoon we met with Dr. Kurt Hartoch and his wife Wilma. Linda Dufurrena was completing an oral history on Dr. Hartoch, and we were eager to renew old friendships and talk with him about his early days in Winnemucca.

We also visited with Pansilee Larson, curator of the North Central Museum. Another history buff, J.P. Marden, was doing extensive research on the history of Humboldt County and was able to give us a good deal of information.

When Linda Dufurrena heard of our plan to look at the Fort Winfield Scott site the next day, she volunteered to pave the way for us by calling the owner of the ranch, Susan Miller Kern, and arranging for us to meet Mrs. Kern in the morning. Without Linda's help, we might well have been denied permission to enter, since the fort is on a private working ranch and is not open to the public. That evening we camped next to a creek just three miles south of Winnemucca.

On November 3, we drove to Paradise Valley, stopping there to look over the old headstones in the cemetery just out of town. Arriving at the Fort Scott site, we were met by Susan Kern and her son, Davey, who graciously showed us what remains of the fort. It is by far the best preserved of any of those we visited. The Kerns are living in one of the original officers' quarters, and a second dwelling, just as well preserved, is nearby. Across the parade ground from these buildings is the remains of one of the enlisted men's barracks. This building was largely intact until a few years ago when about half the roof collapsed. Although we had a map of the old fort, at first, we were unable to locate the site of the hospital. Then, Susan exclaimed: "I never noticed that before!" and pointed out a straight line of obscure foundation stones about 30 inches wide and 40 feet long. They had been driving across those rocks for ten years, the front wall of the old hospital. From Fort Scott we drove to Fort McDermit.

We met with the secretary of the McDermit Tribe at the tribal headquarters and were given permission to look around the site of the old fort there. Only one original building remains, a well-preserved stone building being used as a community center. We were told the physician's assistant at the health center, Rodney Burrow, had a map of the old fort. Referring to his map, we were able to locate the site of the new hospital, some 500 feet up the hill from the existing building. This site had been recently leveled by a bulldozer. And all that remained were two stone and concrete pillars. The old hospital was long-gone.

That night we camped on the road to National Canyon. On Friday November 4, we drove south to Fort Churchill State Historical Park. We explained our mission to the Park Ranger James Prida, and he accompanied us to the location of the hospital.

Fort Churchill has been well cared for after an initial period of neglect, and some renovation and preservation had been done. After looking at the old cemetery (only civilians remain buried there), we retired to the Samuel Buckland Campground near the Carson River to prepare supper and camp for the night.

November 5, we drove to Carson City, where we spent some time talking with Bob Nylen, curator of history at the Nevada State Museum. Next, we visited the Nevada State Library and Archives, where we spent some time poring over microfilm records from Fort Nye. Although we had been told by Bill McConnell that nothing was visible of old Fort Nye, we drove up to the marker on Kings Canyon Road to look at the site anyway, then ate lunch at the end of the paved road. Back to Reno, we had covered over 1100 miles, looked at the sites of six old military forts and identified the locations of five military hospitals. We returned feeling the trip had been most successful. More importantly, we had met and talked with many interesting, helpful, and wonderful people during our trip across northern Nevada.

## Dr. George Martin Kober
## "Blood Ingestion to Cure Tuberculosis," 1870s
# By Dr. Anton Sohn

In the nineteenth century, Nevada frontier life was precarious. The most common cause of death was infectious disease. Cholera, typhoid fever, tuberculosis, smallpox, diphtheria, and scarlet fever were a more serious threat to our citizens than cancer or heart disease. Infant and maternal mortality rates were high. In addition to health concerns, citizens, and travelers worried about Indian raids. (However, we didn't encounter any.)

As a result of this threat, forts were established across the state to protect the populace. The presence of the military not only reduced the Indian menace but brought doctors to the area. The military doctor treated sick and wounded soldiers and supervised the hospital and sanitary conditions of the military post, but also treated private citizens and Indians as well. One such doctor, George Kober, Acting Assistant Surgeon in the US Army, was assigned to Fort McDermit (also spelled McDermitt) on the Nevada-Idaho border in November of 1874.

Dr. Kober, a man of unusual ability, treated all patients, did anthropological studies on Indian skeletons, built a hospital, studied pathological specimens with a microscope and wrote scientific articles while stationed in Nevada. Following his stint in the army he became a professor of hygiene at Georgetown University and became dean of its medical school in 1901.

At McDermit in the mid-1870s, an unusual treatment for tuberculosis was instituted. Lieutenant Kober, with an interest in hygiene and infectious diseases, read an article about the treatment of tuberculosis, advocating the ingestion of fresh blood. Soon an emaciated recruit named Hammond arrived at the fort. A thermometer, recently added to the doctor's armamentarium, revealed fever, while a slight cough and lassitude established for Kober the diagnosis of tuberculosis. Knowing a steer was killed every other day to feed the troops at the fort, Dr. Kober prescribed a pint of fresh blood for young Hammond. The record is not clear as to how long or how frequently the "poor soldier" drank the blood, but it does indicate he regained his health in two months. Much later the bacterial cause for tuberculosis was established and still later an antibiotic was developed, but Dr. Kober used fresh blood to effect what he thought was a successful cure.

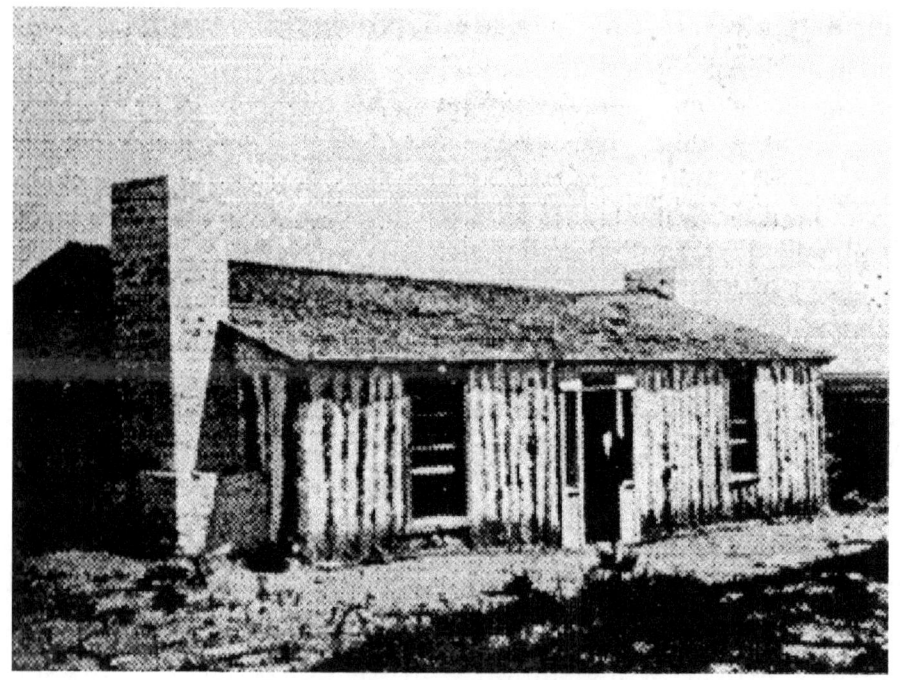

Ft. Ruby Officers' Quarters, 1993

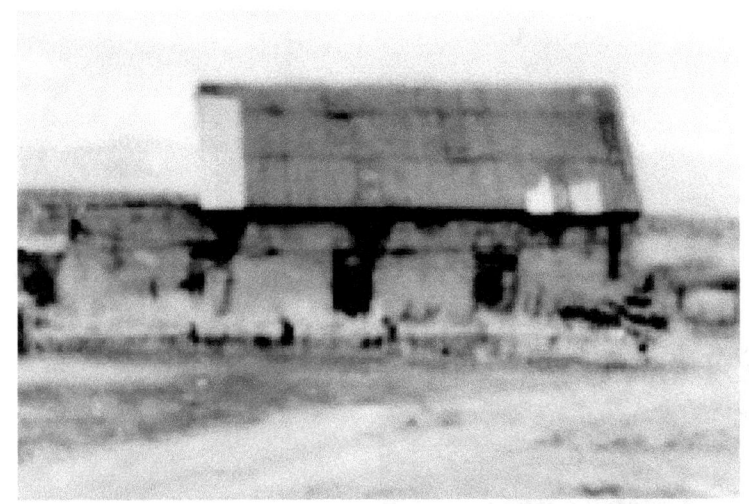

Fort Scott Enlisted Men's Quarters, 1993

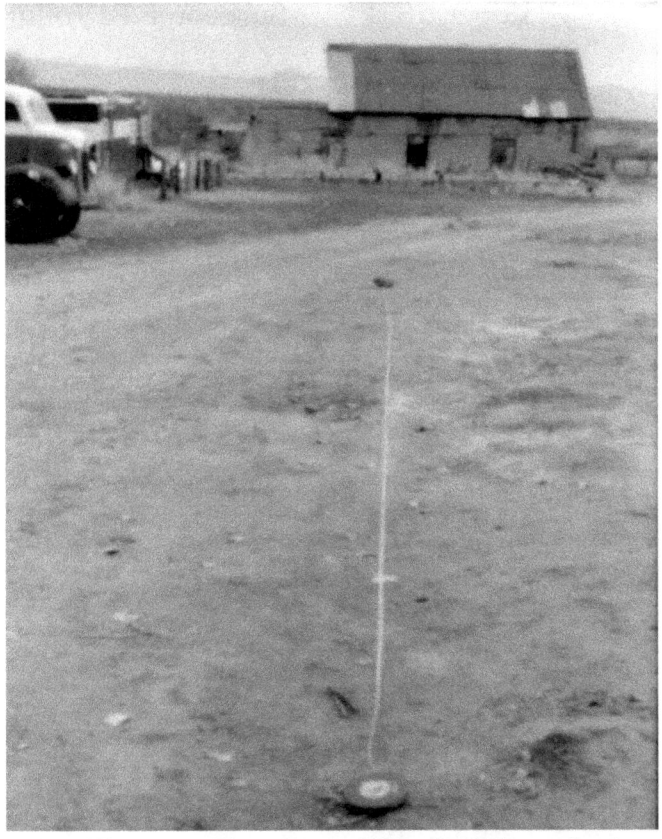

Measuring Tape on Fort Scott Hospital Foundation, 1993

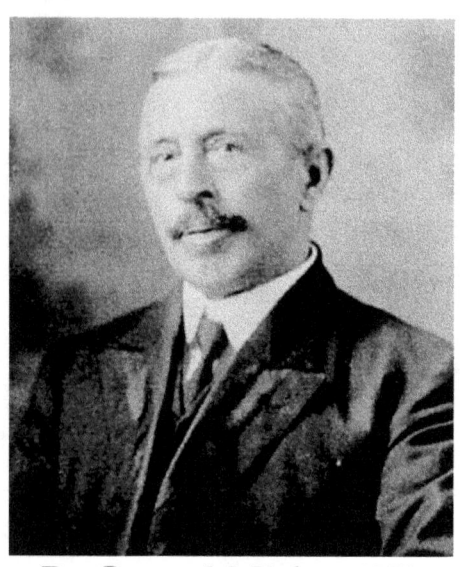 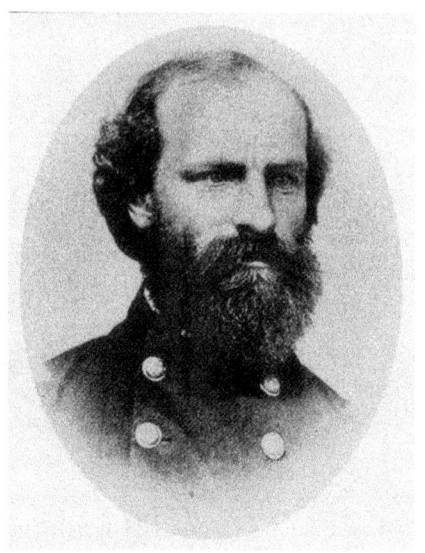

Dr. George M. Kober, 1873   Surgeon E.P. Vollum, 1974

# V

# HOSPITALS
## "TO FIND A CURE"

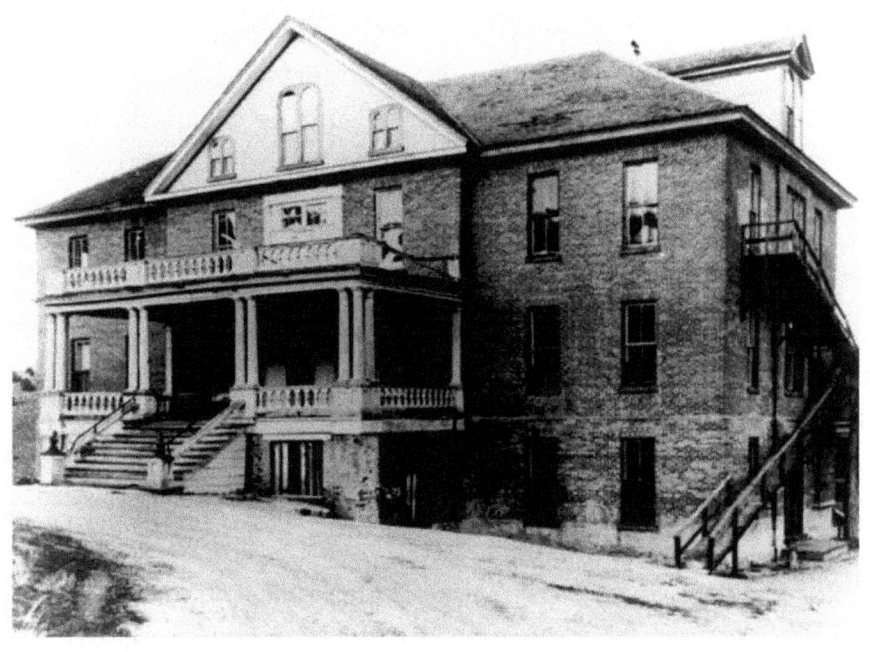

*SAINT MARY LOUISE*
*FIRST HOSPITAL ON THE COMSTOCK 1876*

# Saint Mary Louise, Nevada's First Hospital
## The First Hospital on the Comstock, 1876
### By Cynthia Pinto

Saint Mary Louise Hospital was in the Comstock Historic District, Virginia City, Nevada. This private hospital, including equipment, was completed in 1876 at a cost of $45,000 and was in the final stages of construction when the Great Fire of 1875 broke out, destroying much of Virginia City.

Construction of the hospital was instigated by Father Patrick Manogue, who received substantial backing from a well-known Comstock family. The property for the hospital was purchased around 1874 by Mrs. Marie Louise Hungerford Mackay, the wife of Comstock Baron John W. Mackay. Building the institution was a personal endeavor of Mrs. Mackay, and the project was encouraged by her husband who provided much of the financial support for the construction and operation of the facility.

The hospital grounds, previously known as Van Bokkelen's Gardens, was a prime piece of land facing Union Street. The location of the hospital away from the town, in the eastern suburbs, was a significant factor as it afforded the patients relief from the dust and noise of the mines and mills. This distance proved fortuitous during the fire of 1875 as the hospital was one the few buildings to escape destruction.

Saint Mary Louise Hospital, operated by the Catholic order of the Daughters of Charity, was the Pride-of-the-Comstock. The hospital opened its doors on March 15, 1876, and Dr. John Grant is listed as resident physician, although patients had the option of retaining their own doctors. Sister Ann Sebastian Warns and a staff of five Sisters, as well as additional maids, cooks, and housekeepers, provided patients with the finest medical care available at that time.

The hospital was supported financially by the Miner's Union. Each miner paid one dollar per month to the union hospital fund.

This served essentially as health insurance, providing the miners with prepaid hospitalization and medical care.

John Mackay secretly matched this sum for several years, threatening to withdraw support if the Sisters ever revealed the source of the revenue.

Between 1876 and 1897, more than 1,500 patients were treated at the hospital. Patient records contain a variety of diagnoses ranging from nervous debility and drunkenness to cholera. Many miners were admitted for hot water burns and scalding, an ever-present danger for underground miners on the Comstock. By 1897, Virginia City retained only a fraction of its boomtown population. The once opulent facility was now operated by a staff of only three Sisters who found it necessary to beg for food, clothing, bedding, and fuel to keep the hospital open.

The impending outbreak of the Spanish-American War made it apparent to the Sisters they would have to abandon the hospital, as their services were required elsewhere.

In August 1897, the Sisters were called home to Emmitsburg, Maryland, and the last entry in the patient ledger reads, "*The Sisters of Charity left for good, Sept. 7, 1897.*" So marked the end of the first private medical care facility on the Comstock and Nevada.

## Twenty-Nine Hospitals of West Central Nevada, 1876-1942

Over the years there have been several hospitals established in the Virginia area. Hospitals are created for many reasons, most of which are humanitarian, but teaching, response to epidemics and profit are all motives. When Dr. Bill O'Brien died last year, he left some notes about Virginia area hospitals that had been given to him by the late Silas Ross, Sr. Mr. Silas E. Ross, Sr. a founder of the Ross-Burke Mortuary (now known as Ross, Burke, and Knoble Mortuary) had an abiding interest in the history of medicine in Nevada. While doing research for a volume listing all the physicians who had practiced in this state (which was published in 1957), Ross came across the names of many early hospitals. He gave these notes to Dr. O'Brien with the hope they would someday be of value to medical historians.

The following is a listing of those hospitals, together with the information Mr. Ross uncovered. We have excluded existing hospitals such as St. Mary's, Washoe Medical Center, Veteran's Hospital because their history is well documented.

1. Adventist Hospital—established 1907
   Dr. McCubben, proprietor
   804 Ralston St.—Nathan S. Overton, Supt.
   (Changed to El Reposos Sanitarium in 1912)
2. Allen Maternity Hospital-established 1919
   544 N. Virginia St.
   Established by Mrs. Allen
3. Bond Memorial Hospital-established 1946
   829 N. Virginia St.
   (Closed in 1952)
4. Florence Crittenden Home—established 1913
   (Later became the Wentworth Hosp. at 322 Chestnut)
   937 Forrest St. (now 1000 Plumas)
   (Became the Virginia Platt residence)
5. Royal Hartung Hospital—no date
   71 Ralston St.
   (Old people's home for the I.O.O.F. and Rebecca lodge)
6. Hudson Hospital—established 1942
   43 Virginia Ave
   (Closed in 1945)
7. Invalids Hospital—established 1904
   519 W. Sixth Street
   Cordelia J. Wentworth, Supt.
   (Later became the Wentworth Hosp. at 322 Chestnut)

8. Manitou Sanitarium—no date
   141 W. Fifth Street
   Superintendent Mr. Anderson
   (Closed and the property sold)
9. Mount Rose Hospital—established 1914
   429 Granite (Arlington Ave.)
   Dr. George McKenzie, Proprietor
   (Closed about 1923)
10. Nevada Sanitarium—established 1923
    South Arlington Ave.
    Dr. C.C. Galsgie, Proprietor
    (Closed in 1924)
11. Nurses Hospital—established 1908, site not identified
12. Peoples Hospital—established 1909
    Virginia Street at Fourth St. (2$^{nd}$ floor)
    Established by Dr. J. LaRue Robinson
    Miss Cunningham, Superintendent
13. Red Cross Hospital—established 1908, site not identified
    Alice Hopkins, Superintendent
14. Virginia Hospital—established 1915, site not identified
    Alice Craven, Superintendent
15. Rigelhuth Maternity Hospital—no date
    Lake Street near Sixth St.
    Mrs. Rigelhuth, Administrator
16. Roosevelt Hospital—established 1907
    550 Sierra Street (Later known as the St. George Hospital)
    Frances O'Hara, Superintendent
17. Saint George Hospital—established 1904
    835 Mill Street (Merged with Roosevelt Hospital)
    Mrs. Lissak, Superintendent
    550 Mill St., Frances O'Hara (Superintendent)
18. St. Mary Virginia Hospital—established 1876
    Virginia City (The first hospital in Nevada)

19. A Miner's Coop. Hospital—by the Sisters of Charity
    (Closed in 1897, sold to Storey County)—site not identified
20. Sierra Hospital—established 1905
    507 South Virginia Street
    Pearl Mill and Mrs. Bell Byfers, proprietors
21. Southern Pacific Hosp—established 1909
    Sparks, Nevada (For railroad employees only)
22. Swain Hospital—established 1906— site not identified
    Clement C. Swain, Superintendent
23. University Hospital—established 1902
    On University of Nevada Campus
    (For university students and faculty)
24. Wentworth Hospital—no date
    322 Chestnut Street
    Cornelia J. Wentworth, Superintendent
25. Whitaker Hospital—established 1904
    507 W. Seventh Street
    (Property owned by Drs. Fee and Rulefson)
    Mary E. Evans, Superintendent
26. Emergency Hospital—no date
    Verdi, Nevada (For loggers)
27. Emergency Hospital—no date
    Near Gerlach, Nevada (For the gypsum plant workers)
28. Emergency Hospital—no date
    Gerlach, Nevada (Operated during construction of the railroad)
29. Emergency Railroad Hospital—no date
    Wadsworth, Nevada

## LAS VEGAS HOSPITAL, 1932

### By Dr. Anton Sohn

By 1931, Dr. Royce W. Martin had lived in Las Vegas for several years and had been involved with starting two small, inadequate hospitals that had been converted from small buildings. One of these, the Ferguson-Balcom Hospital, had been remodeled from a private residence and the other, which was called the Martin and Mildren Hospital, had been converted from a small hotel that stood on the site of the present Fremont Hotel/Casino.

Dr. Martin's dream, however, was to build a new, modern hospital of which Las Vegas could be proud. With the assistance of Drs. R.D. Balcom and Ferdinand Ferguson, they acquired some land at the corner of Eight and Ogden Streets and broke ground for the first hospital in Las Vegas.

The building was completed in 1932, and soon thereafter Dr. Martin and Dr. Ferguson turned to other ventures. The newly built hospital was then acquired by Dr. R.D. Balcom, Dr. Clare Woodbury, Dr. Stanley L. Hardy, and Dr. John R. McDaniel. In the early 1930s there was another large construction job underway in Southern Nevada, the building of Boulder Dam.

During the early years of the dam project, sick and injured construction workers were transported by ambulance to the new Las Vegas Hospital for treatment. Within a few years, Dr. McDaniel established a branch of the hospital in Boulder City. By 1943, he discontinued that service and returned to Las Vegas.

During the years of World War II (1941 to 1945), Basic Magnesium Incorporated (BMI) built a plant in the town that became Henderson. Because it was the closest health facility, the Las Vegas Hospital became the chief source of patient care for Henderson community. BMI built a new hospital in the small town of Henderson, while the rapidly expanding population of Las Vegas made it necessary to build a county hospital, and the Clark County Hospital was constructed.

In 1942, the Las Vegas Hospital hired its first full-time administrator, Mr. L.W. Edwards, who continued in that capacity for over twenty years. After the war Dr. Balcom retired and three new partners joined the group. The medical staff consisted of Dr. Woodbury (Surgery and Urology), Dr. Hardy (Obstetrics and Gynecology), Dr. John McDaniel (Cardiology and General

Practice), Dr. W.L. Allen (Ophthalmology and Otolaryngology), Dr. Grant Lund (Pediatrics), and Dr. Gerald J. Sylvain (Obstetrics and General Practice). In 1959, Dr. Erven J. Nelson joined the group, which was known as the Las Vegas Hospital and Clinic.

On the first floor were clinics, doctors' offices, and the emergency and operating rooms. Fifty hospital beds occupied the second floor. The laboratory and maintenance facilities were in an adjoining building. All patients were admitted without regard to race, color, or creed. The hospital had no facilities suitable for psychiatric patient care, and they did not admit patients with tuberculosis or contagious disease.

Hospital charges ranged from $7 to $10 per day, for a private room; $5 per day for a ward bed; $750 for use of the delivery room; $5 to $15 for the operating room and $5 to $10 for anesthesia. Salaries for registered nurses in 1931 ranged from $75 to about $90 per month.

The hospital closed in the mid-1970s. Dr. Gerald Sylvain kept his offices there until 1976, when he moved to West Charleston Boulevard, where he continued to practice.

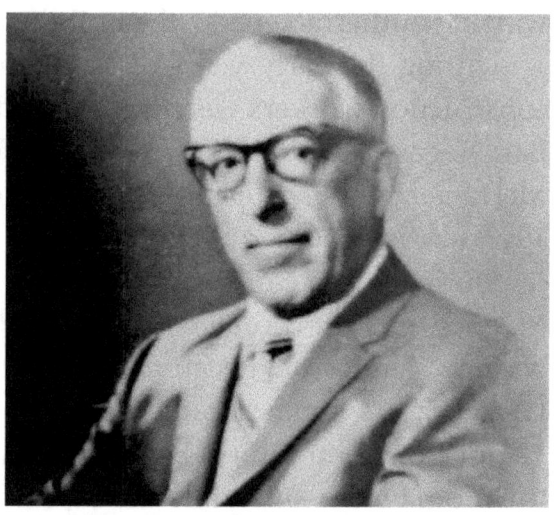

Dr. Gerald Sylvain, 1972

**NOTE:**

Dr. Sylvain is the main source of information about the Las Vegas Hospital. The hospital's first administrator, Mr. L.W. Edwards also wrote about the history of the hospital and clinic.

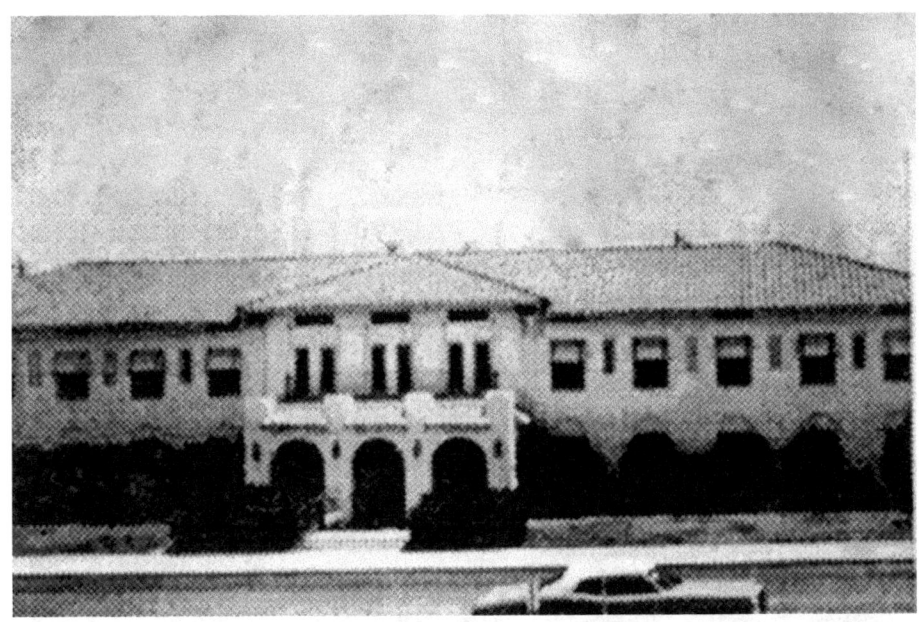

Las Vegas Hospital, 1976

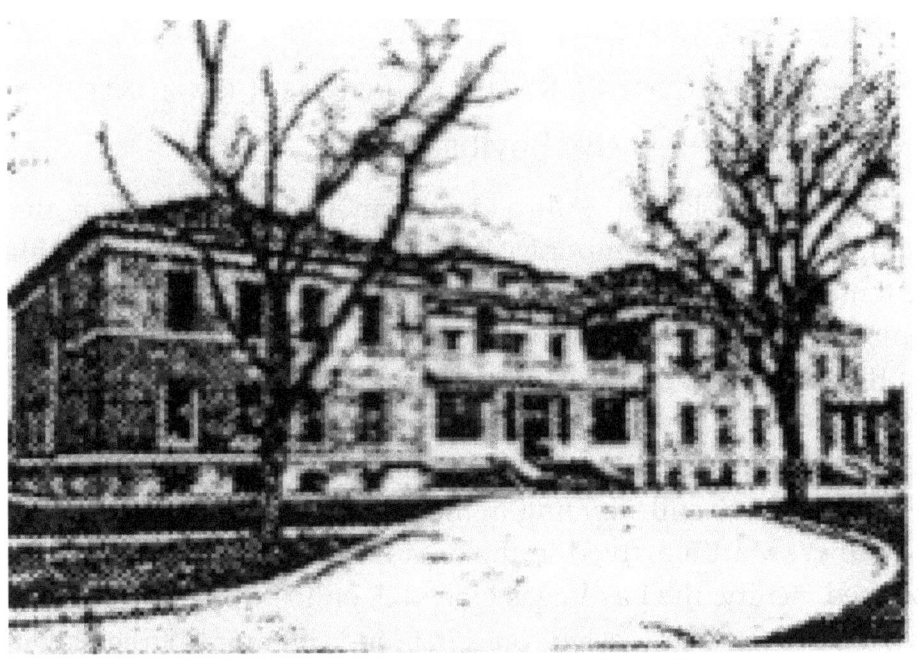

Washoe General Hospital, 1903

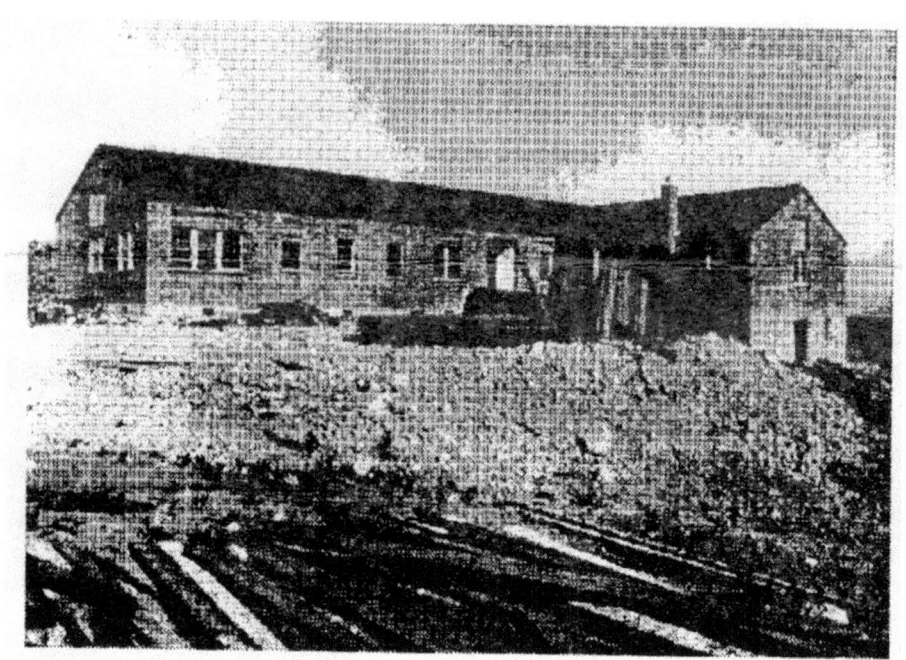

Boulder Hospital under construction, 1931

## CLARK COUNTY HOSPITALS, 1904-1988
### DEVELOPMENT IN A RAPIDLY GROWING COMMUNITY

## By Phyllis Cudek

The Union Pacific Railroad System in Las Vegas laid the foundations for contemporary hospital care in Clark County with a tent community built in 1904 for employees. The company employed Dr. Hal L Hewetson to treat ill and injured employees of the railroad in a four-bed tent located in the railroad yard. In 1905, they replaced the tent with a permanent frame structure. This original building used by Dr. Hewetson for railroad employees was still standing in the railroad yards as of 1948. Dr. Royce W. Martin arrived in the area in 1905 and later opened a six-bed facility, the Las Vegas Hospital, on the upper floor of the Thomas Building located on First and Fremont Streets. Dr. Martin also served a railroad, The Las Vegas/Tonopah Line, but foresaw a great future for southern Nevada and became deeply involved in its development.

There were rumors of a proposed dam on the Colorado River after World War I. This attracted more physicians to Las Vegas, including Dr. Forest R. Mildren, Dr. Ferdinand Ferguson, Dr. R.D. Balcom, and Dr. Sandahl, who was assigned to the Moapa Indian Reservation. Desiring for a "real" hospital, Dr. Martin bought the Palace Hotel on North Second Street and converted it into the Las Vegas Hospital, which opened in 1920. It had eight rooms on the second floor including an operating room. Dr. Hewetson by this time had associated with another physician, Dr. C.E. Bulette. They remodeled a former rooming house for railroad workers and opened the Hewetson Hospital on the corner of Second and Bridger Streets. Equipped with fourteen beds and a nursery, it had additional beds in the rear of the building for indigent patients. Dr. Hewetson lived on the ground floor of the building. The Las Vegas Hospital and the Hewetson Hospital served the community for nearly ten years, until the anticipated dam construction required larger medical facilities.

The Las Vegas Hospital Association was formed by various physicians to construct a more accommodating hospital' at 200 North Eighth Street in 1930. This facility, the new Las Vegas Hospital, remained open until the late 1970's. Dr. Mildren had opened his own Mildren Clinic in his home.

Before the Boulder Dam project brought an influx of workers, Dr. Hewetson died, and Dr. R. Martin retired. Dr. C. Woodbury arrived in 1932, and with other physicians assumed leadership. Eventually the Hospital Association dissolved, and the Las Vegas Hospital and Clinic emerged.

The Federal Government initiated the building of the Boulder City Hospital to care for employees of Boulder Dam and their families. Six Companies, the conglomerate title given to the management sector of the six major construction companies working on the dam, built the hospital at a cost of $20,000. The Department of Interior requested that Federal employees also utilize that facility. Medical and hospital care began August 1931, under the direction of Dr. John R. McDaniel. The hospital building was completed by Christmas. There were twenty beds including an orthopedic ward and a maternity ward. The cost of medical care for employees of Six Companies was $150 per month, which was deducted from their payroll, covering both employees and their dependents. This payroll deduction idea was the origin of today's Kaiser Permanente Plan, as Kaiser Corporation was one of the six companies building the dam.

Boulder City Hospital was located on a hill, while further down the hill a 'pest house' was built for isolation of infectious diseases. The pest house was a single large room filled with cots, surrounded by an eight-foot-high chain-link fence. It provided treatment for diseases such as smallpox, diphtheria, measles, scarlet fever, influenza, and other contagious conditions. The entire complex was closed after completion of Boulder Dam. From 1938 to 1941, the hospital was converted into a National Park Service Museum and Office. It was vacated in 1941 but reopened in 1943 to care for wounded servicemen during WW II. The Bureau of Reclamation took control in 1948, and in 1954, deeded it to Boulder City. There was strong community support, with donation of money and volunteer labor to clean and rebuild used hospital equipment. Citizens organized a volunteer ambulance and the hospital continued to operate until a new hospital was built in 1974. About 1931, Clark County built the Clark County Indigent Hospital to accommodate the indigent patients from Las Vegas Hospital as well as the overflow from the crowded Boulder City Hospital.

For the first two years, the indigent hospital was staffed by a single physician and one nurse, both on duty 24-hours-a day, seven-days-a-week. Dr. Hale Salvin became the county physician. He arranged for the construction of a surgical facility at the county hospital, and soon after the hospital was renamed Clark County General Hospital. In April 1942, Dr. Jack C. Cherry moved from Goldfield, Nevada, to Las Vegas. He was immediately appointed house physician and administrator of the county hospital. As the only staff member, he was paid $150 per month. Soon Dr. Chester George was hired as a surgical assistant to Dr. Cherry.

With establishment of a major military gunnery school in the area and the building of a magnesium production plant, the county transferred ownership of the hospital to the Federal Works Administration in 1943. After the war ended, the county bought the hospital from the government.

The population of Las Vegas increased rapidly after the war and there were several improvements in the hospital during the 1940s and 1950s. In 1956, the hospital was renamed the Southern Nevada Memorial Hospital to dispel any negative connotations associated with a 'county' hospital. In the 1960s, Dr. Harold Feikes, a thoracic surgeon, acquired a heart-lung machine that allowed him to perform the first open heart surgery in Las Vegas. As of 1983, the hospital had a staff of over 300 and the only burn treatment unit in the state. Southern Nevada Memorial, later named University Medical Center, has developed into a major medical center in the Western United States. It was affiliated with the University of Nevada School of Medicine in Reno.

The U.S. Army Air Corps established a gunnery range at the site of the old airport in Las Vegas in 1940. Temporary barracks were erected to care for enlisted personnel training there. This was later relocated and developed into Nellis Air Force Base. In 1963, a permanent structure, the Nellis Air Force Base Hospital, was built in that area to provide medical care for military personnel and their families.

The Saint Rose de Lima Hospital was built in Henderson, Nevada, because of mining activity in a nearby titanium ore deposit. In 1942, the availability of water and power from the Boulder Dam led to the establishment of Basic Magnesium Incorporated (BMI).

The Federal government required BMI to build a hospital for its workers, but by 1949 defense contracts dried up, leaving Henderson with no support for the hospital. A Roman Catholic priest, Father Moran, arranged for purchase of the facility from the government for a token $1.00. The Sisters of St. Dominic, a religious order from Michigan known for their success in hospital management, took charge of the Basic Magnesium Hospital, renaming it Saint Rose de Lima Hospital. The hospital served the medical needs of the expanding community. From 1972 to 1981, it served as a Veterans Administration Outpatient Center.

In 1956, Sunrise Hospital was started as a luxury medical center. Financed by the First Western Savings and Loan, and the Teamsters Union Pension Fun, it opened in 1958, catering to entertainers, gamblers, and wealthy hotel employees. Because the Teamsters continued to fund expansions of the hospital, it was often known as the Teamsters Hospital. Sunrise developed Nevada's first Intensive Care Unit. By 1966, it was one of the largest proprietary hospitals west of the Mississippi River. American Medicorp bought Sunrise in 1969. The management began an advertising program that included charge cards, 5.25% rebates for Friday and Saturday admissions, and recuperation cruises for Friday and Saturday admissions. The medical community had many ethical questions about the advertising campaign. Humana Corporation bought Sunrise in the early 1980s, renaming it Humana Hospital Sunrise. A women's pavilion and neonatal intensive care unit was added in 1984.

In 1960, Dr. Evert C. Freir started the Community Hospital of North Las Vegas to supplement Air Force health services. The hospital provided basic care for military families and hotel workers. After several expansions Huntington Health Services, Inc. bought the center. A new full-service hospital was built in 1971. In 1975, the hospital opened a much-needed alcoholic rehabilitation unit. American Healthcare Management acquired the hospital in the 1980s and added a nuclear medicine facility.

Dr Quincy Fortier and Dr. O'Donnel provided a "birthing center" with the opening of Women's Hospital in 1960. Because of the high cost of new technology and treatment methods, they sold the building to Ramada Inn Corp. in the 1970's. They sold the hospital to Peresellsis Corp. in 1980.

Before 1970, the Desert Springs Hospital was an extended care facility operated by the Four Seasons Corp. Charter Medical Corp. bought it and converted it into an acute care hospital. Dr. Hugh Follmer was the first chief of staff and Star Acuff was director of nursing. Because of its proximity to the Las Vegas Strip, the hospital provided care for many celebrities and entertainers as well as local patients.

In 1971, a group of local investors bought the Nevada Convalescent Center and renamed it Valley Hospital. After some renovations and expansion, the name was changed to Valley Medical Center, and in 1979, it was sold to Universal Health Services. The hospital established an emergency medical helicopter service in 1980. The Las Vegas Hospital closed in 1974 and was destroyed by fire in 1988.

The economic and population growth of Clark County was affected by many diverse factors. The arrival of railroads and the construction of Boulder (now Hoover) Dam, the establishment of Basic Magnesium and other mining developments, the Army Air Corps Gunnery range and later Nellis Air Force Base were some of these factors. The development of gaming and the resort hotel industry contributed greatly to growth. The warm climate, made tolerable by modern air conditioning, provided an atmosphere where people were encouraged to be the "new pioneers." The explosion of medical technology and the arrival of specialized physicians guaranteed good health care for the citizens of Southern Nevada.

**NOTE:**

This article was derived from *A History of Hospitals: Clark County, Nevada* by Sandy Klimek's MA Degree thesis at the

University of Nevada, Las Vegas, Department of Nursing, December 5, 1985. Our thanks to Sandy Klimek RN.

## WMC Administrator Carroll W. Ogren's "Adventures"

# By Dr. Anton Sohn

On reflections and observations over the years, some of this stuff is crazy, but it is of general interest and shows some of the incidents in the life of an administrator of WMC (Now, Renown Regional Medical Center).

Ogren: "I was in the emergency room one day in the early 1960s when two men were brought to the emergency room by the local police department; it seems they had been involved in a jewel heist in the exclusive area of Hillsboro, I, near San Francisco. The perpetrators knew they were being sought and took quick measures to dispose of the jewelry. They each swallowed many of the precious stones, while the remainder were spread out on the floor and sucked up in a vacuum cleaner in the hopes they would get back and get the jewels later. Some sort of chase ensued, and they came to I with two San Francisco detectives hot on their tail.

"The culprits were brought to the emergency room at Washoe Medical Center, where they were both administered Fleet enemas. They both admitted swallowing the jewelry and both were in extreme discomfort with gastritis. The thing that really "tickled" me was when I walked into the emergency cubical where they were being cared for, there were two San Francisco detectives each with a bed pan and a tongue depressor, going through the fecal material picking out jewels. The emergency room personnel, with their usual sense of humor, named it "The 24-Karat Movement."

"I recall vividly another emergency room admission because I happened to be there when a patient was brought in. A young man who was working on a second-floor ladder at a construction project on a motel south of I, fell off a scaffold and landed on a ¾-inch rebar in the foundation. The rebar penetrated under his right axilla and forced its way through his chest and out the left side of his neck. As he came in, he was bemoaning the fact that he was supposed to be married the following I. He was wondering if the injury would interrupt his plans. He was taken to the OR where the rebar was removed. By some miracle, it had not damaged his lungs or heart. He was discharged three days later. I heard no news on his marriage.

"There was another incident in the emergency room with a Skippy Peanut Butter jar. Dr. Gilbert Lenz removed a full-sized Skippy Peanut Butter jar from a man's rectum. I was always amazed during my career in Minneapolis as well as WMC as to the number and types of foreign objects patients inserted into their penis, rectum, and vagina.

"One evening while I was checking out to go home, the switchboard operator told me there was trouble in the delivery room. I took off down the hall and headed for the second south area where the delivery room was located. This was before husbands were allowed in the delivery room. There was always a lot of fuss about this, but the medical staff at Washoe thought it was not an appropriate place for a husband to be. At any rate on this afternoon, the husband of a patient had gone into the delivery room while the staff had their heads turned and handcuffed himself to his wife's ankle. Her bag of water had broken, and she was in the early stages of delivery, so there wasn't much to do but let him stand there handcuffed to his wife's ankle and watch the whole procedure. Characteristic of those days, any incident such as this necessitated a call to the police department. They gave him a dressing-down, and that was the end of it."

**NOTE:**

Information is from *The History of Washoe Medical Center* by Carroll Ogren and Dr. Anton Sohn.

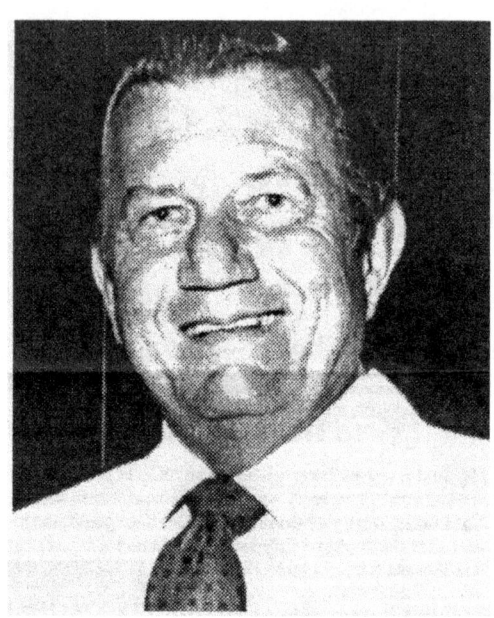
Carroll W. Ogren, 1997

"With sadness we noted the passing of a good friend on February 9, 1999. Carroll W. Ogren expired in a Las Vegas hospital at the age of 72 years. Ogren, a native of Minneapolis, Minnesota attended the University of Minnesota and obtained a master's degree from Washington University in St. Louis. I attended his funeral in Las Vegas.

"He served two tours with the United States Navy, from 1945 to 1946 and from 1950 to 1954 during the Korean War.

"Carroll Ogren first came to Nevada in 1957, serving as an administrative resident at Washoe Medical Center until 1958. In 1958, he became assistant administrator at Washoe Medical Center until he was appointed Administrator in 1964 and served in that capacity until 1978. While Administrator at Washoe, Ogren supervised several expansion projects, including a major $21 million building program. Mr. Ogren served as an assistant manager and administrator of the Jean Hanna Clark Rehabilitation Center in Las Vegas from 1981, retiring in 1992.

"During his career, Carroll Ogren played a role in the establishment of the University of Nevada School of Medicine.

He was a member of the Governor's Advisory Board for the Nevada State Hospital and was vice president of the Association of Western Hospitals. He was a past president of the Nevada Hospital Association and served on the committee on State Hospitals of the American Hospital Association. He was also on the advisory committees of the University of Nevada School of Nursing and the American College of Hospital Administrators."

## FIRST UNIVERSITY OF NEVADA HOSPITAL, 1902
### By Dr. Roderick Sage

Nestled like a house between two hotels on a Monopoly game board, the University of Nevada Hospital graced the campus for sixty years, from 1902 until 1961. In the beginning, it and its larger neighbors, Lincoln Hall, and the Gymnasium, were three of a modest handful of buildings situated on the windy and barren hillside campus just north of the fledgling city of Reno.

In the dozen years since 1885 when the University moved from Elko to Reno, there was minimal organized health care for students. For a few years, a rudimentary first aid station was available in the basement of Lincoln Hall, but in general sick or injured students would visit one of the several Reno physicians, hope for a doctor's house visit to their dormitory, or tough it out.

As the student body grew to nearly 400 members in the late 1890s, the need for an adequate campus infirmary became obvious.

In fact, the Board of Regents had discussed this issue for so many years that it seemed a permanent item on their agenda. In their 1900 Biennial Report, the Regents listed the five most urgent needs of the University:

1) Funds for the endowment of scholarships
2) An astronomical observatory
3) A natural history building
4) A library
5) A small hospital

President J.E. Stubbs recommended to the Regents a hospital construction sum of $1,500, but the state legislature, reviewing the funding needs, realized this was a rather skimpy figure and wound-up appropriating $3,500 which was adequate in that day and age.

The new hospital was placed at what was then the north edge of the campus overlooking Reno. At that time, in 1900, each of the eleven college buildings seemed to stand specter like on the bleak desert landscape—in great contrast to the handsome, modern campus of today.

Preceded by Lincoln Hall and the Gymnasium, which were both completed in 1896, the new hospital construction was finished in 1902. Of the three buildings, only Lincoln Hall remains, still a men's dormitory, and a venerable landmark second only to Morrill Hall in age and length of service to the campus.

The new hospital, upon completion was a 60' x 40' rectangular structure, and was described by the *University Register* as, "one story in height and with six rooms. Entrance is from the south portico into a reception hall. There are four wards, two upon the west for young men and two upon the east for young women. There is a convenient kitchen where food for patients is prepared, and students are cared for by a competent nurse and may have any physician they prefer."

The 1902 yearbook, *Artemisia*, further describes the very hospital as being "cottage like, of pressed brick with exterior trim work painted ivory white, a large door and windows, a sheltered verandah, and an indoor sitting room with an open wood fireplace." The wards for men and women could accommodate five to ten patients each. Architectural drawings for the hospital are not available, but one can view a photograph of its exterior.

Initially the hospital was staffed by a single nurse who conducted sick call and cared for the hospitalized students. After about 1930, two nurses were available to serve the sick and maimed. Students were allowed to stay for up to two weeks as inpatients, after which, if they still needed care, were discharged to their homes or to a local hospital. Students with contagious diseases were not admitted but were sent directly home or to a town medical facility.

Before World War I, a student's personal physician made hospital rounds, but in the 1920s and beyond, a regularly appointed local doctor served as the university physician. In its first year of operation, the little hospital got off to a worthy start, caring for 44 inpatient students, while 87 were treated in the school years 1903-1905.

As the university grew, so did the hospital. In 1918 a basement was added, and just prior to World War II it was again enlarged at a cost of $10,900 to include two new wards, a bathroom, a sterilizer room, a closet, and nurses quarters. About this time the hospital became known officially as "The Infirmary."

Dr. T. Clare Harper, a Reno orthopedic surgeon, was a part-time university physician for years before and after World War II. He describes it as a "jaunty little place," where the young students were well-cared-for, and the nurses were relaxed but always vigilant. His office was an enclosed square in the northwest corner of the central reception room, while the nurses' office was in the northeast corner.

A visit to "The Infirmary" is described by Reno surgeon, Dr. Edwin Cantlon, who as a pre-med student in the early 1930s lacerated his finger in a chemistry lab mishap. The infirmary nurse cleaned the bloody digit, wrapped it in a snug bandage and sent Ed downtown to see Dr. Dwight (Dutch) Hood, who at that time was the part-time university physician. Dr. Hood unwrapped the dressing, gravely examined the injury, then turned to his desk drawer from which he extracted a quart bottle of Old Crow Whiskey. He poured a drink for Ed and himself, noting, "This should make you feel better." After the doctor and patient both ingested the "medicinal libation," Dutch rewrapped Ed's finger and sent him on his way. In the early 1930s and today, Old Crow was (and is) an excellent remedy.

This "Dear Little Hospital" served the university well until the ground that it occupied became more valuable than the structure itself. In 1961, the "Infirmary" and its companion the old gymnasium next door were both flattened to make way for the new Getchell Library and an ever-expanding campus building program.

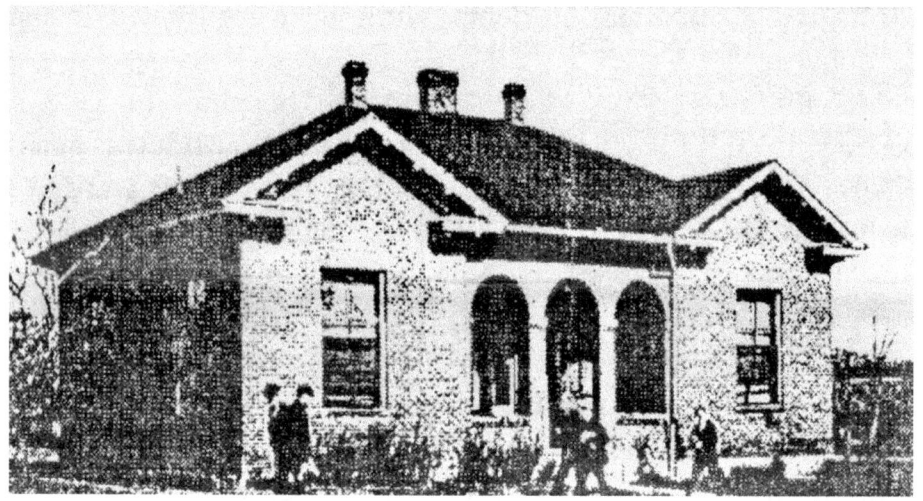

University of Nevada Hospital, 1920

**NOTE:**

Copy of *Reno Gazette Journal* August 10, 1946, article below is from Catherine Magee. It states University of Nevada President John O. Moseley appointed Dr. George R. Magee (her grandfather) as the first fulltime university physician.

### GEORGE R. MAGEE, MD
- Born, California, November 14, 1896
- U.S. Armed Forces, WWI
- University of California, MD, 1923
- Practice, Yerington, Nevada, 1923-41
- President, Nev. State Medical Association, 1941-42
- Ophthalmology specialty training, 1941-45
- Practice, ophthalmology, Reno, 1945-60
- Died, South Lake Tahoe, March 26, 1979

Dr. Gerorge R. Magee
(University of Nevada Reno Archives)

## Name Physician For University
### Full-Time Post For Dr. Magee

Dr. George R. Magee of Yerington, who has practiced medicine in Nevada for a score of years, has been named University of Nevada physician.

In announcing the appointment, President John O. Moseley said that Dr. Magee will be the first full-time university physician in the institution's history.

In addition to serving as director of the university health service, he will teach a course or two in physiology and hygiene, and will serve as head doctor for all university athletic teams.

The new university physician will move to Reno soon and will take over his duties on the campus with the beginning of the fall term in September. His private practice during his spare time will be limited to the care and treatment of the eye.

A graduate of the University of California in 1919, he received his doctor of medicine degree from the same institution in 1923.

Except for four years in graduate study in ophtholmology at Washington university, St. Louis, a clinic of the Dartmouth Eye institute, the University of California, and the University of Colorado, he has resided and practiced in Nevada since 1923.

He is a past president of the Nevada State Medical association.

# VI

+-+-+-+-+-+-+-+-+-+-+-+-+-+-+-+-+-+-+-+-+-+-+-+-+-+-+-+-+

# UNIVERSITY OF NEVADA RENO SCHOOL OF MEDICINE
## "SUPPORTING NEVADAN'S HEALTH"

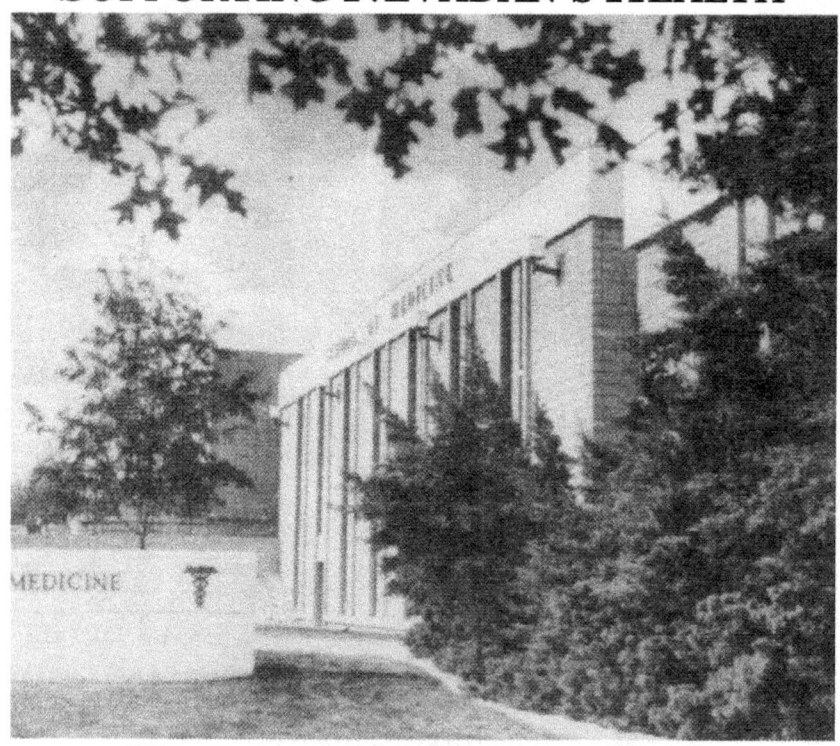

*UNIVERSITY OF NEVADA RENO SCHOOL OF MEDICINE ENTRANCE 1990*

+-+-+-+-+-+-+-+-+-+-+-+-+-+-+-+-+-+-+-+-+-+-+-+-+-+-+-+-+

## Beginning of Medical Education in Nevada, 1969

The University of Nevada has been preparing students for careers in health sciences since college level courses were first offered in 1887, but only in the last 40 to 50 years have health and science programs grown to maturity.

After World War II, there was a dramatic population increase in the State, almost a 100% increase in the 1950s, which lead to the identification of some serious health care deficiencies.

A medical technology program had been established in 1950, and a college program in nursing education had been approved by the legislature. After the university received a gift of $100,000 from Arthur E. Orvis, the Orvis School of Nursing was established, and the first class of nursing students started in 1957.

A study done by the Western Interstate Commission on Higher Education (WICHE) suggested Nevada should begin planning for a two-year medical school to serve the western states.

The proposal to establish a medical school stirred great controversy within the state. Several issues were in contention. First, there was debate concerning the need for more physicians in Nevada. There were arguments as to whether the school should be a two-year school, with students finishing their medical educations in out-of-state, degree-granting medical schools, or should it be a full four-year school in Nevada.

The proposed location of the school in Reno further evoked the long-standing rivalry between northern and southern factions of the state. The largest issue was financial, however, for with a population of fewer than 400,000, taxpayers felt the state could just not afford a medical school.

In February 1967, Reno Philanthropist H. Edward Manville, Jr. announced a gift of $1 million to the University of Nevada Medical School. This offer was later followed by a promise from industrialist Howard Hughes to provide up to $6 million for the medical school.

These gifts broke the deadlock, and on January 11, 1969, the University Board of Regents, chaired by Dr. Fred Anderson and member Dr. Louis Lombardi, approved a two-year medical school for the Reno campus.

On March 25, 1969, Governor Paul Laxalt signed into law AB 130, which appropriated $58,000 for start-up expenses.

March 26, 1969, the *Nevada State Journal* carried the following story: "Governor Paul Laxalt signed AB 130 allowing the Board of Regents to establish a health sciences program, including a medical school, at the University of Nevada, Reno. The issue had split the legislature and the Board along sectional lines since a feasibility study was proposed in 1967. That battle ended when Howard Hughes pledged up to $6 million over 20 years to the school. Strong opposition remained as the plan was broadened from the original two-year medical school concept to include related studies and fields. It squeezed through both houses with supporters saying the plan would fill a big need in the State and opponents saying the State could not afford it.

"The bill would appropriate about $58,000 from the State general funds to get the program off the ground. It also would authorize the

Regents to spend about $480,000 in University fees and grant to remodel two old buildings which have been scheduled for demolition.

"The first dean of the School of Medical Sciences was Dr. George T. Smith, a pathologist who had been Director of the Laboratory of Pathophysiology at the Desert Research Institute based at WMC. Dr. Smith had been involved in studies and planning for the new school."

The initial proposal for a two-year medical school had been broadened by the Board of Regents to provide two-year basic science education to a variety of pre-professional students. These included pre-dentistry, medical technology, health education, physical therapy, speech pathology, pre-pharmacy, and audiology; therefore, the institution was named the School of Medical Sciences. Within a few months the school had received grants totaling more than $900,000 from the Commonwealth Fund and the W.K. Kellogg Foundation.

In 1967, foundation grants totaled $1.2 million, and more than $1.4 million was secured from a variety of federal agencies, in addition to nearly $400,000 raised from local sources.

The charter class of 32 students began studies in the fall of 1971.The initial faculty numbered nine full-time and five part-time instructors. This slim cadre was supplemented by many local physicians who volunteered their time. During the first few years, more than 200 practicing physicians from throughout the State participated in the teaching program, and 20 additional basic science faculty were recruited.

During the first five years of operation, the School of Medical Sciences admitted 221 students, 19 from out-of-state and the remainder from Nevada. During those first five years, there were only six dropouts or failures. The remaining 215 transferred to degree granting medical schools for two years of clinical studies, and all 215 were granted MD degrees.

**NOTE:**

Source of information was abstracted from *School of Medical Sciences, University of Nevada,* article by Drs. T.J. Scully, and George T. Smith.

## NEVADA SCHOOL OF MEDICINE COMES OF AGE, 1990

### By Lynne D. Williams

On March 25, 1969, Assembly Bill 130 establishing the two-year school was signed into law. The charter class entered the program in 1971, and, with four succeeding classes, completed their basic science studies in Reno. Those students then transferred to four-year programs in other medical schools for their clinical studies.

According to Dr. Fred M. Anderson, during those years the

government changed its attitude about support of two-year programs and offered $2.5 million to the medical school to help in its conversion to a four-year, degree-granting institution. The legislature approved the change on April 14, 1977, and the school's first class of physicians trained entirely in Nevada graduated in 1980.

The school became a thriving institution with an annual operating budget of $21 million, approximately half of which is appropriated from the legislature and half is generated through research grants and other contracts.

Making good on its pledge to serve the needs of the entire state, the school is continually expanding its educational and outreach programs.

Although the basic sciences facility and a Family Medicine Center were located on the University of Nevada-Reno campus, four departments are based in Las Vegas.

A second Family Medicine Center was housed in a Clark County Community College building. Additionally, a Genetics Network was established with offices in both Reno and Las Vegas, and (as of 1990) the school is planning to buy or construct a building to house the Las Vegas based programs and medical school faculty members.

In 1989, Nevada's first kidney transplant program was established in Las Vegas. This program was developed in a collaborative effort by UNSOM and University Medical Center in Las Vegas.

The rural communities are also an important part of the school's programs. Its Office of Rural Health works with several communities to assess their health needs and to help recruit medical health care professionals. The Area Health Education Center (AHEC) also boosts the health care of rural communities. AHEC is a federally funded program that allows the medical school to offer continuing education programs for physicians, nurses, and allied health professionals, and to encourage students from rural areas to pursue careers in the medical profession.

There are approximately 150 full-time faculty members and more than 600 community physicians who serve as clinical faculty throughout the state. Faculty researchers compete successfully for federal research dollars totaling approximately $3 million each year to investigate some of the most pressing scientific mysteries: AIDS and the infections that kill AIDS patients; stress; hypertension; cancer; Alzheimer's disease; diabetes; and gastrointestinal disorders.

New equipment and facilities, such as a transmission electron microscope (one of only 20 of its kind in the nation), a DNA synthesizer, a monoclonal antibody laboratory, and a fluorescence imaging system (one of only 13 in the world), allow Nevada's scientists, who have been recruited from prestigious institutions around the country, to continue their research work.

Finally, its students, the proudest measure of the school's success, are meeting all-and exceeding some-national academic standards. As graduates and fully trained physicians, they also are filling Nevada's need for doctors, especially in the rural communities.

What is the most satisfying to planners is the conspicuous absence of the question that plagued them in the early years: "Well, do you think the school is going to make it?" The answer is a resounding, "Yes"—The dream is a reality.

**NOTE:**

The article was published in *SYNAPSE*, School of Medicine publication, November 1990. As of March 1991, the University of Nevada School of Medicine had granted MD degrees to 724 graduates. Of those graduates, 212 had returned to practice medicine in Nevada after completing their residency training.

# Nevada Health Service Corps, Established in 1989
## By Dr. Robert Daugherty

After the 1989 session when Senate Bill 87, authorizing and funding the Nevada Health Service Corps, was passed, Caroline Ford and I thought it would be a nice gesture to ask Joe Dini to go with us to give the first Nevada Health Service Corps recipients their checks.

Initially there were five recipients. We asked Mr. Joe Dini to accompany us because he was instrumental in passing the bill creating the service corps. We decided to use the state plane to accomplish the grants in one day. Thus, Caroline and I drove to Carson City and flew to Yerington to pick up Mr. Dini. Halfway there, Caroline realized she did not remember to bring the checks!! So, we landed in Yerington, and she ran inside to call her office to get the checks. This was before cell phones. Caroline, Mr. Dini, and I then flew to Reno where Caroline's staff person met us with the checks. The rest of the day went as planned.

The first recipients of the Nevada Health Service Corps were:

| Physician | Town | Current Location |
|---|---|---|
| Rodney Phillips, MD | Eureka | Unknown |
| Allan Burnside, MD | Lovelock | Colorado |
| Cheryl Winder, MD | Fallon | Deceased |
| James Winder, MD | Fallon | Reno |
| Richard Ingle, MD | Winnemucca | Winnemucca |

## School of Medicine Psychiatry Residency
## By Dr. Robert Daugherty

After many days, weeks, and months of explaining why we needed a psychiatry residency program, AB 345 was introduced in the Assembly Ways and Means Committee, chaired by Marvin Sedway. Marvin was a tremendous supporter of the School of Medicine and its mission, but he always wanted more programs in Las Vegas. I had assured him a part of the psychiatry residency would include rotations in Las Vegas. Only after such assurances did he agree to introduce and support the bill.

Thus, the morning agenda in Ways and Means included psychiatry with Dr. Ira Pauly, Chair of Psychiatry, members of the psychiatry department faculty, and me in attendance. Only Dr. Pauly and I were to testify and explain the training program. Dr. Pauly went first and gave, as I recall, a very succinct explanation of the program. I followed with the budget explanation and justification. In the discussion, Chairman Sedway asked me about the possibility of the residents rotating in Las Vegas. I assured him they would. At that moment, a member of the department jumped up and said he wanted to testify. Remember that any citizen can testify before legislative committees. Mr. Sedway recognized him, and the member immediate outlined why the program would not be accredited if residents rotated to Las Vegas. He quoted from the accrediting body's policy regarding continuity of care.

Chairman Sedway immediately adjourned the committee meeting and announced there would not be a residency. I waited for 20-30 minutes and then went into Chairman Sedway's office to try to mend our fences. As I walked into his office, he said, "Get out, get out, I don't want to talk to you. Get out!!" What a day!! The bill died in the Ways Means committee. The residency was started three years later with funds from the Department of Mental Health.

# Fourteenth School of Medicine's Anniversary, 1983
## By Anne McMillin

The final week of September witnessed a flurry of celebratory activity aimed at recognizing the fourteenth anniversary of the University of Nevada School of Medicine. School of Medicine founding Dean George Smith MD invited all thirty-two members of the charter class, which entered in the fall of 1971, to gather at the home of Mrs. Nena Miller, widow of Jim President N. Edd Miller when the School started, to get reacquainted and discuss their medical careers and life paths since completing their first two years of medical school basic sciences in 1973. About a dozen members of that class, their spouses, and inaugural and current faculty members attended the September 23 reception.

The next night, the 28th Annual University of Nevada, Jim Foundation Banquet turned its focus to health sciences with a record crowd of nearly 1,000 people coming out to honor the University of Nevada School of Medicine's fourteenth anniversary at John Ascuaga's Nugget in Sparks.

University President Milton Glick delivered the big announcement when he revealed the William N. Pennington Foundation committed $10 million for the purpose of the planned Health Sciences Building which would allow for the eventual doubling of both the nursing and medical student class sizes with it is completion in the fall of 2011. The building would be named the William N. Pennington Health Science Building and would sit just east of the current Pennington Medical Education Building.

President Glick also mentioned the gifts provided for the building from the Nell J. Redfield Foundation, the Thelma B. and Thomas P. Hart Foundation, many people, and organizations that helped the University reach its $15 million fundraising goal for the facility.

President Glick also recognized George Smith MD, the

founding dean of the medical school who was in attendance and Susan Desmond-Hellmann MD, 1982, chancellor of the University of Jim San Francisco, the recipient of the School of Medicine's first Outstanding Alumni Award from the School's Alumni Association, which was presented earlier in the evening at a reception.

Distinguished surgeon, teacher, and writer Atul Gawande, staff member of Brigham and Women's Hospital in Boston, gave the keynote address, noting the challenge for the medical profession today is to make the medical experience better for patients who have long struggled with medicine.

Legislators Joe Dini, Don Mello, and Virgil Getto, who helped establish the school were recognized with plaques at the reception before the banquet.

Dr. George Furman, the first OB/Gyn chair in Jim, as well as Ron Pardini PhD, who taught biochemistry to the first class, attended the festivities. Ted Bacon and Janice Goodhue, two of the original members of the School Advisory Board, were at the banquet. Charter faculty member Jim Gillette as well as Georgia Fulstone and Andrea Pelter, who were early strong supporters of the school attended. Former Deans, Robert Jim, and Jim McFarlane attended the event.

Charter Class members Patrick Colletti, Jim Noble, Jerry Calvanese, Henry Prupas, Jim Moren, Ed Piercznski, Ronald Ainsworth, Richard Priest, Jay Chamberlain, George Manning, Henry Nelson, and Mark Rhodes attended some or all the week's events.

The week's festivities concluded at the September 25 event in the Manville auditorium at which current School of Medicine faculty members gave presentations for continuing medical education credit to the attendees.

# Founding Dean Dr. George Smith
## By Dr. Robert Daugherty

Dr. Joan Brookhyser (class of 1975) spearheaded a drive to establish a Student Scholarship in memory of Dr. George Smith.

George had been a successful cardio-vascular pathology research faculty member at Harvard before he arrived in Reno to begin research at the Desert Research Institute. He came to establish Nevada residency to finalize his divorce. Little did he realize he would leave Reno ten years later, having provided the leadership to create Nevada's School of Medicine.

The historical accounts of the activities from the 1965 feasibility study by George to the bill signing creating the School by Governor Paul Laxalt in 1969 are well documented. However, the stories surrounding George Smith's personal and professional life during that time are less well documented and border on becoming folklore.

Rather than recount history or folklore, we thought it more fitting to remember George as the individual who worked with many to create the School. Thus, we will share with you the personal recollections of this man by those with whom he worked.

**Tom Hall MD,** Pathologist: I had the good fortune to be associated with George Smith in the very early days before the Medical School came into being. Although it is rightly said that Doctor Fred Anderson is the Father of the Medical School, it was through the efforts of George Smith that the concept was realized.

It is hard for most of us to understand how much work George had to do, largely on his own, to first build acceptance and then support for the School. There were countless meetings with physicians, legislators, and community leaders. I remember him coming to our pathology group to ask for our financial aid in setting up a chair of pathology. Initially we had certain skepticism. Ultimately, we were quite willing to comply, in a large part because of the respect and affection we had for George. When it became evident despite many obstacles, the School would indeed be set up, he approached again to ask that we free up one of our members for three years to set up and head the pathology department.

I was pleased to be named to this post and to know George as an administrator and dean. His style came as no surprise. He would choose staff that he trusted and then allow them to do their job with no unnecessary interference.

When I reflect on the qualities that made George so successful in this remarkable undertaking, I realize it was not primarily his intelligence and ability to work very, very, hard. Rather it was his unquenchable optimism and personal warmth. It was a pleasure to teach with George and to have him as a friend.

**Miles Standish PhD,** Physiologist and Administrator: I was one of the new faculty recruited to the School of Medical Sciences in the early 70s. We were mostly young, without much experience, and too few for the job at hand. I taught physiology and worked with Dean Smith to develop programs and funding, and later convert it to a four-year medical school.

George was certainly one of a kind; he was the perfect dean for difficult, exciting, and usually fun times. I still don't know what it was about George that made him what he was: the perfect person to start a medical school in Nevada. For our small faculty, one of the things that made George unique was his ability to make his goals our goals, and we gladly worked long days, often nights, and sometimes 7-day weeks to get the job done.

After George left for Alabama, I realized that in all the years I worked with him he never once thanked me for anything I did. If he had, I would have felt insulted: after all, I didn't work FOR him, I worked WITH him.

We were a team that worked as hard as we could to accomplish the same thing. All of us who were there while George was dean will tell you the story of those years would make a good movie. But Hollywood would never have cast George as the star. He wouldn't be at all right for the part. Maybe Harrison Ford, but never George Smith. Without that one very special man, though, I don't think there would be a Nevada School of Medicine.

**George Furman MD,** First Chair of OB/GYN: George Smith was engaged in practicable cardiovascular research, including work on an implantable cardiac pacemaker, after arriving in Reno. His paper entitled Slot Machine Stasis called attention to pulmonary emboli as the result of prolonged lack of leg movement while gaming. With only a tiny budget for the new two-year medical school, he managed to recruit an outstanding full-time faculty and a volunteer clinical faculty. George was a good friend, and I couldn't say no to him-even when he asked me to teach anatomy to undergraduates.

**Tom Kozel PhD,** Microbiologist: George was a master at representing the medical school to various stake holders. Whenever he met with legislators, foundation representatives, or donors, he always brought along a student and a junior faculty. These students and faculty were the face of the future of the medical school. It was a very effective and very attractive presentation. Regardless of the audience or the topic, George would say, "I have three things to say about this." It was always three; never one; never four. George would go on at length about the first point. He might touch on the second point. He never got to the third point.

**Bud Baldwin PhD,** Administrator: George was an amazing and somewhat unlikely paradox; on one hand a brilliant and talented leader with great instincts and inclusive ideas, yet he often affected an air of vulnerability, and even helplessness, that made some people underestimate him and want to help and protect him. I can't tell you how many times I would drop in on Friday evening to say good night, looking forward to a restful weekend, and he would say, "Bud, I wonder if you could help me with this problem." I was stuck working for the weekend. You simply couldn't refuse him-a quality, I believe, that was essential and worked wonders in the early days of the school.

He had great ideas of his own yet felt free to entertain those of others and then gave them the space to develop their ideas without needing to claim credit. He was a generous, fun-loving man and a good hands-off leader who was able to inspire great loyalty.

**Malcolm Edmiston MD,** First Chair of Surgery: George did an incredible job. I think part of his success was because he involved community doctors in the school. Community Drs. Jerry Dales, Frank Roberts, Robert Myles, Bill Tappan, and Tom Scully were involved.

He only had eleven full-time faculty and had to create a curriculum based on the systems and not departments. I was really impressed how he and Phil Gillette were able to manipulate finances. They had little money, but they moved it around to keep the school going. They were magicians in finances. George was an effective leader.

**Joan Brookhyser MD,** Member of the 1975 Class: I have some very clear memories of Dr. George Smith- particularly from early August of 1973.

The class was gathered in the biggest meeting room we had at the time-in fact, in the only building, overlooking a pasture with cows.

We were in an orientation session in which several members of the faculty came to welcome my class of forty-five men and five women. We were eagerly getting to know each other, 'scoping out the situation' and listening very carefully to what was being told to us by Dr. Scully, Dr. Kozel, Dr. Smith, and others. I remember Dr. Smith saying two things to us. FIRST, He spoke for a few minutes about the struggle and history of the creation of general and CONCLUDED BY SAYING, "Medicine is a very demanding mistress."

I was a bit taken aback at the construct, but after thirty years of training, professional opportunities, and 'teaching moments,' I understand. Medicine is the most demanding, the most rewarding, the most exhilarating, the most heartbreaking, and the most thrilling thing I have encountered in my life. Without George Smith and his commitment to opening the University of Nevada School of Medicine, our lives would be different, and Nevada would be much the poorer.

As a result of his efforts, I, and countless others like me, would walk through its door and impact thousands of lives. You were right about Medicine, George, and we thank you from the bottoms of our hearts.

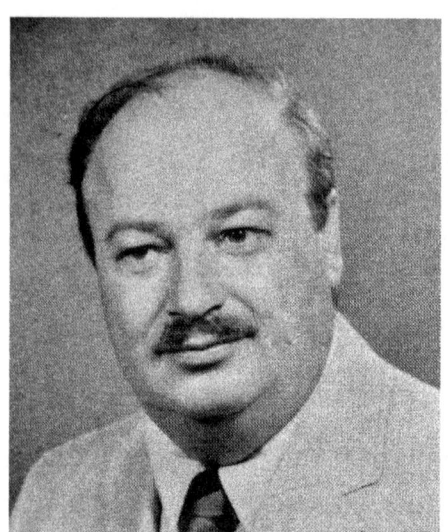 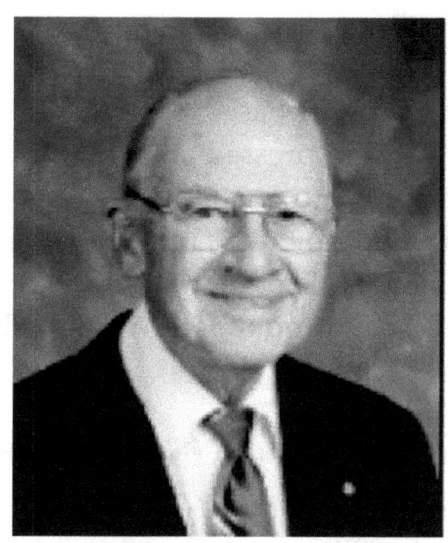

Dr. George Smith             Dr. Bill Tappan, 1976

**Jim Moren MD,** Member of the Charter Class: As a teacher, George was not a great lecturer-dry without much intonation. Obviously smart and well-educated, he was always there supporting the faculty and students while working hard behind the scenes to garner support from the Legislature and the medical community.

A smoker despite the known health risk, he had a gravelly quiet voice and firmly talked us through two years of medicine.

He prepared us well before we transferred for the last two years at an MD granting medical school. He shared a beer or two with students, and then met with heads of state, cajoling and finessing them with his vision of a top community medical school, which our School has become.

George kept our letters of our third and fourth-year medical school experiences and returned them to us in 2009. So, for thirty-six years, George kept these reports of how we were doing, with particular attention to how we compared with our peers at established medical schools. The fact that George kept these papers indicates his interest in our class and his long-term commitment to the students and their successes. The first class was special in so many ways, and we were treated with respect, and dare I say, loved by George and the faculty.

The image on a banner to characterize George would be him in a black suit, white shirt, thin tie, cigarette in hand, and a look mixed with pride and curiosity beneath a balding head. George, the faculty, and the medical community groomed us for success, and the success of the University of Nevada School of Medicine is a tribute to George and the standard he set.

## Dr. Sandra Daugherty, SOM's First Female Professor

It is with great sadness that we noted the passing of Dr. Sandra Daugherty.

Dr. Daugherty died May 30, 2000. She spent her medical career as a clinical researcher and epidemiologist, earning a national reputation for her work in hypertension, chronic fatigue syndrome, and women's health issues. She was also a teacher and mentor, often publishing with medical students and faculty colleagues who collaborate don her studies.

After graduating from Kansas, where she was one of four women in her class, Sandra was a Health Service physician in Oklahoma.

After she earned her doctorate in Public Health at the University of Oklahoma, her academic career took her to Michigan State University, Wyoming, Indiana, and finally to the University of Nevada School of Medicine, where she was on the faculty for nineteen years. Here, she was the first woman to earn the rank of Professor in the School of Medicine.

Dr. Sandra Daugherty was responsible for securing the largest grant ever awarded to Nevada's university system: $8.5 million for the Women's Health Initiative Study. Begun by the National Institute of Health in 1993, the Women's Health Initiative was a national twelve-year study of 160,000 women to examine risk factors involved in heart disease, breast cancer, and osteoporosis in older women.

While on the faculty at Michigan State, Dr. Daugherty was the first woman in the country to be principal investigator of a National Institute of Health clinical trial; she worked from 1971 to 1976 on a hypertension detection and follow-up program. This study led to the awareness that physicians need to actively treat high blood pressure. Due to the success of this trial, Dr. Daugherty was awarded the prestigious Albert Lasker Award for Outstanding Medical Research in 1980.

She spent many years working with the National Heart, Lung, and Blood Institute and the American Heart Association on review committees, study sections, and conference planning committees.

She was one of the first women to assume a leadership role with the American Heart Association, serving on the executive committee and a chair of the council on epidemiology.

Dr. Daugherty's scientific investigations were without end: she investigated the effects of treatments on reduction of death among patients with high blood pressure and heart disease; she studied mercury levels in Dayton, Nevada, and evaluated its effect on residents' health status. She also conducted an epidemiological study of the outbreak of Chronic Fatigue

Syndrome (CFS) at Lake Tahoe and concluded that CFS was, in fact, a disease and not a psychological malady. In addition, the Nevada chapter of the American Heart Association established the Dr. Sandra Daugherty Award for Excellence in Cardiovascular Disease to be given to promising young researchers.

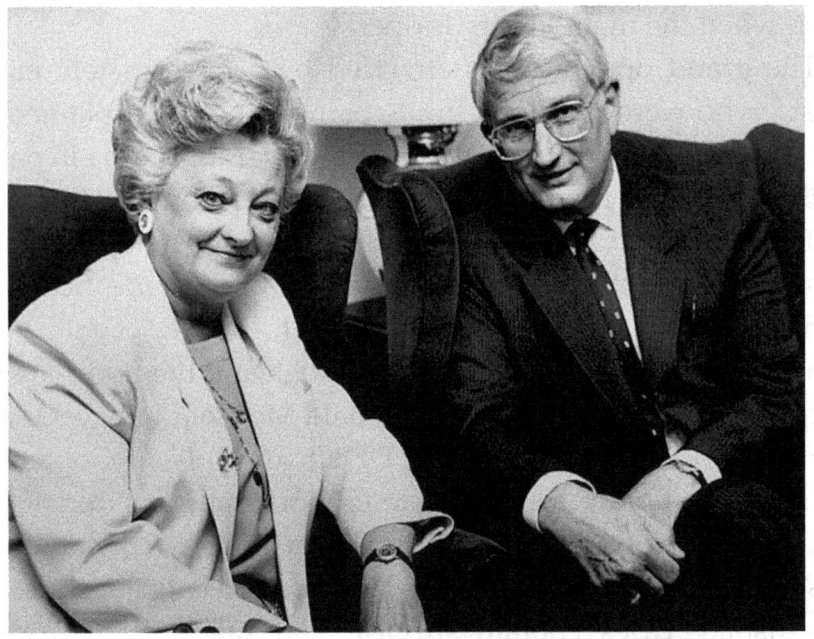

Drs. Sandra and Robert Daugherty, 1990

Dr. Sandra Daugherty had many talents outside of the field of medicine. She was a music and literature major at the University of Kansas before she entered medical school. She was a gifted singer, seamstress, and art collector. Her first love was her husband and their three children. Dr. Bob Daugherty was dean of the University of Nevada School of Medicine from 1981 to 1999. Allison and Doug Smithson lived in Reno and have two children, Bob and Kim Daugherty also lived in Reno and have two children.

Dr. Christopher and Karen Daugherty lived in Chicago with their two children. Dr. Sandra Daugherty is missed by us and her many friends.

# History of Medicine Museum/Library Opening, 2002

May 7, 2002, the grand opening of Nevada's first and only library and museum dedicated solely to the health sciences. Located in the new Pennington Education Building on the Reno campus of the School of Medicine, the Doctors Hood History of Medicine Library and museum is open to the public during the hours when the main library is open.

The grand opening was attended by approximately eighty guests, who were provided guide pamphlets that explained the significance of the thirty-one framed photographs hung in panels on the walls. The photographs depict scenes from the history of medicine dating back to the 1400s; however, most of the pictures illustrate the history of the University of Nevada School of Medicine, which opened its doors in 1971.

The walls are constructed from red oak and the floors are oak parquet. Each of three areas, Dr. Donald Mousel Lounge, Dr. Bob Daugherty Reading Room, and Dr. Owen Bolstad Conference Room, in the library are delineated by oriental rugs donated by Drs. John Iliescue and Anton Sohn. Dean T. Schwenk named the museum Anton & Arlene Sohn History of Medicine Museum. The display cases contain surgical and medical instruments collected by Nevada physicians, and most were used in the Silver State. Some of the surgical instruments were used at the time of the Civil War.

The museum collection includes Dr. Fred Anderson's, Father of the Medical School, medical artifacts, and herbs from Nevada Indians. Museum artifacts are also located in the Pennington building, in the entry of the Savitt building, and in the Nevada State Laboratory.

The oldest artifact in the library is a marble column from the ancient city of Byblos, Phoenicia. The column is approximately 3,500 years old. It has a carving of a snake, the emblem of medicine. Other exhibits include Dr. Donald Mousel's collection of over seventy historic spectacles dating back to when Benjamin Franklin invented bifocals in 1784.

We want to thank the following individuals whose donations made the library a reality: Dr. James Barger, Eileen Barker, Dr. & Mrs. Glen Biddulph, Dr. G. Kim Bigley, Dr. Harold Boyer, Dr. Thomas Brady, Dr. Curtis Brown, Gussie Burgoyne, Dr. and Mrs. H. Treat Cafferata, Dr. and Mrs. Edwin Cantlon, Dr. A.W. Carlson, E.P. Charleton II, Dr. G.N. Christensen, Dr. Robert Clift, Walt Collins, David Console, Phyllis & Dr. Ronald Cudek, Dr. Robert Daugherty, Dr. John M. Davis, Dr. Art DiSalvo, Barbara & Dr. Wm. Feltner, Dr. Quincy Fortier, Teresa Garrison, Dr. and Mrs. Joseph George, Dr. and Mrs. Jay Gibson, Mrs. Kurt Hartock, Dr. and Mrs. Tom Hood, Kevin and Frances (Massoth) Hull, Dr. John Iliescu, Dr. Wm. King, Dr. and Mrs. Leonard Kreisler, Dr. Colleen Lyons, Doris Hawn Manville, Dr. Harry P. and Grainelle Massoth, Patricia Massoth, Louise Massoth, Lynda Mulvey McLellan, Dr. Hoyt Miles, Carol Mousel, Dr. Frank J. Nemec, Dr. Fred Newman, Dr. Sam Parks, Dr. Roger Ritzlin, Jean & Dr. Frank Roberts, Dr. Rodney Sage, Todd L. Savitt PhD, Arlene and Dr. Anton Sohn, and Dr. Gerald R. Sylvain.

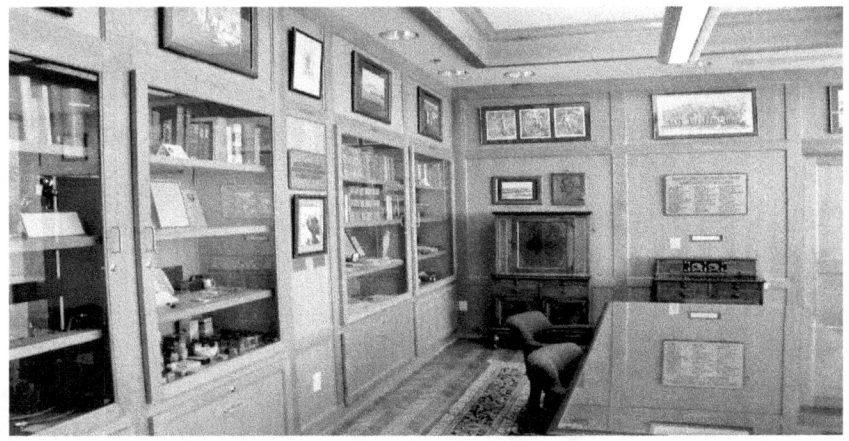

Doctor Robert Daugherty Reading Room
in the Dr. Anton and Arlene Sohn Great Basin History of Medicine Museum, Univ. of Nevada Reno School of Medicine

# Dr. Fred Anderson
## Father of the School of Medicine
# By Dr. Anton Sohn

Fred Anderson was born in 1906 and raised in eastern Nevada on a ranch in the Ruby Mountains. He related that he was a cowboy before working in a pharmacy in the small town of Ruth.

According to his oral history, recorded by the University of Nevada Oral History Program, he passed the state pharmacy board examination and worked one day as a pharmacist.

He attended the University of Nevada in Reno. There, he came under the influence of Professor Peter Frandsen who persuaded him to study medicine.

After graduation in 1928, he was awarded a Rhodes scholarship at Oxford University in England. Fred returned to the United States and went to medical school at Harvard where he graduated *cum laude*. He was a military veteran and returned after WW II to his roots in Nevada.

In the early 1960s, he was chairman of the University of Nevada Board of Regents and a member of the West. Interstate Commission for Higher Education.

The commission was composed of three representatives from each of the western states without a medical school. It initiated a feasibility study for a medical school in one of these states, and Nevada, under Dr. Anderson's leadership, was selected. The finished feasibility study was presented to the University's Board of Regents in a contentious meeting on February 11, 1967. Chairman Fred Anderson relinquished the gavel, stepped down, and fired the shot-heard-around-the-state. His motion fueled the north-south fight that would haunt Nevada for years. It pitted the surging growth of Las Vegas and Clark County against the established tradition of the north.

Dr. Anderson moved to "form a two-year school of basic medical sciences, taking the first class in the fall of 1971 or 1972."

It passed six to two. There might have been others who earlier thought Nevada should not have a medical school, but Fred had the position to make it happen.

Southern Regents Dick Ronzone and Dr. Juanita G. White expressed doubt whether the state could financially support the school and voted against it. Their real reason might have been resentment that Reno preempted Las Vegas. This information is from the book, *Better Medicine: The History of the University of Nevada School of Medicine*.

For his role in the drama of creating the University of Nevada School of Medicine, Dr. Anderson was named the "Father of the Medical School." Furthermore, the first building in the school's complex is the Fred M. Anderson Building.

In addition to his role in education, Fred had a sense of history that was uncommon. As he traveled around the state consulting on medical cases, he amassed a collection of 19th century medical instruments, antique books, Indian artifacts, and items related to ranching. Fred never forgot his ranching background and time-in-the-saddle.

His extensive collection of Nevada branding irons was on exhibit at the Nugget Casino in Sparks. It has been said that when Dr. Fred Anderson asked for an artifact to be donated for historical preservation, it was not refused.

The History of Medicine Library in the new Pennington Education Building on the Reno campus also exhibits some of Anderson's collection. The exhibit case in the entrance of the building houses memorabilia related to Dr. Anderson's life. It would be incomplete to relate the above information without saying something about Dr. Anderson as a physician. Attorney Ralph Denton who practiced in Las Vegas and served on the advisory committee to the dean of the medical school was a good friend of Dr. Anderson. Mr. Denton recalled when his son had a fatal burn and Dr. Anderson heard of the accident, he immediately traveled to Las Vegas to comfort the family and help treat the boy. He wouldn't take a penny in payment. Governor Mike O'Callaghan summed it by saying, "Anderson was extremely intelligent but also compassionate."

## SCHOOL OF MEDICINE'S SECOND DEAN, DR. THOMAS J. SCULLY

It was with profound sadness to receive the news of Dr. Thomas Scully's death in September 2008. He had been involved in the School of Medicine since its inception and was one of its most inspiring teachers. A native New Yorker, Dr. Scully began his career in Nevada as a pediatrician in Las Vegas. After a two-year stint in a New Jersey heading a residency program, he returned to Nevada in 1969 to be a founding faculty in the new School of Medical Sciences. Appointed dean after Dr. George Smith resigned, Dr. Scully's career as dean was cut short by bad health.

Dr. Scully was involved in numerous facets of medical education and service to the profession, both on a local and statewide level, but he is best known as one of the School of Medicine's best teachers.

He had a unique way of relating to students and teaching them how to be a caring physician. A recognized expert on medical ethics, Dr. Scully and wife, Celia, authored a book, *Playing God*.

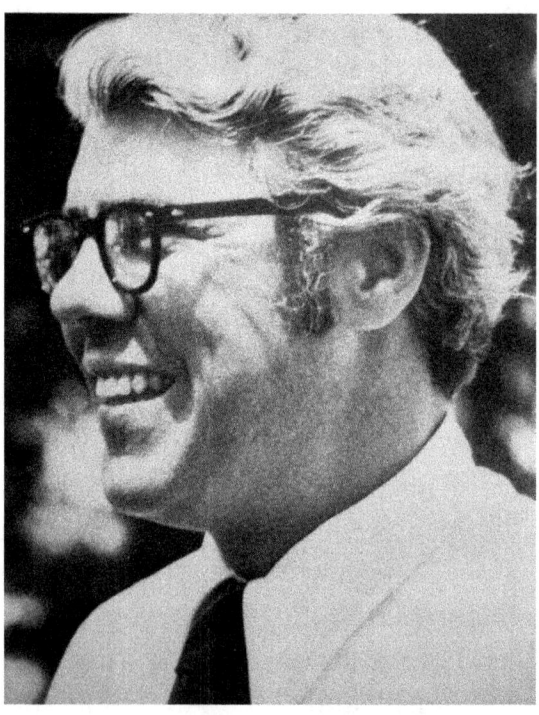

Dr. Thomas J. Scully

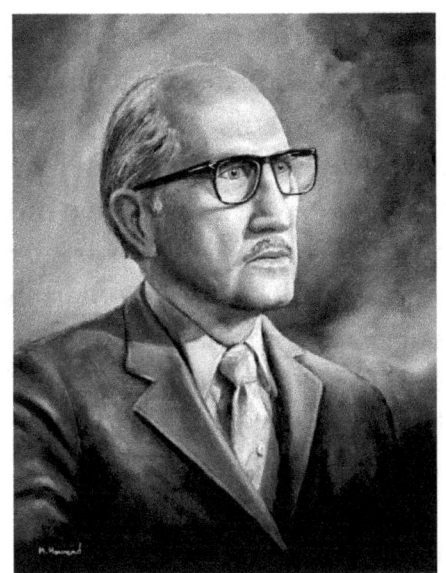 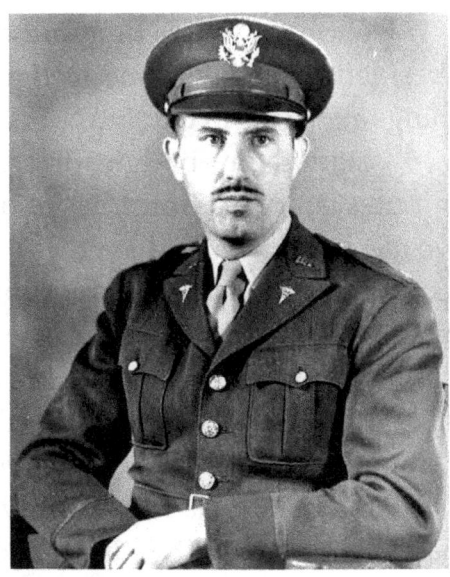

Dr. Frederick Anderson

## SCHOOL OF MEDICINE'S BUDGET CRISIS OF 1981

### By Dr. Robert Daugherty

January 1981 commemorated the fortieth year since Governor Paul Laxalt signed the bill on March 25, 1969, establishing the medical school. Since that time, we had eight deans with tenures varying from two years to Dr. Bob Daugherty's nineteen years. The following article is Dr. Daugherty's reminiscence about his first year at the School of Medicine and the challenges.

Dr. Robert Daugherty: "Twenty-eight years ago in January 1981, I flew into Reno on a sunny cold Sunday from Indiana to meet with acting Dean Mazzaferri and his staff including financial officers, to review the School of Medicine's 1981-83 budget request to the legislature. The state budget office had already reduced the budget, and we knew a fight was coming. Like the 2008-9 financial situation, 1981 was a time of economic recession. The following Monday at 6:00 AM, President Joe Crowley and I drove to Carson City for my presentation of the medical school's budget to the Nevada Assembly Ways and Means Committee.

"Chairman Roger Bremner called the meeting to order, and President Crowley introduced me as the new dean. He said nicer things about me in that introduction than he would ever say again.

"I started my budget presentation, and no more than two minutes later I was interrupted by someone, who said, 'When did we decide to have a medical school?' This was followed by Committee Member Robert Robinson, 'This medical school is an albatross around the neck of the state. We would save money by buying every medical student a Ferrari and sending them out of state.' He was quickly followed by Member Jack Verglies, 'Dr Daugherty, I sure hope you haven't sold your house in Indiana.' This statement was followed by the chairman, 'I sure hope you haven't bought a house in Nevada.

"Without hesitation, Mr. Bob Cashell, Chairman of the Board of Regents at the University stood and said, 'If I was in the legislature, I wouldn't have voted for the medical school either.' I heard the quiet voice of President Crowley behind me, 'Bob, sit down, Bob, sit down.' I sat down and chairman Bremner adjourned the committee. Everyone in the room left except me. I sat there somewhat amused by what had happened.

"I have told this story to several folks over the years. They often look horrified and comment, 'How awful, how devastating.' However, this experience reminded me of my Wyoming experience some five years earlier. I was hired by the University of Wyoming in 1976 to start a new medical school in Laramie. In my experiences with the Wyoming Legislature, I found many of the legislators were surprised to learn the University of Wyoming had approved the funding of the new school. That experience taught me there is always another day in dealing with the legislative process.

"Thus, as I sat in the Nevada Assembly committee room that cold January 1981 day, I reflected on my political education in Wyoming. I realized the next step was going to be up to me and me alone. After all, the President and the Chairman of the Board of Regents not only had not defended the medical school, but they had left the room. What should I do? In the preceding six months, as I visited Reno and the state, I met many physicians, legislators, and community leaders.

"I had accepted the deanship because I felt there was sufficient support of the school despite much vocal opposition. On one of these visits, I met Mr. Bob Barengo, Speaker of the Assembly from Reno. Dr. Bob Clift, a local Reno physician on the search committee, introduced me to him. In fact, Dr. Clift was the only community physician on the committee. He described himself as the 'token doc' on the search committee. Dr. Bob Cliff and I developed mutual respect, which was assisted by the fact that we had both graduated from the Kansas University School of Medicine.

"Furthermore, I knew from my Wyoming experience that the speaker of the assembly appointed the standing committees of the assembly, which include the Ways and Means Committee where I had just met my apparent demise!

"Therefore, I decided to pay Speaker Barengo a visit. In those days in the Nevada Legislature it was easy and comfortable to walk into a legislators' office and visit or seek help.

"As I walked into the speaker's office, he met me with a smile and a hearty, 'Hi Dean, how are you and welcome.' I responded that I was fine, but I had a question. 'It is my understanding that you, as Speaker, appoint the committee chairs in the assembly. Is that correct?' Mr. Barengo responded, 'Yes.' I immediately responded, 'I think you owe me one.' I then described what had transpired in the Ways and Means Committee hearing.

"The Speaker looked at me and asked with a slight smile, 'Do you need any funds for Las Vegas?' I responded, 'Yes, what should it be?' Bob Barengo, 'You decide but get it to me by tomorrow.' I presented a Las Vegas budget of $400,000 to him. When I returned, he said, 'Dean, your budget will be approved, all of it, including the Las Vegas funds.'

"I learned my first and most important political Nevada lesson. Always include both Reno and Las Vegas in my requests to the legislature. I also learned rural Nevada was another priority. On the other hand, by the time I left my deanship, nineteen years later, rural Nevada was my priority, but it no longer was the legislature's priority.

"In the remaining days and weeks of the 1981 legislative session, I spent much face-to-face time with members of the Ways and Means Committee.

"As a result, by the next legislative session, Mr. Bremner had become supportive of the school. However, it was not always evident because he had his own way of helping.

"Another member also had a unique way of helping. Mr. Jack Vergiels, never voted for us, but he never voted against us. Other members were never supportive. For example, Mr. Robert Robinson was consistently against any of our proposals for the length of his legislature tenure. Little did I realize this initial Nevada political education would carry me through nine more sessions.

"The School of Medicine and I enjoyed good support from succeeding legislative leaders over the following nineteen years, giving us the opportunity to provide Nevada's best and brightest students an excellent medical education—second to none in the country."

## School of Medicine's First Financial Officer
## Phillip J. Gillette

Phil Gillette died January 4, 2010. He had many titles and duties over his forty years of dedication to the School of Medicine. He was the first financial officer when the school was created in 1969, but none of Phil's titles could adequately describe his dedication and commitment to the School nor describe his valuable advice to many of us during our time with the school. He was tireless and always available when called upon.

**Bob Daugherty MD:** "Indeed, I was surprised to note he had retired in 1987 after I had been Dean for six years. During the subsequent years before my retirement in 1999, I don't think Phil missed a day of working for the school. His knowledge on the history and mission of the school was critical in reminding us on a day-to-day basis of our priorities. To say Phil Gillette will be missed does not begin to describe the void left by his death. Below are comments from former colleagues and his children, who give us a reminder of the caring nice person many of us had the opportunity to know and work with. We all have lost a piece of our soul."

**Tom Kozel PhD,** former Chair of Microbiology: "My memory about Phil from the early days was the graciousness of him and his wife Geneva in welcoming new faculty to the medical school. The faculty was small at that time, and we were in a precarious situation. There was a tremendous need for everyone to hang together.

"Phil and Geneva provided much of the glue to make that happen. As the newest and youngest faculty in 1971, I, along with my wife, Pat, appreciated the warmth with which we were brought into the Reno community."

**Mike Reed PhD,** former Dean of the School of Business: "My recollections of Phil begin with recalling the way he would come to the office to talk about health issues. He was an incredibly cheerful and graceful man who was dogged in his determination to build a relationship between the School of Medicine and the College of Business. I also recall his way with students while he taught in the college. I recall Phil's gentle nature and smile- always the smile. I recall the way he would prod me to get something accomplished.

"And while I can't recall particulars, what I do know is he would smile across the table, verbalize the idea, and remark that the initiative was something that would be of substantial benefit, involve little work and be quickly attained. I also recall being amazed at how such a slight person could be, and remain, so vibrant."

"Phil exuded a positive energy every time I saw him, especially when he and John Bancroft would approach me. Their presence together scared me in a good way because I knew I was about to get an important lesson I would realize and appreciate later."

**George Hess MD,** former Chair of Family and Community Medicine: "The thing I remember most about Phil was that he always seemed to have a smile and a positive word no matter how grim the situation. He loved teaching and sharing his knowledge, while he actively taught in the schools of Business and Medicine. He coordinated the Practice Management Course for our residency and made it invaluable to the residents with his many contacts and guest speakers. He never seemed to hesitate to volunteer if a job needed to be done. This was true at our church, in the community, and, as well, at the University. Lastly, as a green Department Chairman, I found Phil extremely helpful as an advisor and as a friend."

Sam Parks MD: "Even though Phil was retired, he functioned as the secretary of the committee during my years as chairman. He was invaluable because of his knowledge and history with the School.

"He never missed a meeting and was responsible for disseminating the minutes to the school's faculty. Despite his declining health he was always cheerful and ready to help with any task. The School will miss Phil."

**Jerry May PhD:** "Phil was always a delightful positive man who loved the School of Medicine. He was always raising his hand to help the school in any way. We were both from the State of Washington and we would reminisce about old times. Phil was also avid golfer, and we would bring each other up to date on national tournaments and our game. He and I knew early on that we would need to keep our day-job' as we would not be professional golfers.

"He kept up on the progress of the School of Medicine, and I am not aware of anyone who was more dedicated to see the school succeed. I wish I had one more chance to say to Phil: Thank You!"

**Denise and Rick,** Phil's Daughter, and Son: "Our dad not only had passion for his work but also for so many other things. He had such great love for his family and especially our mom, Geneva, during their nearly sixty years together. He devoted most of his extra time to several charities and volunteered his services to many organizations. He loved food, sports (football), investing in the stock market, and was very interested in business and politics. He loved to travel, and wherever he went he truly appreciated the beauty of that area. His favorite places were the states of Washington and Hawaii. One of our fondest memories is when our family took a month to travel throughout the United States seeing museums, national monuments, and several other sites in about twenty-five states -very memorable! If all of us could even live half as much as he did, how lucky we would all be. Wish we could have just one more of our two-hour phone conversations. Dad, we miss you so much!"

## Former Dean Dr. Ernie Mazzaferri

Former Dean of the University of Nevada School of Medicine, Ernest Mazzaferri died at home in Henderson, Nevada, on May 14, 2013, after fighting Alzheimer's disease. Ernie graduated from Ohio State School of Medicine, served in the U.S. Air Force, and taught briefly at Ohio State before he came to Nevada in 1978. As chairman of internal medicine, the School and its students recognized him as an outstanding teacher.

In 1979, Dean Tom Scully became ill, and Ernie became the interim dean for two years. Dr. Mazzaferri was recognized nationally for his research and teaching abilities. Ohio State recruited him from UNSOM to be chairman of internal medicine, and he remained there until he retired in 1999.

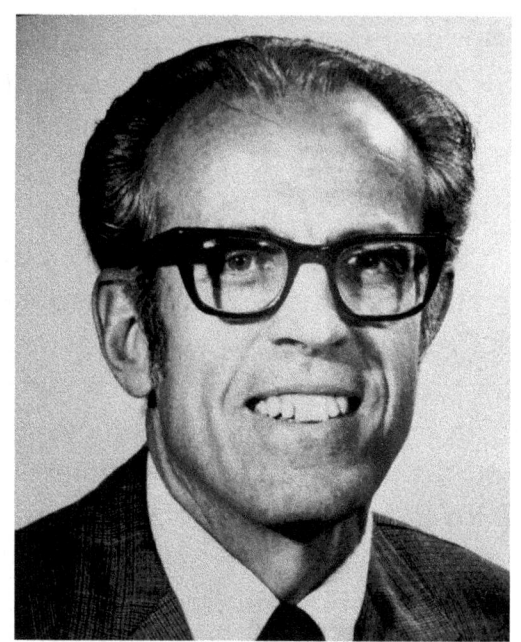

Phillip John Gillette

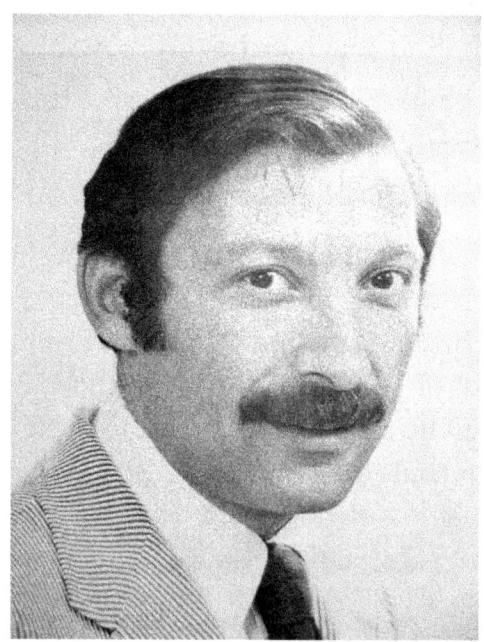

Dr. Ernie Mazzaferri

# VII

+_+_+_+_+_+_+_+_+_+_+_+_+_+_+_+_+_+_+_+_+_+_+_+_+_+_+

# DENTAL CARE
## "Promoting Health"

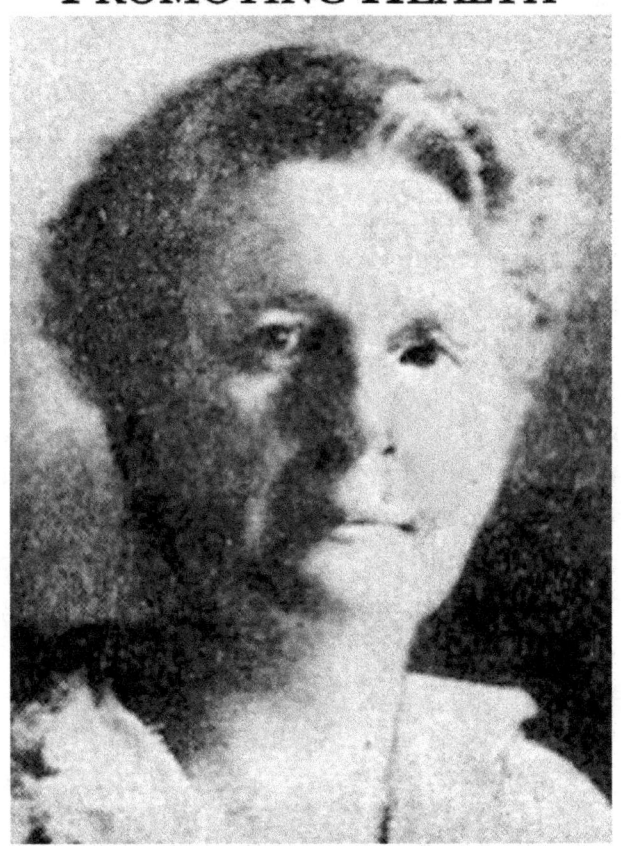

*Helen R. Shipley, Nevada's First Female Dentist 1905*

+_+_+_+_+_+_+_+_+_+_+_+_+_+_+_+_+_+_+_+_+_+_+_+_+_+_+

# Helen Shipley DMD,
## Nevada's First Female Dentist, 1905

A true native daughter of Nevada, Helen Rulison Shipley was born in Dayton, Nevada, July 23, 1870, where her father, Charles Rulison, earned his living as a millwright on the Comstock Lode. She received most of her schooling in the Dayton schools. When the mining boom declined, Helen's family relocated to Reno during her senior year in high school. She graduated in 1888 at the top of her class, despite the disruption of the sudden move.

That year Helen, or "Nellie" as she was called during her youth, enrolled at the University of Nevada School of Business, graduating on June 13, 1889. With limited vocations available to women in the late 19th century, she chose to become a teacher and soon was teaching thirty-seven pupils at the South Side School across the Truckee River from Reno. During her first year as a teacher she received a salary of $65 per month.

When Helen's older brother, David, graduated from the University of California Dental College in 1891 he opened a practice in Reno. He advertised he was "the only graduate in dentistry in Reno." Influenced by his success, Helen retired from the teaching profession, moved to San Francisco, and enrolled at the University of California in 1894, graduating as a Doctor of Dental Surgery in 1896. Three years later, her younger brother, Fred, also graduated from California Dental College. By the year 1906, there were three members of the Rulison family practicing dentistry in Reno, a community of about 4,500 people.

In 1905, Dr. Helen Rulison was appointed to the Nevada State Board of Dental Examiners. She was the first woman to practice dentistry in the state, and the first woman to serve on the Dental Board of Examiners. Late in 1906, she moved her practice to Goldfield, Nevada, following the gold and silver discoveries there. She opened her office in the San Jose Hotel, advertising herself as a specialist in crown and bridge work. Within a few years, Goldfield began to decline, and in 1912, Dr. Rulison moved to Tonopah as the population there was more stable and there were fewer dentists. At the age of forty-six, Helen married Robert H. Shipley and continued to practice in Tonopah until 1926 when they moved to Reno.

She opened an office at 126 Ridge Street, where she practiced until her retirement in 1946. Nevada lost its first female dentist when Helen died on June 6, 1955, at age of eighty-five. Dr. Helen Rulison Shipley cared for the people of Nevada for over a half century.

**NOTE:**

The material contained in this article was excerpted from a story in the *Washoe Rambler* published by the Washoe County Historical Society in 1978. It was written by Guy Louis Rocha, Historian and State Archivist for the Nevada State Library and Archives. Our thanks to Mr. Rocha for permission to use this most interesting story.

### HARRY MASSOTH DMD, FORENSIC DENTIST, 1945

Supported by a grant from the Northern Nevada Dental Society, and individual gifts from Dr. Peter M. DiGrazia and Dr. Rafael Gamboa, a series of oral history interviews was completed with Dr. Harry Massoth, a well-known dentist who has practiced in Pioche, Ely and in Reno, Nevada for 49 years. The interviews were done by Eileen Barker, manager department of pathology at the University of Nevada School of Medicine. An edited and annotated transcript of this oral history was early in 1995 and released at the meeting of the Northern Nevada Dental Society on September 14, 1995.

Dr. Harry Massoth, a 1939 graduate of the University of Buffalo School of Dentistry, came to Pioche, Nevada, in 1945. He moved to Ely in 1947 and later to Reno in 1955 where he practiced until his retirement. He was active in the affairs of Nevada Dental Association and Nevada State Board of Dental Examiners.

A pioneer in forensic dentistry in Nevada, Dr. Massoth has been called upon on many occasions to assist authorities in identification of unknown deceased individuals. Dr. Massoth served as Dental Consultant for the Nevada Medicaid Program and assisted the Washoe County Medical Examiner to identify teeth impressions. He was one of only four original oral surgeons to practice in this state. Dr. Massoth was used on several occasions at the Washoe County Coroner's office to identify bite marks on deceased individuals.

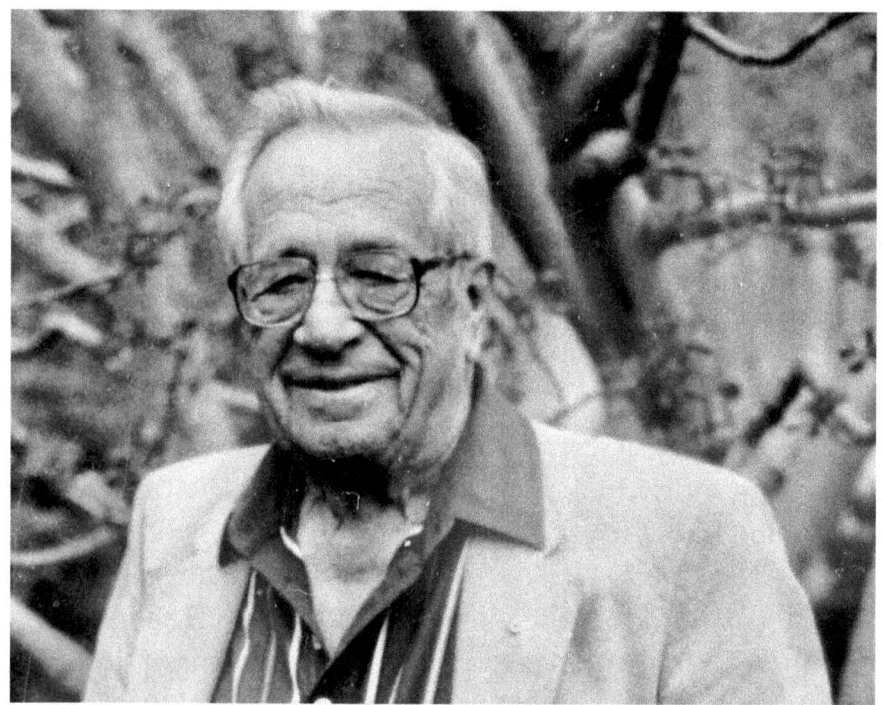

Harry Massoth DDS, Oral Surgeon

## HERMANN SEYFARTH DMD, 73 YEARS A DENTIST

There may be other individuals who have been involved in the field of dentistry for more than 73 years, but Dr. Hermann B.F. Seyfarth is one of a very few who have been in practice that long. Born in Thuringia, Germany, in 1903, Hermann apprenticed to a Swiss dentist when he was 14 years of age. Because he was a neutral alien, the Swiss dentist was able to continue working after

Germany became embroiled in the first World War, but both Hermann's father and his brothers were drafted into the German army.

The apprenticeship as a dental technician was long and difficult, with laboratory and formal studies occupying six days a week for three years. After working for four years with the Swiss dentist, Seyfarth worked as a certified technician for two other dentists, who were in a partnership. During that time a dentist from Boston, Massachusetts, visited with the men with whom Seyfarth was working.

He showed them some new methods and advantages in dentistry, and while working with the Bostonian, Seyfarth asked him, "why don't you take me back to America with you?" Surprisingly, the American agreed to do just that. So, at the age of 19, although he spoke no English and had no money, the young German found himself in the United States. He had borrowed money from the Boston dentist for the cost of the trip, to be repaid as he worked as a laboratory technician. First, he had to learn English, then he enrolled in night school to earn high school credits.

Within three years, he entered Harvard College and three years after that entered Harvard University School of Dental Medicine. At about that same time (1928) Hermann Seyfarth became a naturalized American citizen. He graduated from Harvard Dental School in 1932, with the degree of DMD and was appointed to the teaching faculty at Harvard, where he remained for the next ten years while also maintaining a private practice. During this period, he was invited to give a demonstration of dental techniques at the International Dental Convention in Vienna, Austria.

With the bombing of Pearl Harbor on 7 December 1941, Dr. Seyfarth volunteered for service with the Sixth General Hospital, which was made up of doctors and nurses from the staff of Massachusetts General Hospital. He was granted a commission as Captain in the Dental Corps and in 1943 was shipped to Casablanca, Morocco.

During the ensuing four years his hospital unit followed the Allied troops as they advanced through North Africa and Italy. While in Italy, he had a truck outfitted as a dental laboratory and operatory, together with an assistant and two laboratory technicians, they went out into the field to provide services for his patients. So little room remained in this unique "dental office" that the patient was forced to sit with his feet projecting out the rear of the truck.

Dr. Seyfarth returned to the United States in October 1945 with the rank of Major. Distrustful of the uneasy post-war period (the Cold War) he joined the army reserve, where he served 15 years, attaining the rank of lieutenant colonel. Practicing in Boston, he re-entered private practice.

He served on the teaching faculty of Tufts University and the staff of Massachusetts General Hospital in Boston.

In 1955, Dr. Seyfarth, at an age when most professional would consider retirement, removed his practice to Reno, Nevada, where he continued practice until his retirement in 1991 at the age of 87 years. After 73 years in dentistry, he has certainly contributed a great deal to his chosen field. In April 1998, Dr. Hermann B.F. Seyfarth DMD celebrated his 95th birthday with his many good friends-still enjoying life to the utmost.

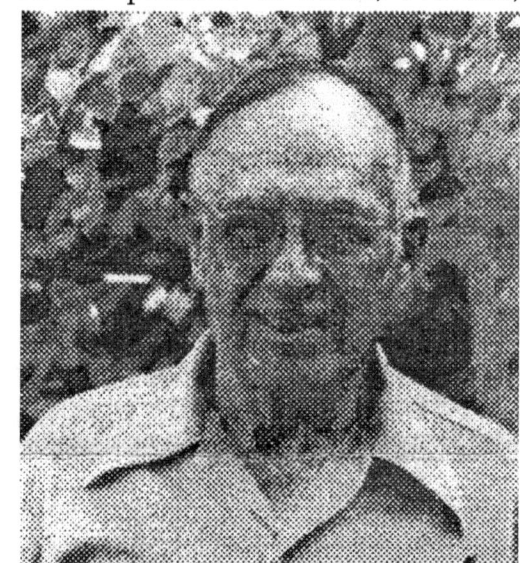

Hermann Seyfarth DMD

# VIII

+_+_+_+_+_+_+_+_+_+_+_+_+_+_+_+_+_+_+_+_+_+_+_+_+_+_+

## Epidemics
### "Scourge of Mankind"

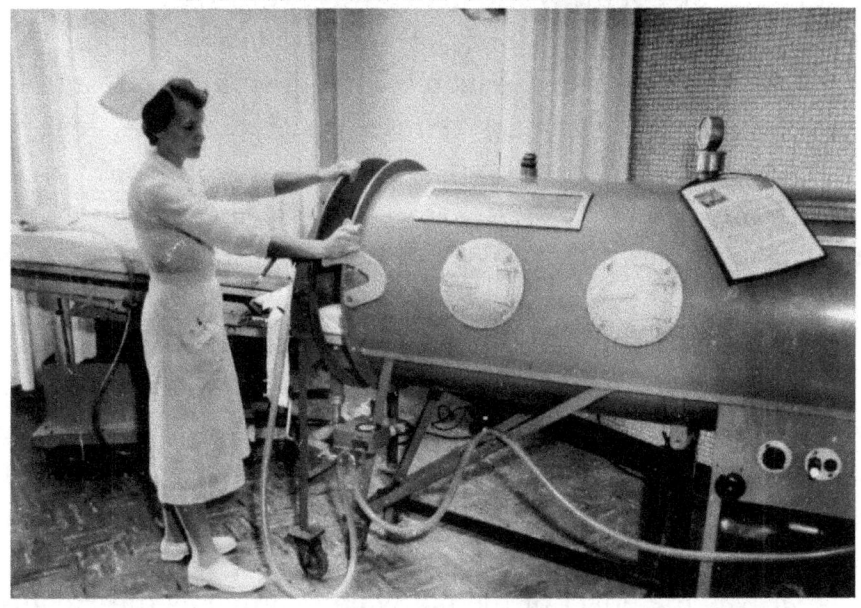

*Nurse Lawson, Iron Lung 1950*

+_+_+_+_+_+_+_+_+_+_+_+_+_+_+_+_+_+_+_+_+_+_+_+_+_+_+

# 1918 Nevada Flu Epidemic
## By Dr. Anton Sohn

The flu outbreak during World War I was probably the most explosive and devastating disease of the twentieth century (COVID-19 came later). AIDS might be more disastrous. but it certainly didn't circle the world as fast or kill as many in as short a time as the flu. Interestingly, both diseases are caused by a virus and have targeted the young adult. It is postulated that older individuals in 1918 had some immunity to the influenza virus.

Influenza swept the world in two waves during 1918. The first wave started in early March at Camp Fuston, Kansas. The second-more deadly wave began late August in France and was spread by ocean shipping and returning servicemen. As many as 25 million and possibly as high as 40 million people died. In the United States alone, at least 550,000 people died of flu and its complications, more than five times our military losses in the war. Because of the sudden onset of symptoms and the virulence of the unknown organism, many experts suggested a bacterium, or a combination of bacterial etiologies; at that time little was known about viruses. Even if the cause of the highly contagious malady had been established, the treatment and preventive measures probably would not have changed, thus the outcome would have been the same.

What was the effect of the fall wave, known as the 'Spanish Flu' because the disease was uncensored in Spain and therefore more publicized, on Nevada citizens? We cite newspaper narrations of the flu in Fallon, *The Fallon Eagle*, Las Vegas *The Age*, Reno *Evening Gazette*, and *The Nevada State Journal*, Sparks *Tribune*, Carson City *Daily Appeal*, and the University of Nevada *Sagebrush*.

In Fallon, about a dozen cases were mentioned October 5, 1918, and the first death, Hall Sumner, age 37, was recorded on October 19. By the end of the month, citizens were concerned about prohibition and the menace of alcohol. "Saloons a menace to society, a parasite on the industry of others and aid to the Kaiser."

In December, preventive measures such as face masks became mandatory in the schools. Public gatherings were banned. By December 14, servicemen were returning home and the epidemic was waning.

Las Vegas was harder hit and panic soon ensued. Although the flu arrived in mid-September, by mid-October there were 140 cases with five new cases a day. The symptoms were headache, backache, fever, and bronchitis. Pneumonia was a dreaded complication. Doctors were overworked, hospitals were full, caskets were in short supply, and the local undertaker, C.B. Faust, was in bed with the flu. By the end of November, new cases were ten per day and schools were closed. Flu masks of ·four to six layers of fine mesh gauze were recommended to control the spread. By December 14 when the "Dry" law was scheduled to become law, approximately fifty people had died in the Las Vegas area.

Panic was also the order of the day at the University of Nevada in Reno. On October 15, 1918, even before there was an outbreak, a quarantine was posted. By the end of the month there were 45 cases and one death, Private Wilbourn Stock. The second death was Coach Ray Whisman, and the girls of Manzanita [Hall] were making flu masks. By November 12, the situation had quieted down enough for the military companies wearing flu masks to march in a parade in downtown Reno, commemorating the end of the war.

Off campus, in the Reno-Sparks area the first cases were reported on October 12 and a flag parade was called off. It was reported that eating "plenty of raw onions and food seasoned with red peppers" was a good preventive. Because the odor caused people to keep their distance.

This was probably excellent advice! Within one week,

everything was closed except saloons. October 14 was "Sermonless Sunday" and ministers were advised to use "unpreached sermons" on the next Sunday. Nurses wanted more money for their "increased risk" while on duty. Milder than onions, sagebrush tea-an old Indian remedy which breaks fever in hours was recommended to fight *la grippe*.

At least sixteen dead were reported by the *Sparks Tribune*. *Carson City Daily Appeal* reported calomel, citrate of caffeine, along with well-lighted and ventilated rooms with wide open window might be effective. Dr. W.H. Hood of the State Board of Health promised help from the state if needed.

One can see confusion and panic was the order of the day during the epidemic. The flu pandemic of 1918 is remembered in this country as much as is the horror of WW I. We can readily understand the concern of Nevadans in 1918 if we consider deaths due to influenza, with its cause unknown, outnumbered combat fatalities.

A study published by the Armed Forces Institute of Pathology (AFIP) for the first time demonstrated the organism responsible for the death of 20 million people worldwide. Although the organism is closely related to that causing the swine flu, its genetic make-up is distinct, and it had never been seen previously. This difference apparently accounted for the lack of cross immunity with other influenza viruses and the resulting profound effect on its victims.

Using lung tissue recovered from victims of the epidemic 79 years ago that had been preserved in formaldehyde and paraffin, the researchers were able to recover enough of the virus to study its genetic make-up and concluded it did not match any virus that had been seen since that time.

Dr. Jeffery K. Taubenberger, the leading scientist of the team from the AFIP warned the disease could strike again. It has been postulated the virus evolved from an infection in American pigs and was carried around the world by U.S. Servicemen serving during World War I. Dr. Taubenberger proposed naming the virus Influenza A/South Carolina because much of the autopsy material originated from Fort Jackson, South Carolina.

For the many years since World War I, the epidemic has been known as the Spanish flu. If Taubenberger is correct, the Spanish got a bum rap, and it should more logically be called the American flu.

**NOTE:**

Phillip I. Earl of the Nevada Historical Society determined the Flu Masks picture was taken near the Washoe County Courthouse on Virginia Street in Reno and that the poster probably depicts the commander of Field Marshal Ferdinand Foch of France. The original photograph which provided the stimulus for this article, was provided by Dr. Frederick Elliott, retired Reno internist. He dated the back of the photograph, November 12, 1918.

## 1952-'53 POLIO EPIDEMIC
## By Dr. Anton Sohn

Prior to the development of the polio vaccine by Jonas E. Salk in 1955, poliomyelitis was a dreaded disease of children, who were usually stricken between four and fifteen years of age. It was recognized there was a greater incidence of polio infection following tonsillectomy, and this operation was frowned upon during the summer season. Public gatherings were discouraged, and organized summer sports were virtually banned. The polio virus was endemic worldwide and occurred in epidemic proportions in the United States during the summer months.

Reno was no exception and as the result of two near fatalities from bulbar spinal poliomyelitis in 1952 and 1953, a team was formed by the Washoe County Medical Society to manage future cases since there were no available facilities between Los Angeles and Salt Lake City. The team included representatives from many disciplines.

Maida Pringle represented nursing with nurse "Red" Johnson and Nurse Cunningham. Later, Renee Quinn RN, a recovered victim of bulbar polio, returned to work on the hospital team. All the nurses did yeomen's duty and, in a sense, pioneered in the development of the first real intensive care unit.

Mr. Clyde Foxx was the hospital administrator, and Ed Sontag was hospital engineer. The first two patients treated with iron lungs were housed in the administrator's office, gaudy wallpaper, and all.

Drs. Ken Maclean, Fred Anderson, Bill Tappan, Frank Russell, Wes Hall Sr., Ed Cantlon, and Vernon Cantlon were all general surgeons on the team, and Drs. Bob Locke, Peter Rowe, and Fred Elliott were the representatives from internal medicine. Pediatricians on the team included Drs. Jack Palmer, John Scott Sr., and Emmanuel Berger. The ENT staff consisted of Drs. Joe Elia and Olin Moulton. There were also people on the team from neurosurgery, orthopedics. otolaryngology and anesthesiology.

Anesthesiologist Dr. William O'Brien III spearheaded the project. The Washoe County program, which became a nationwide model, included training, fundraising, transport, ventilation, respiratory assistance—tracheostomy when necessary—and supportive care. The program is described by Dr. William A. O'Brien III and his associates, Arthur E. Scott, Robert C. Crosby, and William E. Simpson in a book *Diagnosis and Treatment of the Acute Phase of Poliomyelitis and its Complications*, published by The Williams and Wilkins Company.

As the first order of business, a Polio Equipment Fund was established by the Washoe County Medical Society and a panel of its members appeared before service clubs in the area requesting support.

Funds were badly needed to purchase 'iron lung type respirators,' which at that time were the only thing available to care for patients with respiratory paralysis. Multiple sets of tracheostomy tubes and similar special equipment were needed to deal with the numerous cases seen in an epidemic. Civic leaders were taken to the wards of Washoe Medical Center to be shown the status of care and the need for equipment. The needed funds were quickly raised.

One person who was particularly successful during the fundraising drive was Mrs. Barbara Savoy, who at that time was the office manager for the partnership of Drs. O'Brien, Scott, Crosby, and Simpson. She was able to scrounge equipment from all over the United States. Mrs. Savoy was active in both the local and state March of Dimes organizations and was able to arrange financial assistance from that organization as well.

Washoe Medical Center was designated as a regional polio treatment center, and accepted patients from as far away as Grass Valley, California and Las Vegas, Nevada. At one time the hospital cared for a maximum of 18 patients in respirators, along with several other polio victims who did not require assistance breathing.

Some of the funds were used to equip the transport team which consisted of an otorhinolaryngologist, anesthesiologist, and hospital engineer. Forty-one patients were transported from 33 to 300 miles by air, ambulance, or car. The ages ranged from seven weeks to 59 years and there were few complications associated with the transport.

A brother and sister about 5 and 7 years of age from Grass Valley, both about one-week post-op after a T&A, were stricken with polio. Since no care was available in the entire Sacramento area, they had to be transported to Reno, no easy task since U.S. #40 over Donner Summit was virtually closed by a blizzard. The boy expired during the trip.

The desperately ill girl, although she required tracheostomy and respirator care for a long time, eventually did make a good recovery. For the most part, many lives were saved by earlier respiratory assistance.

The success of the team is demonstrated by the statistics from the first two years. During that time 137 patients with polio were admitted to Washoe Medical Center and 40 required a respirator. During the first year, the mortality rate for those patients on the respirator was 30% while the second-year mortality rate dropped to 17.3%.

The success of the polio team, in response to this medical emergency, was due in part to the efforts of the community and medical profession. The various agencies worked together to identify, finance and fight what had been a hopeless medical entity-respiratory paralysis due to polio.

**NOTE:**

This story had a great deal of assistance from Dr. W.E. Simpson, a retired anesthesiologist now living in St. Helena, California. Dr. Simpson was one of the authors of *Diagnosis and Treatment of the Acute Phase of Poliomyelitis*. Dr. Simpson was one of the anesthesiologists on the treatment team at Washoe Medical Center during the poliomyelitis epidemic in the early 1950's prior to the availability of vaccine.

Dr. Simpson: "One of our problems was high vs. low tracheostomy. The surgeons had all been taught to do low tracheostomies—to keep the tube as far away as possible from the vocal cords. However, a high tracheostomy made respirator care much easier, for suctioning, cleaning etc. We, the anesthesiologists, preached for a high trach. One day, we got a patient, I believe a serviceman, from the Las Vegas area, who arrived with a tracheostomy in place. He made a good recovery but was still unable to talk. After quite a while, Dr. William O'Brien did a direct laryngoscopy and found, indeed, the tracheostomy was high.

"We also had an infant who required tracheostomy and respirator use. After a couple of weeks, the baby started having periodic episodes of respiratory distress. It finally dawned on all the fancy specialists, anesthesiologists, pediatricians, surgeons, etc. that the baby was still growing and had outgrown the tracheostomy tube. At least twice it was necessary to replace the tube with a longer one. The press soon learned we were caring for an infant, and we received a donation of a baby sized iron lung. I believe it was from either Harold's Club or Harrah's. It may still be rattling around in the basement or attic of WMC.

"I was on call when we admitted a husky, strapping, red haired young man who had been deer hunting in the early California season when it was still quite warm. He had shot a small buck and had carried it on his back several miles to his car. He was admitted with minimal symptoms of spinal polio in his legs. Over the next 10 or 12 hours the disease rapidly overcame his entire nervous system.

"Tracheostomy and respirator care were to no avail, and he died around 4:00 or 5:00 am. I thought this young man's worst luck was shooting that deer and the extra exertion from packing the animal out, for I thought the exertion made his disease worse.

"I recall a patient that Dr. Elmer Hanson flew over from Hawthorne. Elmer had gotten a large plane from the Navy Air Station near Hawthorne. He had hand pumped the respirator all during the flight. We met the plane at the Reno airport and transported the patient to WMC, but despite all of our efforts, he died within a short time."

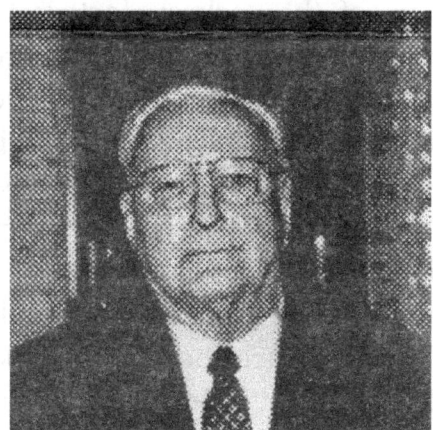 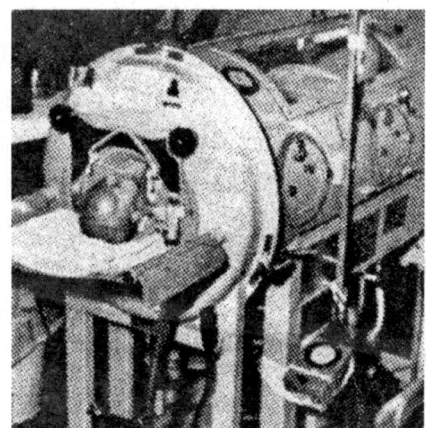

Dr. William E. Simpson     Seven-week-old baby with Polio in an Adult-Iron-Lung

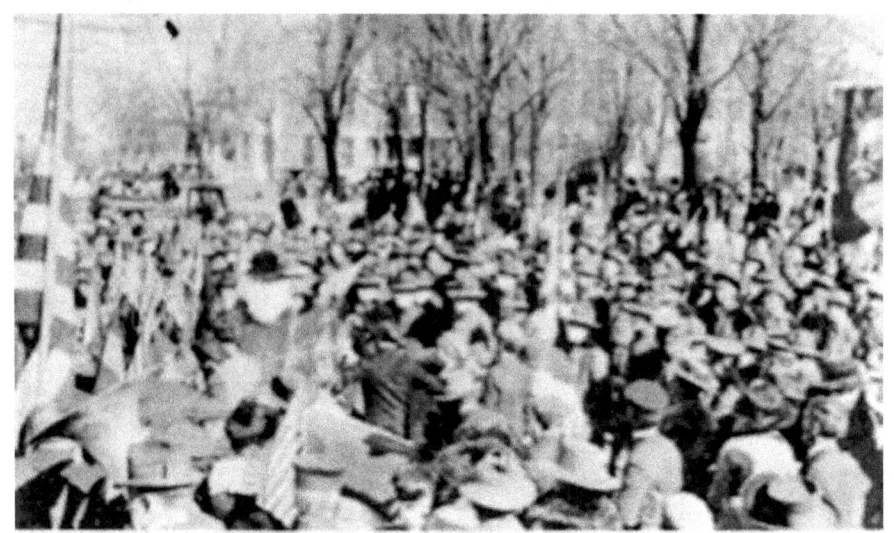

Reno Flu Masks on Soldiers and Citizens, 1918

## DEALING WITH SMALLPOX IN THE OLD WEST, 1863

Smallpox was just one of the devastating infectious diseases immigrants introduced into the West, and it was introduced into native Paiute and Washoe tribes. When it appeared the Department of the Interior provided funds for vaccination. The U.S. Army was expected to provide the service free of charge, but when the disease outbreak was not near a military base, the Department hired civilian physicians to do the vaccinating.

Dr. George Munckton was one of the earliest doctors to practice medicine in Carson City. Dr. Munckton practiced there from 1859 until 1879. He was also a volunteer surgeon at Fort Nye (near Carson City) in 1864. During the period from 1863 until 1865 he vaccinated 416 Indians to protect them from smallpox. The local Indian agent submitted a request for payment to Dr. Munckton in 1868—three years after Munckton's treatment.

The following letter to the commissioner accompanied a bill to pay Dr. Munckton $916, one dollar for each Indian and $500 for the service. Letter to Hon. N.G. Taylor, Commissioner of Indian Affairs, Washington, D.C. from Dr. Jacob T. Lockhart, July 21, 1868: "Sir, I have the honor to submit herewith a subsequent account for the consideration of the Department. I designed to have this account accompany my final account submitted and settled during the past month. Unfortunately I do not have this account with me. I had ordered it sent here in time for it to make a part of the former account spoken of, but it did not reach me as soon as I expected it would and desiring to settle my affairs to stop the suit that had been commenced against my Bondsman, I proceeded to settle the account then on hand. The account against the Government arose in this way. The 'smallpox' which was communicated to the Indians in their wearing cast off clothes, worn by persons afflicted with this disease. In this way the disease was very generally spread throughout the Pah Utah and Washoe tribes. The Commandant at Ft. Churchill was induced to employ his Sergeon [sic] to vaccinate the neighboring Pah Utahs, which he did, and afterwards presented a bill of some $2,000, which I refused to pay.

"I told him he was employed by the Government and being in an Indian Country he should treat the Indians free of charge. Dr. Moncton [sic] visited the different Indian camps and make and exceedingly low charge for his services. The necessity for incurring this expense will be understood better when I stay [sic] that the Indians were dying at a fearful rate, more than one hundred died at the Truckee Reservation. And in many other parts the disease was only arrested by vaccination."

**NOTE:**
Mr. Bob Ellison provided a copy of this letter.

## STEVE ST. JEOR PhD, AND BRIAN CALLISTER MD, "HANTAVIRUS"
### By Chelsea Isom, UNSOM Medical Student

Disease with symptoms like the present-day Hantavirus has been described in China since 1000 AD. It manifested in frightening ways, with conjunctival hemorrhages, petechial rashes, edema, cutaneous flushing, renal failure, and death. Even with high mortality and unknown cause, the disease was thought to be self-limiting and not spread by human contact. In the 1950s, this ancient disease probably reappeared in 3,200 American soldiers in Korea. Doctors described it as Hemorrhagic Fever with Renal Symptoms (HFRS). It would be over twenty-five years before its cause, Hantavirus, would become elucidated and found in the United States. The virus was named after the Hantan River in Korea, the site of the 1950s outbreak, but when much later, it occurred in the United States, it became the "New World Hantavirus." This disease presented with pulmonary symptoms and not renal symptoms, and hence the name, Hantavirus Pulmonary Syndrome (HPS). By 2009, over 700 people were diagnosed in America.

Dr. Brian Callister documented Nevada's first case, and Dr. Stephen St. Jeor at the University of Nevada School of Medicine led the way with research. The following narrative tells the history of Hantavirus, reviews Callister's patients, and details St. Jeor's research.

In the 1950s, American soldiers stationed in Korea became ill with hemorrhagic renal syndrome with 20% mortality. Doctors recognized all the soldiers had the same disease, but efforts to identify its cause was unsuccessful. In 1978, Hantavirus was isolated from a striped field mouse, and doctors concluded Hantavirus had caused HFRS in the American soldiers. A survey of rodents in the United States determined different rodents were hosts to different strains of Hantavirus. The common rat carried Seoul Hantavirus, and the meadow vole carried Prospect Hill Hantavirus.

The survey suggested Hantavirus in the U.S. had evolved within separate rodent species.

After these revelations, researchers reviewed patients in the Centers for Disease Control and Prevention (CDC) database and found three patients in Boston with a mild hemorrhagic disease, and several patients on dialysis with antibodies to Hantavirus.

This was just the beginning.

On May 14, 1993, the New Mexico Department of Health reported three unexplained deaths among previously healthy individuals. Two were engaged to be married to one another and died within days of each other. Later, the Indian Health Services identified five patients who died from acute respiratory failure in Four Corners, where New Mexico, Arizona, Utah, and Colorado meet. Investigating agencies could not find the cause, like the situation that had occurred in Korea. However, within eight weeks, ten people died from acute pulmonary failure in Four Corners. All tests were negative, but CDC scientists using a test developed by the U.S. Army found antibodies to the Hantavirus. Researchers also found the virus in mouse excrement, and Hantavirus nucleic acid sequences were then detected in a deer mouse in the home of the first deceased couple. The new world virus was named Four Corners where it was discovered, but residents rejected the notoriety. The virus was subsequently renamed Hantavirus Sin Nombre, which translates to "Hantavirus Without Name." Once the infectious agent was discovered, CDC researchers took steps to determine risk factors and focused on patients in Four Corners with unexplained acute respiratory distress or pulmonary interstitial infiltrates.

Less than three months after the 1993 cases in Four Coroners, Dr. Callister reported two patients with Hantavirus in Nevada were treated by him, Chris Ward DO, and Hank Hayes PA.

The first Nevada patient in July 1993 was a 24-year-old housewife from Round Mountain, who presented in Tonopah with acute respiratory distress. She had a one-week history of fever, myalgia, nausea, and malaise. When admitted, she had bilateral interstitial infiltrates consistent with Adult Respiratory Distress Syndrome (ARDS). In addition, she had antibodies to Hantavirus. Up until then, clinicians treated Hantavirus with intravenous fluid and antiviral Ganciclovir, but they had 90% mortality.

On the other hand, Callister felt this disease was secondary to an overactive immune response, and treated his patient with high flow oxygen, aggressive diuresis, and high dose corticosteroids.

One month later, a 51-year-old man from Tonopah developed fever, myalgia, nausea, and vomiting over six days. Within twelve hours after admission, he had rapidly 'progressing interstitial infiltrates', shortness of breath, and hypoxemia. He also had high levels of antibodies to Hantavirus. Once again, Dr. Callister treated the patient with oxygen, diuresis, and corticosteroids. Both patients fully recovered.

Dr. Callister related the following noteworthy facts about his patients:
1. Both were treated at Nye Regional Medical Center in Tonopah, even though physicians in Arizona and New Mexico criticized Callister for not referring them. Yet, both patients survived while referred patients had 90% mortality.
2. Both patients lived in filthy living conditions conductive to mice propagation.
3. A guiding principle for Callister's treatment was his opinion that adults with intact immune systems develop ARDS, and
4. For example, babies, elderly people, and 340 immune-compromised individuals rarely develop the syndrome suggesting the life-threatening complications of ARDS are indeed due to an overactive immune response rather than viral toxemia. National guidelines now include corticosteroids as a treatment option.

After Dr. Callister's experience, by December 1994, there were 108 patients with HPS, and over one half were from Four Corners. Most of these illnesses appeared in spring/early summer, which suggested environmental/seasonal factors. Researchers did not know whether this was a new disease or reemergence of an old disease. It turns out the second hypothesis is true.

In 1994, Dr. Stephen St. Jeor at the School of Medicine became interested in Sin Nombre Hantavirus. He learned about the virus from a friend, Dr. Stuart Nichole, who was in the special pathogen branch of the CDC. Dr. Nichole and colleagues discovered the virus in a deer mouse.

St. Jeor and Nichole received a grant to determine virus transmission and investigate a possible vaccine. St. Jeor found the virus in 40% of deer mice in Nevada. Truckee Meadows Community College in Reno had a terrarium of deer mice in their lunchroom. Approximately 20% of the mice harbored Hantavirus; however, not one worker had the virus antibody even though a ventilation fan blew across the terrarium into the lunchroom. Even more interesting, the deer mice had been together for several months, but they did not have close to a 100% infection rate as might be expected in animals living together in a cage.

In a closer-to-home tragedy, in the early 1990s, two faculty members in the College of Agriculture at UNR contracted HPS; one recovered but sadly the other died. When one looks at the difference in transmission statistics in the United States, the presence of Hantavirus in individuals (forest workers and mammologists) is very low compared to the carrier rate of the virus in deer mice. However, at-risk-individuals in Europe have a much higher infection rate than U.S. workers adding to the mystery in differences in spread and immunity. Initially, evidence of the virus was found in salivary glands and kidneys of the rodents, but it could not be grown in the laboratory. Later, CDC scientists were able to isolate Hantavirus from deer mice but not from humans.

Dr. St. Jeor's study of the New World Hantavirus stretched from Reno's San Rafael Park to an Argentinean ski resort, Baraloche, where the strain is known as the Andes Hantavirus. It is the only Hantavirus is proven to pass from human to human. St. Jeor worked to discover why the virus only occasionally affects humans and determine how the virus is spread between rodents. In the U.S., the total number of reported cases is approximately 400, the number of cases in South America is over 1,000, and worldwide there are about 100,000 cases per year. Dr. St. Jeor is also worked on the development of a vaccine, but because of the small number of human cases, pharmaceutical companies considered it to be financially impractical.

On another level, researchers questioned why the 1993 Hantavirus had reemerged in greater numbers than in previous years.

They desired to determine factors that would predict future outbreaks. It was discovered rain enhanced food supply producing an increase in deer mice. In 1997, there was a significant early rainfall, suggesting to scientists the possibility of a Hantavirus outbreak. The department of health warned Four Corners authorities about the increased risk.

Despite these warnings, the number of patients increased from six in 1995-97 to thirty-three in 1998, which supported the precipitation theory. The Sin Nombre strain of Hantavirus is present in the United States, and while it may not be widely reported in the news, it is still taking lives. In 2010, five children from Four Corners developed HPS and one died. All five lived or played in areas near deer mice.

The Sin Nombre virus is in Nevada, but if it will ever cause many infections like the Old World HHRS strain is uncertain. One thing is clear, to prevent this disease one needs to avoid areas where rodent's droppings are present or can be aerosolized. The <u>HPS-virus-carrying-deer-mouse is brown, unlike the common gray-colored-house-mouse</u> found in homes throughout the world. On the other hand, there are other rodents that carry Hantaviruses associated with human infections, such as the Prospect Hill virus that is found in meadow voles throughout the world. The best advice is to avoid contact with all mice and voles.

After Dr. Brian Callister finished his residency at UCLA Nye Regional Medical Center recruited him with financial aid from the Rural Nevada Health Service Corps to relocate to Tonopah. He knew Tonopah from re-fueling stops in the small airplane when he flew as a child with his surgeon father. During four years of practice in Tonopah, he cared for the patients with Hantavirus and became friends with physicians from Reno. When he decided to move to Reno, it was because of his relationships and respect for those Reno physicians, some of whom had flown into Tonopah regularly to see patients for him.

Dr. Stephen St. Joer, a graduate student at the University of Utah, studied mechanisms by which arthropod-born encephalitis viruses, after being dormant reappear in the spring. This research was instrumental in stimulating his interest in viruses found in nature.

He worked with human herpes viruses for 30 years, both at the Pennsylvania State University's Hershey Medical Center and later at the University of Nevada School of Medicine, where he was working when the outbreak of Hantaviruses in Four Corners renewed his interest in the spread of viruses. When his colleague, Stuart Nichole, who had worked at UNR's College of Agriculture and the School of Medicine, moved to the CDC, St. Jeor remained friends with him. They later agreed to jointly study the new Hantavirus, which reignited Dr. St. Jeor's interest in the survival of viruses in nature.

## Infectious Diseases in 1800s Frontier Soldiers
### By Dr. Anton Sohn

During the early years of military presence in Intermountain West, 1861-1865, Civil War Years, servicemen in the East had a higher mortality and morbidity rate from disease than soldiers and male civilians in the West. The health conditions in the East reflected inadequate sanitation and poor hygiene due to crowding and poor conditions during the Civil War. In the West, living conditions were more healthful due to less contamination of the environment and good climate.

Later, military surgeons commented on the salubrious effect of the climate and altitude on the health of the command. For instance, Surgeon Edward P. Vollum at Fort Douglas, Utah, in 1874 noted he and the local physicians observed the beneficial effect of Utah's climate on phthisis (tuberculosis) and asthma. In a report to the Surgeon General Vollum stated, "There were no cases of phthisis unconnected with heredity transmission. Furthermore, early cases of tuberculosis get well spontaneously from the beneficial effects of the altitude and the inland dry character of the atmosphere." He continued, "The beneficial influence of this climate on asthma is decided and deserves a prominent mention."

On the other side of the Great Basin similar comments were made. In June 1867 at Fort Independence, California, Assistant Surgeon Washington Matthews stated there was one trifling case on sick report during the month. In 1873, at Fort Warner, Oregon, there were 3-6 on sick report a month and an average strength of 50 men. In all, most soldiers enjoyed good health at the Great Basin commands.

Sanitation, hygiene, and adequate food supplies were still a problem for the soldiers stationed there. Doctors did not understand the role of the mosquito in malaria and the role of fomites in the spread of some disease had not been elucidated. As a result, food, water, and utensils were sometimes contaminated; bad habits extended and increased the risk. In this environment epidemics of dysentery or diarrhea caused by cholera, typhoid and other enteric diseases were a threat to military camps and the civilian population.

Other diseases such as rheumatic fever spread in epidemic proportions through the West partly because the importance of the 'contagious' sore throat was not associated with the severe arthritis. Frequent questions on the military examination for doctors emphasized concern about these issues. Thus, poor hygiene, uncleanliness and spread of contaminated material were the most important factors in the spread of infectious diarrhea, the most prevalent disorder on the frontier.

After diarrhea and other epidemic diseases, the surgeon spent most of his time treating more mundane problems. By reviewing the hospital records one can get an idea of the day-to-day practice at Forts Churchill, Bidwell (California), Halleck, Independence (California), McDermit and other Great Basin posts. During 1860 and 1861, the aggregate strength of Fort Churchill varied from 182 to 284 while admissions to the hospital varied from 23 to 70 per month. For one month an outbreak of diarrhea and other diseases hospitalized 34 percent of the command, with an average length of stay of three days, leaving no doubt the hospital was full, and the strength of the command was depleted.

Between 1870 and 1874, a four-year period, health conditions at seven Great Basin forts, Cameron (Utah), Bidwell (California), Douglas, Halleck, Harney (Oregon), Independence (California) and McDermit, were reported to the Surgeon General. At Fort Cameron, the mean strength of the command varied between 181 and 215 men and upper respiratory infections led the list with eleven cases.

Although respiratory infections were, from time to time, a problem in the Great Basin, diarrhea was a greater threat to life.

Fort Douglas had an average of 364 men and diarrhea was the most common disease with 836 cases over a four-year period. Trauma from accidents with 671 cases, malarial fever with 472 and rheumatism with 400 were next in frequency. Later in the 1890s when 600 were stationed at Fort Douglas, Assistant Surgeon Deshon reported, "The hospital averaged about twenty patients, the commonest causes of admission being tonsillitis, rheumatic affections, venereal [disease] and trauma."

At Fort Halleck with a mean strength of 99 men and four to six officers, the most common cause for sick call was trauma (152 cases during the same period). Harney had mean strength of 56 and trauma was also the most common disorder with 176 cases.

Independence had a mean strength of 48-63 and rheumatism and accidents were equal with 40 cases each. For the same period at McDermit the mean strength was 59 men with two to three officers and fever led the list with 103 cases. Thus, each fort had unique problems, but none was immune to alcoholism, intestinal disorders, and other disease that from time to time occurred.

Over the four-year period there were 1,477 men per year on sick call (not including trauma) at the seven bases (Cameron, Bidwell, Douglas, Halleck, Harney, Independence and McDermit). The average number of men stationed at these combined bases was approximately 969 producing a sick rate of 1,524 per1,000 men. During this period the sick rate for the whole United States Army varied from a high of 2,087 in 1871 to a low of 1,561 in 1873. Therefore, the military sick rate on the Great Basin appeared to be at the low end of the average for the Army. If trauma is included the rate was 1,824 per 1,000 men.

A further breakdown of the specific illnesses during this early period reveals diarrhea accounting for 18.4% of the cases. Trauma accounted for 18.2% of the cases; malarial fevers were 12.1% and rheumatism resulted in 9.5% of the entries. Although alcoholism accounted for a high percentage of the admissions on occasion, overall it was 3.6%. Another social problem among soldiers was venereal disease. It was less than one half as prevalent as alcoholism.

In an interesting observation, Dr. George Martin Kober, in unpublished memoirs from Fort Bidwell, estimated as high as 15% of the soldiers who reported for sick call would not have complained of their illness in civilian life.

A word of caution is necessary about prevalence of disease in the 19th century because some diseases were confused with others. The diarrhea seen with scurvy was confused with the diarrhea of gastrointestinal disease. Scurvy associated arthritis was confused with other causes of joint pain and stiffness of the lower extremities. Also, fever and malaise associated with many infectious diseases sometimes overshadowed the more diagnostic features, resulting in misdiagnosis. Thus, malaria in camps during the Spanish-American War of 1898 was often confused with typhoid fever.

## DR. EDWARD JENNER, THE FIRST VACCINATION, 1796

In one of the most significant experiments in the history of medicine, on May 14, 1796, Dr. Edward Jenner confirmed cowpox inoculation conferred immunity against smallpox. Using an eight-year-old boy as a subject, Jenner proved his treatment-called vaccination (after the *Latin* for cow) could be used as a safe alternative to inoculation using the matter from smallpox pustules. Some physicians who had lucrative clinical practices providing inoculations went so far as to suggest not only was vaccination ineffective but \ its recipients would develop bovine features. Children were the preferred source of scabs since they reduced the chances of receiving sexually transmitted diseases during inoculation. The very real hazards of inoculation such as the development of full-blown smallpox or transmission of other diseases made vaccination attractive and ultimately successful. English country doctor Jenner's observation that milkmaids seldom fell victim to smallpox but did display symptoms of milder cowpox, led to a classic leap of scientific insight which was confirmed by his experiment.

**NOTE:**

Source of information was U.S. Army Medical Dept. (AMEDD) *Museum Notes,* May 1995.

## "RABIES IN NEVADA, MUZZLES AND BULLETS..., 1915"
### By Reuel Jake Measom, School of Medicine Medical Student

Outside the pages of fiction, the losses to the state, which depended largely on commercial livestock, were significant. Over the course of a twenty-month period conservative estimates placed the loss of livestock at over $750,000 (which adjusted for inflation is just over $17 million today). The severity of this disease, and the subsequent catastrophic industrial losses, prompted an organized effort that could be argued as one of the greatest public health successes in Nevada's history.

Rabies or hydrophobia is a particularly sinister and well-known condition, the course of which has been popularized in both literature and film. The disease is spread by the bite of infected animals as the virus is transmitted through the saliva. The bullet shaped zoonotic virus then invades the peripheral nerves and makes it way to the brain where it settles into the hippocampus and causes anxiety, paranoia, agitation, and hallucinations. The later stages progress to the classic hydrophobia, where the patient is unable to drink despite crippling thirst and from there into delirium, coma, and inevitably death.

The fear of impending death, and grueling symptoms that precede it, prompted many victims to commit suicide. The hysteria that precipitated this practice was quite prevalent even into the late 19th century when Louis Pasteur first developed a treatment in France. The initial product, while crude, found itself to be quite effective and the first use of which was well documented. In 1885, Pasteur performed the first successful post-exposure prophylaxis on a young boy named Joseph Meister, following an attack by a rabid dog. The resulting method, though initially frowned upon by mainstream science (many contested it was over applied and caused rabies in originally uninfected persons, the so-called *'rage du laboratoire'*), soon became the standard of care for rabies and was known appropriately as the Pasteur treatment.

Time of the Rabies, by Robert Laxalt, "If there's rabies out there, they'll show up. If they're sick, they won't be afraid of a man or his gun."

"So what am I supposed to do?" Ramon asked.

"Shoot-and-shoot-and-shoot…" Cade replied.

In the early 1900s, an old-world malady was introduced to the western United States. The disease was rabies, an ancient misery making fresh tracks on a landscape that had never known its flavor of cruelty. The disease made its way from California in 1909 and slowly worked into the surrounding states where it established itself. This epidemic in Nevada was sufficiently terrible to prompt famed Basque-Nevadan author Robert Laxalt to pen the novella, *Time of Rabies*, which fictionalizes the account of a family of Basque ranchers as they cope with the losses and the dangers of living and working in the heart of the epidemic.

Pasteur Institutes were set up throughout Europe and North America to prepare and administer the lifesaving vaccine. The vaccine was made by infecting rabbits to produce the virus. Once they were noted to exhibit rabid symptoms and perish in a uniform time frame, the spinal cords were removed and dried for varying periods with potassium hydroxide. The drying time was the key to the dose to produce immunity. The cords were ground up and placed in a solution of broth or saline for administration. Patients received injections from cords dried for 14 days and injected sequentially until a "two-day cord" dried for two days was used (immunity was built by giving serial vaccines with an increasing viral load).

The procedure was reputed to be only slightly less terrible than the disease. It included 21-25 subcutaneous abdominal injections over a period of 18-22 days, with three doses given on the first day. Despite the crude nature of the treatment, it was highly effective. There is no known case in Nevada where the prescribed treatment failed. One doctor noted that with the addition of proper dog laws, rabies is one of the most preventable of diseases.

In Nevada, public officials had been able to track the progress of the disease through the neighboring states but could not prevent its inevitable entrance beyond its own borders. It started in California, appearing as early as 1909, then, making its way into Oregon by way of a sheepdog in 1912.

The sheepdog is thought to have spread the disease into the wild through a fight with a coyote, which then propagated the epidemic. The first known case of rabies in Nevada occurred in April 1915.

A band of coyotes came into Humboldt County from southern Oregon. Soon afterward the disease passed into Washoe County from eastern California, and into Elko County from Idaho. Radiating out from three different routes the full force of the epidemic was fast approaching.

Nevada health officials led by Dr. W.B. Mack at the Nevada State Hygienic Laboratory recognized entrance of the disease was only a matter of time and thus took preemptive action for public health measures. They obtained a sample of virus from Dr. W.A. Sawyer at Berkeley to begin preparations of the Pasteur treatment previously described. In addition to the medical prevention measures, the state formed the Nevada Rabies Commission. This was the first organization of its kind, an entity dedicated entirely to the control of rabies.

In September 1915, the executive office of Nevada issued a public service announcement, printed in newspapers statewide describing the threat, modes of spread, and the methods to be used for containment. By that time, the federal government had become involved. The U.S. Biological Survey and the state entered into a cooperative agreement to hire men 'to hunt, trap, and poison' animals, namely coyotes, with a propensity to be vector for the infection. In addition to wild animal control there were strictly enforced police regulations requiring the muzzling or destruction of all dogs. It was noted one of the most serious obstacles in the control of rabies was the degree of affection many people exhibit towards dogs. The rule was stern and enforced. Dogs found without a muzzle, even while on a leash (and in one case while in a fenced yard) were shot on sight. In terms of the wild hunt, death tolls were significant.

From October 1915 to December 1916 over 8,800 coyotes, 1,300 badgers, 1,200 bobcats, and 100 mountain lions were shot or trapped. Two hundred and fifty thousand poison traps were also set that may have killed an additional 25,000 coyotes. The degree of success on the campaign was such that many of the men who worked as fur traders began selectively leaving females alive to sustain a future livelihood.

Despite the aggressive animal control, the cost in livestock losses remained tremendous (though likely mild compared to what could have been).

The true success of the public health measures undertaken by the state can be appreciated by examination of human rabies cases, or lack thereof. Since the introduction of rabies to Nevada in 1915 until the epidemic tapered off around 1920 there were a total of 186 persons administered the Pasteur treatment by the Nevada Hygienic Laboratory. Although no exact figures exist, it is estimated that greater than 200 other persons received some form of anti-rabies treatment by private physicians in the state. Not a single person who received the vaccinations was known to have suffered the full course of the disease. In fact, according to the modern Nevada Public Health Department there has never been a verified human rabies death in the state.

There are, however, two notable exceptions as described by Edward Record DVM: "In 1932 ...so far as known, at most only two persons have died of rabies because of exposure to infection in Nevada. Neither of these patients received preventive treatment. One died in an isolated location during a storm-bound period without medical attention, but the history and the symptoms reported leave little doubt as to the diagnosis. The other case was a man bitten by a dog, which afterward proved to be rabid, who left Nevada and was lost track of. This man was reported to have died of rabies later."

The first Nevada rabies epidemic posed a very real threat to the health and safety of the population. With quick action, the concentrated efforts of public officials resulted in what could be considered a near best case scenario outcome.

Rabies still exists in Nevada but is rare. The most common culprits are bats, an occasional ground squirrel, and even more rare, dogs. The State Hygienic Laboratory is now known as the Nevada State Public Health Laboratory at the UNR School of Medicine. As previously mentioned, there has never been a single documented human rabies death in Nevada, a statistic not shared by surrounding states. Whether or not the continued success of rabies control is attributable to the original epidemic and the implemented control measures is uncertain. What is certain is that Nevada set the bar for rabies control at that time.

## "Animal House"
### Yosemite Hantavirus Infections, 2012
### By Sally Higgins

Winner History of History of a Disease Essay for Second-year Students in Pathology Awarded the Measom Family History of Medicine $1,000 Scholarship. Dr. Higgins graduated May 18, 2018, and is a lieutenant in the United States Navy Medical Corps. She trained in emergency medicine at Naval Station Norfolk, Virginia.

> *One impulse from a vernal wood*
> *May teach you more of man*
> *Of moral evil and of good*
> *Than all the sages can.*
> *—William Wordsworth—*

In 2012, a strong smell of pine filtered through the trees along with rays of late summer sunlight. It was a beautiful day to be in Yosemite, the press of early summer over, but the chiller evenings of autumn still at bay. A small group of outdoor enthusiasts was where they most wished to be at the end of a long day, ready to settle in for the night in a much-coveted tent camp in Yosemite's Curry Village.

Curry Village is a mere mile southeast of Yosemite Village with unparalleled views of Half Dome and Glacier point. It was difficult to reserve a cabin, and individuals paid more than $140 per night depending on the accommodation type. There were two kinds of cabins available in Curry Village—regular cabins and signature cabins. Both were made up of simple wooden frames, elevated off the ground and covered by sturdy canvas. The signature cabins had a distinct feature that made all the difference for its guests: a hefty layer of foam insulation between the canvas and frame. This insulation provided superior temperature control and was found in no other cabins in Yosemite. Our small group of hikers that night all stayed in signature cabins, falling asleep, taking in the cool night air of the High Sierra, and dreaming of their grand and dusty adventures the next day.

About one month later, after returning to their respective homes in California, Pennsylvania, and West Virginia, each visitor began to develop unseasonal flu-like symptoms: chills, backache, and fever. Five days later, their respiratory function declined, then failed. Emergency chest x-rays showed pulmonary edema. The patients were admitted for respiratory failure, some were intubated, all underwent a battery of tests. Providers were mystified—they might still be if not for a critical clue, two of the patients from California presented simultaneously and both shared a history of recent travel to Yosemite. The patients' serum was tested for many pathogens and came back positive for one in particular—IgM antibodies against a strain of hantavirus. The California Department of Public Health, the CDC, and the National Park Service (NPS) Office of Public Health began an investigation of a possible Hantavirus outbreak in Yosemite.

Hantavirus is a large genus of over 200 single-stranded negative sense RNA viruses in the Bunyaviridae family. Unlike other viruses in that family, Hantaviruses are unique for being carried by rodents, not insects. Hantavirus is a particular virus. Only eleven of the two hundred Hantaviruses are known to cause human disease, and each is selective for rodents and regions. Each virus also inflicts a slightly different clinical form of the disease. The most common and well-known form is hemorrhagic fever with renal failure. This course of classic or old-world hantavirus has been well known, even if the virus- was later revealed to be the disease-causing agent during the Korean War, and so named for Korean's Hanta Valley.

Classic or Old World Hanta virus has a well-characterized natural course. First, a patient inhales aerosolized droppings of urine of a rodent carrying the virus. One to six weeks later, the victim presents with flu symptoms: fever, backache, and chills. Almost immediately after flu onset, the patient experiences abrupt hypotension, shock, and one out of three—death. Those who do survive go on to develop oliguria and renal failure, and half eventually perish.

Hemorrhage from Disseminated Intravascular Coagulation (DIC) and thrombocytopenia occur concurrently in the skin (petechiae), lungs (hemoptysis), and intestines (melena), engendering the term hemorrhagic fever.

The variant that struck Yosemite did not follow this pattern. It was a new type of virus, discovered a mere twenty years before—it was carried by a novel host, the deer mouse, and it targeted the lungs, not the kidneys.

The virus was called Sin Nombre (No Name). In 1993, a cluster of twelve people under age 40 died of unexplained respiratory failure in the Four Corners region of the United States. All presented with a febrile illness, respiratory symptoms, and progressive low platelet counts. The illness followed a rapid course; 75% of the patients died. Unlike the fever, hemorrhagic signs, and renal failure of classic Hanta, this variant presented more like unprovoked and rapidly fatal Acute Respiratory Distress Syndrome (ARDS). The one uniting factor for both types of Hanta infection? Rodent exposure. This called for a serious investigation.

So the outbreak of disease was met by an outbreak of research. Scientists soon discovered a horde of new hantaviruses. These so-called New World hantaviruses were associated rodents in the Americas, from territories as far north as Alaska and as far south as the Andes mountains. Overall, twenty new viruses were discovered and nearly all that caused human disease did so by infecting the lungs. A new term was born for this disease process, Hantavirus Pulmonary Syndrome (HPS).

Sin Nombre Virus (SNV) causes HPS by infecting vascular endothelium in the lungs. First, inhaled virus gains access to the lungs by infecting circulating dendritic cells or alveolar macrophages. This causes upregulation of special receptors in the infected cells. Once in contact with the lung microvasculature, the hijacked cells latch onto endothelial cells via integrins, and the virus payload makes contact. Once the virus is inside the endothelial cell, three units of single stranded RNA are transcribed by host polymerases into mRNA: each has a different role in replication, protection, encapsulation, and release from the host cell. Newly synthesized virus's bleb off the apex of the endothelial cells to infect their neighbor, and more alveolar macrophages in the airway.

The direct blebbing, along with the inflammatory and cytokine response, leads to severe microvasculature leakage in the lungs and progressive pulmonary edema. An average of two weeks (but up to six weeks) after the initial infection, flu-like symptoms develop. Five days after flu symptoms start, the infection can cause pulmonary edema, hypotension, and shock.

Thrombocytopenia occurs in almost all cases. The kidneys are rarely involved. Overall, 35% of those with HPS die, a case fatality rate on par with Ebola and smallpox. As in most viral infections, treatment is symptomatic.

The California Department of Public Health and the National

Park Service (NPS) had access to this earlier research. They knew the heaviest concentration of HPS was in the southwestern U.S. and HPS was caused by SNV from deer mice. When they investigated Curry Village, they found evidence of hundreds of Peromyscus leucopus, <u>(white footed brown deer mouse)</u>, living in the insulation of the signature cabins. <u>(The common house mouse is black.)</u>

Of the seventy-three deer mice captured near the signature tent cabins, ten had confirmed antibodies for SNV.

While the guests slept in the cots, the deer mice slept, ate, and bred in and around the specialized insulation of the signature tents. The mice also defecated and urinated, shedding virus in their droppings. When desiccated, these viral-laden droppings aerosolized and were inhaled by unsuspecting campers. Additionally, the specialized insulation protected the virus from denaturation by UV light, enabling it to survive for up to two weeks outside its mouse host. The insulation worked too well—it warmed the clients, housed the mice, and protected the virus.

The California Department of Public Health, NPS, and the CDC now had a clear picture of the Yosemite Hantavirus Pulmonary Syndrome: bilateral diffuse interstitial edema and respiratory distress within three to five days of hospitalization in an otherwise healthy person who had visited Yosemite. The patients essentially had fever with ARDS and a recent trip to the park. Yosemite officials acted quickly, coordinating with the National Park Service to minimize risk and warn those who may have been exposed.

Campers who had visited Yosemite that summer received pamphlets explaining the signs and symptoms and urging them to seek care if they manifested. All ninety-one of the signature tent cabins in Yosemite's Curry Village were closed. Over one thousand additional buildings in the park were inspected for rodents, and precautions were made to avoid infestation. The park began an intensified trap and surveillance program, particularly in Yosemite Valley. Ultimately, the NPS closed Curry Village, rechristening it as Half Dome Village in 2016. It is still the park's largest lodging area, but all traces of the signature tent cabins are gone.

Of the ten people diagnosed with HPS that year, nine had visited Yosemite National Park, eight had been infected in Curry Village, and three had died of HPS. Most experts agree the true case rate was higher than nine, as some individuals exposed to the virus likely suffered from a nonspecific febrile illness but recovered on their own. Serendipitous timing gave a critical clue to the California Department of Public Health, and thanks to the coordinated efforts of three major agencies, an investigation was underway quickly. Prior scientific research had already characterized HPS, elucidating the symptoms, identifying the host rodent, and improving serologic testing. A less publicized, but no less important lesson learned was how even seemingly benign interactions with animals—and the human alteration of their habitat—are not without risk. For those living in the Sierra Nevada, and for anyone who enjoys the outdoors, this may be the most important lesson of all.

# IX

+_+_+_+_+_+_+_+_+_+_+_+_+_+_+_+_+_+_+_+_+_+_+_+_+_+_+

# MEDICAL EVENTS
## "SUPPORTS NEVADA MEDICINE"

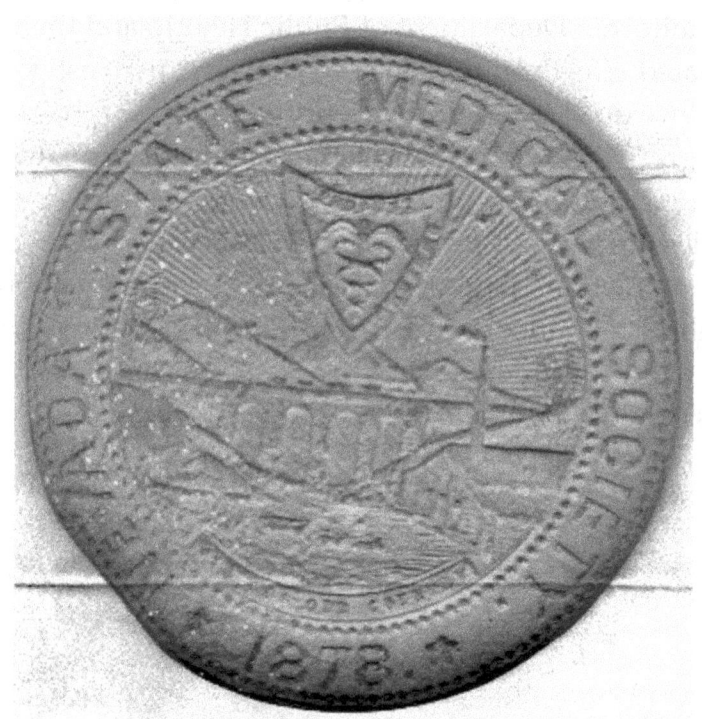

*1878 NEVADA STATE*
*MEDICAL SOCIETY MEDALLION*
FOUND IN VIRGINIA CITY DUMP 1930

+_+_+_+_+_+_+_+_+_+_+_+_+_+_+_+_+_+_+_+_+_+_+_+_+_+_+

# WASHOE COUNTY MEDICAL SOCIETY FORMATION, 1907

The following is a transcript of the organizational meeting of the Washoe County Medical Society, Reno, Nevada, May 25, 1907. An earlier attempt by Dr. Bergstein in 1872 was unsuccessful. The Washoe County (Nevada) Medical Society was duly organized on this date by the following named Physicians at the Elks Home, Reno, NV.

| | |
|---|---|
| C.H. Woods | C.E. Mooser |
| John Lewis | W.H. Hood |
| M.R. Walker | S.K. Morrison |
| L.J. Richie | R.L. Rice |
| B.F. Cunningham | J.L. Robinson |
| C.H. Francis | Washington Kistler |
| B.D. Bice | Roberts |
| R. St. Clair | R.Mc.W. O'Neal |

On motion duly made, seconded, & carried, Dr. Woods was elected temporary president, Dr. John Lewis temporary Vice-President and Dr. C.E. Mooser temporary Secretary. It was moved, seconded, and carried that the temporary officers be elected permanent officers.

Dr. Ben F. Cunningham moved that a committee on by-laws consisting of 3 members be appointed by the chair. Motion seconded and carried. The president appointed the following: Dr. Cunningham, Dr. S.K. Morrison, and Dr. M.R. Walker. Dr. W.H. Hood moved that the board of censors, consisting of 3 members be appointed by the chair. Motion seconded & carried. The president appointed the following: Dr. W.H. Hood, Dr. Washington Kistler, and Dr. C.H. Francis.

Owing to the intended departure from the State of our newly elected President, Dr. Morrison moved, seconded by Dr. R. St. Clair that the following resolution be adopted, and a copy be presented to Dr. C.H. Woods. Resolved: That the Secretary of the Washoe Co. Medical Society is hereby instructed to furnish our departing president, Dr. Woods with a letter of introduction to the San Diego County Medical Society in token of the esteem in which he is held by the members of this Society—motion carried unanimously.

## PETER FRANDSEN, A TEACHER TO REMEMBER, 1900-'42

The members of the selection committee of the Great Basin History of Medicine met with senior physicians from Nevada to select subjects for its continuing series of oral history studies. After interviewing a number of these candidates, we noticed an unusual coincidence. In conversations with these older doctors, almost without exception, the name of Dr. Peter Frandsen was mentioned.

Peter Frandsen, a native of Denmark, came to Reno with his parents at an early age. He was granted an AB degree from the University of Nevada in 1895, where he studied human anatomy, physiology, and histology with the intent of studying medicine. After graduating from Nevada, he took a job with a borax mining company, locating borax and soda deposits in the deserts of northwestern Nevada. Later, he found a job teaching in an ungraded school in central Nevada to save money for his further education.

One of his instructors at the University of Nevada, Dr. Cowgill, urged Frandsen to apply to Harvard University and secure a degree there before entering medical school. Dr. Cowgill's letters to Harvard gained Frandsen admission to that University as a sophomore without examination, and at the end of his first year, he advanced to senior standing. This was truly remarkable, since at that time the University of Nevada had not received full academic recognition, and Frandsen had no high school credentials.

Graduating from Harvard with an AB degree, he intended to study medicine. but was persuaded to continue graduate work at Harvard with the offer of a teaching fellowship. He served for some time as a laboratory instructor in comparative anatomy at

Harvard and in general zoology at Radcliffe College. He had completed some 30 units toward a PhD at Harvard when, in 1899, Dr. J.E. Stubbs, the president of the University of Nevada, visited Peter Frandsen in Cambridge, and offered him a vacant position.

To fill this position, Frandsen needed to acquire some experience with animal diseases, and arrangements were made for him to study at the Bureau of Animal Industry in Washington, D.C. during the summer.

Frandsen returned to Reno in 1900 during an anthrax epidemic in the Truckee Meadows. Fortunately, with the experience he had gained in Washington, he was easily able to diagnose the disease with his microscope and cultures in his laboratory.

He became assistant professor of zoology and bacteriology. For at least four summers, he and another biology professor spent weeks gathering botanical and zoological specimens. These expeditions, for the most part were spent on horseback and with pack train in Elko County. It was during these trips he developed his deep appreciation for Nevada. He was also teaching psychology. In 1909, he traveled in Europe for a year.

During those early years, Professor Frandsen developed a close association with the medical profession. Many the local physicians felt the need for help in diagnosing infectious diseases and pathology, and turned to Frandsen and his laboratory, where microscopes, slide preparations, cultures, and laboratory animals were available. Frandsen worked closely with local doctors and developed many close friendships.

He mentions many of the early doctors in his reminiscences but singles out Dr. W.H. Hood as perhaps his closest friend. Dr. Hood was the holder of Nevada State Medical License #1. Frandsen went on frequent vacation trips with Dr. Hood and his wife. They loved to go camping, fishing, or simply travelling. On these trips they met many old friends and made many new friends. Frandsen tells of one trip when a filling station attendant came limping out with his hand on his back.

Dr. Hood asked the man what his trouble was, and he replied his kidneys were hurting. Hood told him to raise his arms and began thumping on the man's back. Soon Hood exclaimed, "Kidneys nothing! What you have is a low-grade pneumonia from the flu. Here, make up this plaster. Put it on your back when you go to bed, and you'll be all right." "Are you a doctor?" The man asked, "What do I owe you?" "Not a damned cent, I'm on vacation," Dr. W.H. Hood replied.

There was a typhoid epidemic in Reno which was later traced to a dairy. The epidemic caused great alarm in the community.

Professor Frandsen, together with Dr. O.P. Johnstone of the State Hygienics Laboratory, prepared a vaccine against typhoid and announced it to the public to allay the concern. To prove the safety, they gave each other extra-large doses, and promptly suffered rather vigorous reactions.

Frandsen was a member of the National Social Hygiene Association, lectured frequently against the anti-vivisectionists, and gave lectures on venereal disease. As one of his duties with the Animal Experiment Station, he visited Farmers' Institutes all-over Nevada, and became acquainted with physicians, farmers, and ranchers statewide. He was a director and almost perpetual vice president of the Nevada Tuberculosis and Health Association.

Frandsen continued to be active both in scholastic and medical affairs. He was instrumental in the formation of the Student Health Service at the University, and together with LeRoy Fothergill, organized a pre-medical honorary society called Omega Mu Iota. This society later became affiliated with the national pre-medical honors society, Alpha Epsilon Delta. He gave several scientific papers before the Washoe County Medical Society and was invited to attend their meetings.

After returning from his sabbatical in Europe, he lectured to the Washoe County Medical Society about insect-borne protozoan diseases, with slides collected from laboratories in Rome, Paris, Berlin, and London. He was invited to present several papers at the Nevada State Medical Association meetings about hemophilia and on another occasion about the *Mendelian Inheritance of Night Business*. In 1924, he was granted an honorary Doctor of Law by the University of Nevada.

Peter Frandsen rather drifted into the directorship of the pre-medical program at the University of Nevada, and because of this program Dr. Frandsen became best known. Since 1895, several hundred pre-medical students from the University of Nevada have graduated from his program, and most of them have become physicians. A number became dentists, some veterinarians, several morticians, and many others have gone on to earn degrees in biology.

His students have earned positions in the Biological Survey, the National Park Service, and the U.S. Forestry Service.

Dr. Frandsen, to whom his students fondly referred "Professor Bugs" was widely known throughout the academic world. He took a personal interest in each of his students, carefully evaluating their abilities and guiding them in their studies. When he wrote a letter of recommendation to a specific medical school, the student could be virtually assured of acceptance. His students have received MD degrees from at least 21 medical schools in the United States. Frandsen was particularly proud of the fact that at least 12 sons of local physicians took their pre-medical studies with him and went on to become doctors.

Many testimonials to the great influence of Peter Frandsen can be found within the memoirs of his students. In his honor, the agriculture building, constructed in 1918, was named the Peter Frandsen Humanities Building.

A bronze plaque in his honor, commissioned by his former students, is inscribed with the names of 71 of those students. Most of these students are well known and respected physicians in the community. This plaque now resides at the University of Nevada School of Medicine History of Medicine Museum. Among his many other honors, he was given the Distinguished Nevadan Award in 1958. On several occasions, Dr. Frandsen was offered positions at other institutions, with the promise of higher pay and greater research opportunities, but his love of Nevada led him to decline the offers. Dr. Frandsen retired in 1942 as Professor of Biology and Head of the Department of Zoology. He moved to Oroville, California and operated an olive orchard until his death in 1967.

**NOTE:**
Some information is from an undated letter, Dr. Owen C. Bolstad.

## Persia Bowers, "1874 Mystery"
### By Eileen Barker

*Nevada State Journal,* July 15, 1874: "Died... In Reno, July 14th, Persia Bowers, age 12 " One hundred and eighteen years later the cause of this child's death remains as much a mystery as the circumstances surrounding her birth and adoption.

No official records of her death can be found, and sources of information are few and mostly unreliable. The story begins in 1859 when Lemuel Sanford "Sandy" Bowers, a miner in Virginia City, Nevada, met and married boardinghouse owner Alison "Eilley" Cowan. The two held interests in adjacent mines. The mines struck silver and the money poured in. They amassed a fortune reported to be $4,000,000.

In 1861, construction of a home suitable for the new millionaires was planned in Franktown, a lush valley lying between Carson City and Lake's Bridge (also known as Lake's Crossing, later renamed Reno). At this point, fact, and legend merge. It has been written that the Bowers traveled to Europe, and for two years, cut a wide swath shopping for and shipping home expensive furniture for the new home.

The story continues with the return trip aboard the USS Persia of the Cunard Line. While traveling from Liverpool to New York City, Eilley took as her own child the infant daughter of a woman, Margaret Wixson, who had died and was buried at sea. Eilley named the child Margaret Persia. Four years later in 1868, following the untimely death of Sandy Bowers, the widow was engulfed in financial difficulties. Creditors and bill collectors descended on the heavily mortgaged mansion and chaos ensued. To remove her from the daily upheaval, Persia was sent to Reno, twenty miles to the north.

Reno was incorporated in 1869. On Persia's arrival, the town was still in its infancy. Persia found in Reno a flourishing clutter of saloons, stables, blacksmith shops, hay yards, stores, hotels, restaurants, several churches, a schoolhouse, a theater, a weekly newspaper, and a fire department.

A handful of streets formed the town's business core, with residential neighborhoods clustered nearby. Persia boarded on West Street at the home of N.J. Roff, a harness maker, who also gave music lessons and played in the Reno Municipal Band. At the Roff home, Persia studied music and prepared her school lessons. She was a good student at the four-year-old Reno Public School.

On December 20, 1873, *Nevada State Journal* reported: "The usual closing examinations of the Reno Public School were held yesterday."

The examinations were under the supervision of Mr. Orvis Ring, the very efficient teacher. The average attendance for this term was about fifty.

Miss Persia Bowers recited her composition "Darwinism in the Kitchen."

As had been their plight in previous summers, during that hot summer of 1874, the citizens of Reno were plagued with fevers. Winds stirred clouds of dust from the primitive streets and rains turned the streets into quagmire. Most townspeople took untreated water from the Truckee River into which sewer lines emptied or drew water from the irrigation ditches which lined most of the streets

The fevers—typhoid fever, military fever, swamp fever, typhus, cholera, diphtheria, and malaria—were treated with mercury compounds like Calomel, with doses of quinine, or with sweating the patient. Patients were dosed with sulfur and molasses, herbal brews, lard, or even axle grease. Despite the crude therapy, some of them did recover, but many did not. The doctor's office of that day was simple and plain. Prescriptions were compounded by hand. Surgery was performed in the patient's home, and asepsis was often ignored.

The 1874 V&T Reno City Directory listed four practicing physicians and surgeons—Drs. William Bergman, Simeon Bishop, H.S. Brower, and C.W. Friedriechs. Dr. H.H. Hogan was the County Physician with an office at the newly built county hospital and poor house, a facility for the indigent sick.

The first general hospital in the state was St. Mary Louise Hospital, 20 miles away over Geiger Grade in Virginia City. In 1874, it was still two years away from completion. Much earlier, in 1861, a Dr. Joseph Ellis had taken over a cluster of hot springs at Steamboat Springs, a few miles south of the Truckee River and built a 34-bed facility which was a favorite place for miners from the Comstock to cure hangovers. It was not a general hospital in the usual sense, and in 1867, under suspicious circumstances that place burned to the ground.

Hospitals generally were greeted with suspicion and fear by the people of that time, for being sent to a hospital was a death sentence.

It would not be until 1903 that a general hospital would be "attempted" when an undertaker and veterinarian renovated and remodel the old Whitaker School for Girls on Ralston Hill. This proved to be an unsuccessful venture. In 1905, the Dominican Sisters would remodel their old schoolhouse, Mount

Saint Mary's Academy at 6th and Chestnut streets into the hospital (St. Mary's Hospital) that operates there today.

But for Persia Bowers on that hot day in July 1874, no such medical amenities were available when, in that little house on West Street, she developed a high fever, suffered intense pain, and quickly died. Her mother, summoned from the mansion in Franktown, was unable to reach her daughter's bedside before she died.

What caused Persia's death? No certificate of death can be found, for the state of Nevada did not require the recording of births or deaths until thirteen years later. The popular belief is that little Persia died of scarlet fever, but certainly a multitude of other possibilities exist. With better medical treatment, could she have survived to relate the intriguing story of her family? It shall probably remain a mystery.

## Professor Nathanial Wilson IV, "1899 Diabetes Guinea Pig"

### By Barbara Parish

In 1922, Nathanial Wilson IV was given the diagnosis of diabetes. At that time diabetes was almost always a fatal disease. Wilson was a chemist by profession and moved to Nevada in 1889 to become a professor of chemistry at the new land grant university in Reno, Nevada.

In 1922, dietary management was the only known method of treating diabetes mellitus. His family relates how he would sit at the kitchen table with his scales, carefully measuring every gram of food that he consumed. At the onset of his illness, he had been a short man of stocky build, but he soon became thin and gaunt from his limited diet.

He would test his urine for sugar by placing a specimen into a test tube, adding Benedict's reagent (*a copper reduction test*) and heating the test tube in a double boiler. The test tube would almost always turn from green to brown, an indication of high glucose. He would then attempt, by dietary management, to lower his glucose enough to enable him to function.

In 1927 or 1928, he was approached by Dr. Dinsmore, of the Nevada State Hygiene Laboratory, and was asked if he was willing to be a "guinea pig" in an experiment. Two of Dr. Dinsmore's associates from Canada, Drs. Banting and Best, were attempting to develop insulin for human use. Wilson, by then tired of the strict dietary constraints immediately agreed to participate in the experiment and became one of the first humans to receive insulin therapy. He remained insulin dependent until his death in 1961 at the age of 92 years.

Many of the local physicians referred their diabetic patients to Professor Wilson for help in managing their disease. He was acutely aware of the difficulties these patients would experience with wound healing, and was quick to provide them with Unguentum, a salve he had concocted and patented. He took great care with his own skin, especially the skin of his feet, and was quick to treat any injury he might sustain with the same salve. At the time of his death he suffered from some loss of vision, but otherwise had none of the other usual complications of diabetes.

Professor Wilson, together with one of his colleagues, did work on the early development of X-ray. They tested the effects of the machine by holding their little fingers under the machine. Eventually the repeated exposure to uncontrolled doses of X-ray caused great tissue destruction, with resulting atrophy so the fifth fingers looked like "a dried-up claw." Wilson refused to allow amputation of the digit, fearing that due to his diabetes the wound would not heal.

On one occasion, the professor came staggering home with the assistance of a neighbor, who assumed he was drunk. Although his daughter did not realize he was suffering from insulin shock, all she could think of to do for him was to give him a piece of chocolate cake and some apple sauce she had just made.

After this very effective treatment the professor rallied. He asked his daughter how she knew what to do, and all she could tell him was, "It just seemed to be the right thing to do."

**NOTE:**

This interesting look at the early treatment of diabetes mellitus was taken from an essay written by student nurse, Ms. Barbara Parish.

Her instructor, Susan Ervin RN, encouraged her to submit her essay to *Greasewood Tablettes*. According to Ms. Parish Nathanial Wilson IV was her great grandfather. His son, Nathanial Wilson V, was a 1913 University of Nevada graduate, who became a pharmacist, working in pharmacy until well into his 80's. One of Nathanial's sons, Frank (Tim) became Nevada State Drug and Dairy inspector, and his only surviving child is Ruth, the widow of the late James "Rabbit" Bradshaw, a Hall of Fame football player for the University of Nevada. Professor Wilson lead an active and productive life. He achieved some measure of fame when he and his wife took their 3-year-old son (Nat V) on a 12-day bicycle trip from Los Angeles to San Francisco in 1894 with Miss Bertha Bender.

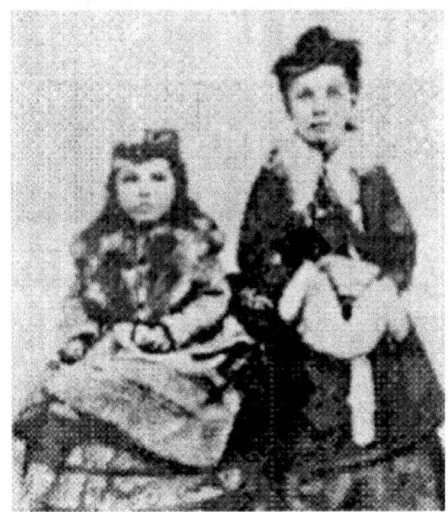

Persia Bowers (standing)

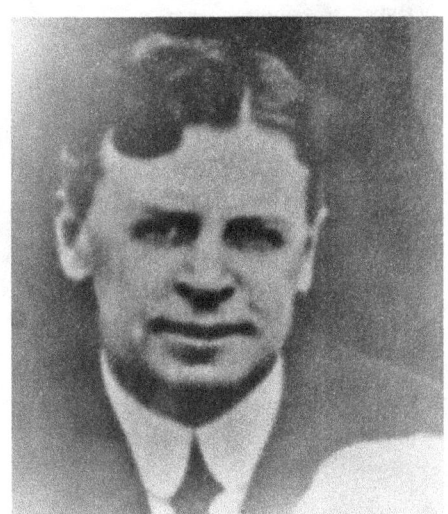

Dr. Ben Cunningham

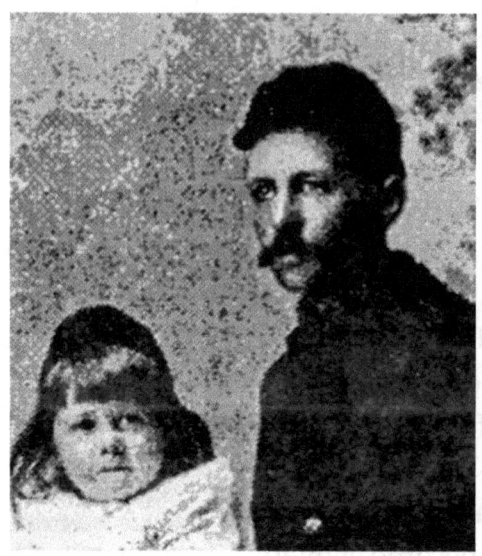
Prof. Wilson IV & son, Nathanial

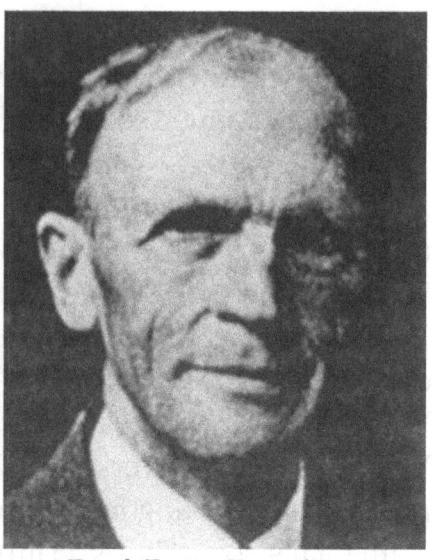
Prof. Peter Frandsen

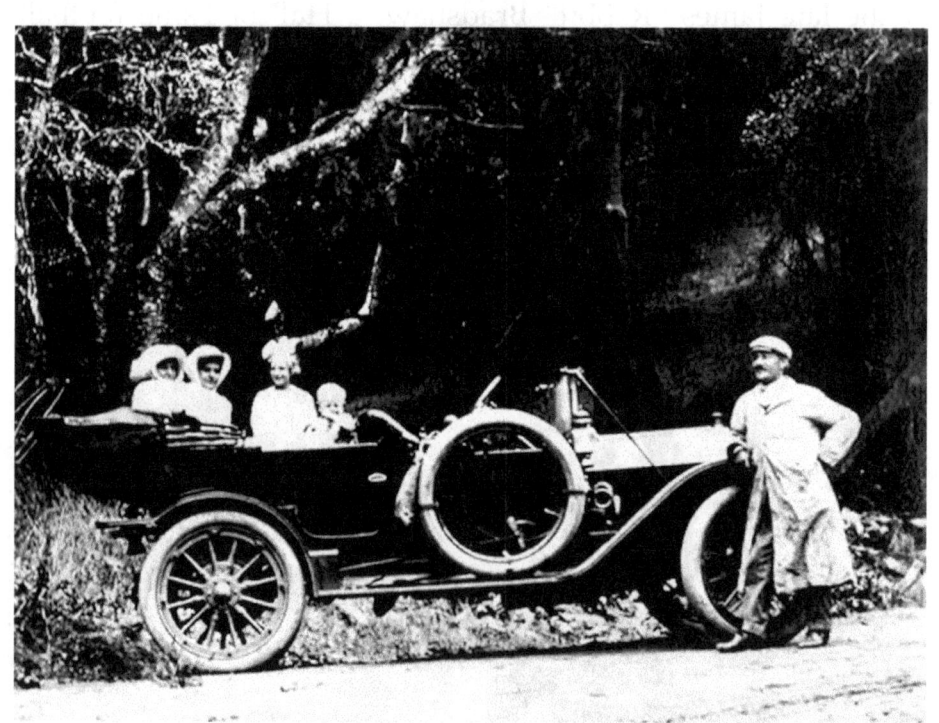
Dr. Raymond St. Clair and Family, 1925

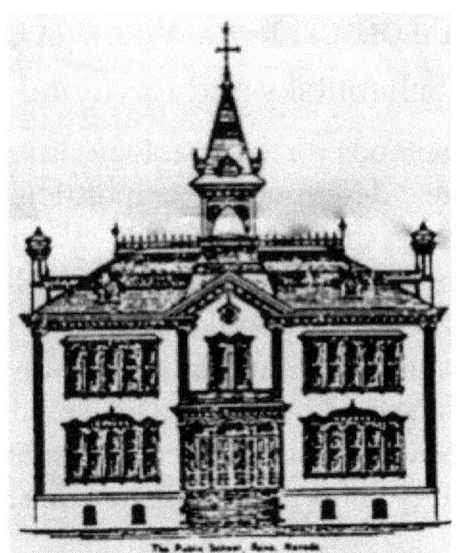

Reno Public School, 1874

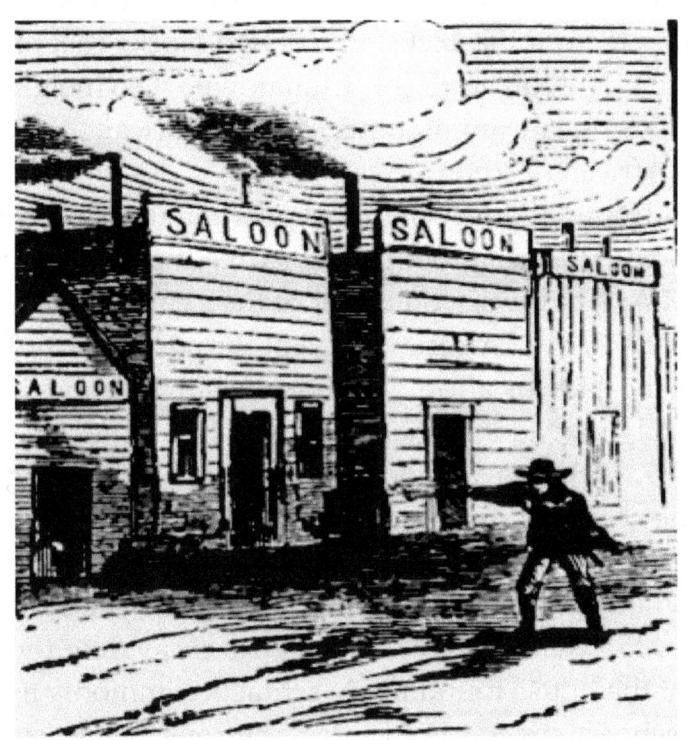

"Hamilton Main Street" in Harper's Weekly, 1869

# Medical Archaeology, 1870s Virginia City Artifacts
## By Julie M. Schablitsky and Raymond A. Grimsbo

Traditional methods of archaeology involve analysis of artifacts by date, description, composition, function, and location. A difficult challenge for urban archaeologists is to assign ownership to artifacts recovered from household refuse where there is high-density population.

Julie M. Schablitsky from Portland State University and Raymond A. Grimsbo of Intermountain Forensic Laboratories, Inc., utilized DNA analysis in the new subfield of forensic archaeology to study items recovered from an archaeological dig in Virginia City.

During excavation of a working-class neighborhood, they found the remains of a nineteenth century dwelling. The house was situated in a densely occupied, ethnically heterogeneous neighborhood from the 1870s. It was two blocks east of the red-light-district and adjacent to Chinatown. The neighborhood included European immigrants and Americans along with people of African descent.

The address, 18 North G Street, recorded in the Virginia City land deed book, appeared in 1873 as a dressmaker shop operated by Mrs. M.A. Andrews, a daughter of the Temperance Society.

In July 1873, Mrs. Andrews died at the age of thirty-five, and based on the lack of affordable housing in Virginia City, new tenants likely moved into that address that summer.

By 1875, a British family, the Coopers were living in that house. The crowded dwelling also contained Carpenter Thomas Cooper, his wife Eunice, and three children. In October 1875, a large fire that razed central Virginia City destroyed the house.

Almost 125 years later, archaeologists excavating the charred remains of the house found many artifacts commonly associated with households such as bottle glass, buttons, beads, stoneware, and straight pins. However, there was an unexpected find.

Discarded beneath the floorboards was a glass hypodermic needle. Within proximity were six more hypodermic syringe needles.

The discovery of drug paraphernalia prompted the questions: Who used the syringe and for what purpose, and what was injected? The hypodermic injection of medicines, particularly morphine, became widely accepted across America during the 1860s and 1870s. Although other drugs such as quinine, caffeine, atropine, and strychnine were used, morphine was injected about ninety percent of the time.

Morphine and syringe kits were available in local pharmacies. Easy access to drugs gave rise to nonmedical drug use. Injection of morphine was more potent and less expensive than opium smoking. The effect of morphine on the body included a warm glow of benevolence, a disposition to do great things, and a mental calmness. The low cost and the sense of euphoria may have encouraged the social use of morphine. Dr. F.E. Oliver observed in 1872, "The sulphate of morphia seems to be growing in favor, its color and less bulk facilitating concealment, and being free from the more objectionable properties of opium."

No social strata were untouched by morphine use and addiction. Examination of four of the needles recovered during the excavation demonstrated human DNA in two of them. The STR (Short Tandem Repeat) technique suggests multiple users of the hypodermic syringes and associated needles. Additionally, both male and female DNA were found in at least half of the samples. Most intriguing is the presence of three loci most common in the populations of African descent. These findings show at least four different people used the syringe.

Schablitsky and Grimsbo suggest a likely scenario was a social gathering of at least four adults where morphine was injected for euphoric effects, as recreational drug use was common on the Comstock.

Forensic science has proved to be an invaluable tool to

archaeologists. DNA analysis and the STR have found historic data unattainable by the archaeologist and historian. The discovery of drug paraphernalia in the archaeological ruins of a house opened the door into the past, and forensic science has taken us through that door. What could never be found in history books is the physical profile of the drug user and the social setting in which the activity took place.

The discovery of multiple users, presence of both male and females, and a probable link to people of African descent on the hypodermic syringe boldly illustrates the need to incorporate forensic science into the field of archaeology.

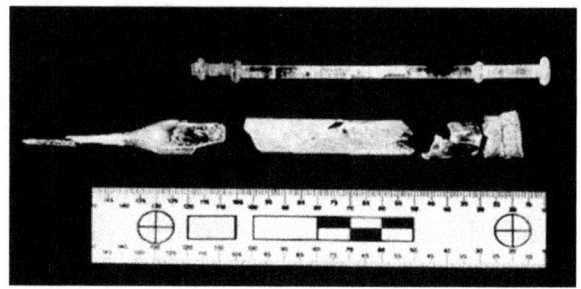

Virginia City Needle and Syringe, 1800s

## WEST'S PREMIER SURGICAL SOCIETY
## HISTORY OF RENO SURGICAL SOCIETY (RSS)
### By Phyllis Cudek

By 1960, members of RSS numbered 44, and membership required board certification or equivalent training-and that 60% of one's practice be surgical in nature. Originally only one dissenting vote was needed to block membership; this was subsequently changed to 90% approval of the polled membership.

Perhaps the 1960s, 1970s, and 1980s can be defined as a somewhat "golden age" in the history of the group. Reno grew in population, but not so rapidly that medicine and its personality was compromised. Meeting places varied to include Coney Island Restaurant, Peppermill Casino, Hidden Valley

Country Club, Johnny's Little Italy Restaurant, and Yen Cheng Restaurant. The tradition of cigars for everyone after dinner continued, and Dr. Fred Boyden continued to tell his well-known "shaggy dog" stories. The order of the evening was cocktails, a thirty-minute speaker, and then dinner.

Sadly, however, as the years passed, interest dwindled among the Reno physicians and good medical programs were harder to arrange.

However, eventually membership was expanded to include family practitioners, In 1961, continuing medical education credits were offered for the first time. However, the annual meeting was discontinued. At a later meeting, Governor Grant Sawyer would praise Reno's physicians, noting they had dispensed approximately $2,000,000 in free care to residents.

Reno became the center of American medicine in the 1970s when Dr. Wesley Hall, Sr. past president of Reno Surgical Society and Nevada State Medical Association became president of the American Medical Association. Yet, Reno Surgical Society attendance declined.

So, to stimulate interest, prominent speakers were invited to some monthly meetings. Thus membership increased to over 100 members. This increased popularity of monthly meetings and led to the adoption of two hosts to divide the cost of meetings.

A few of the subjects presented over the years at Reno Surgical Society meetings included: metal prosthesis in orthopedic surgery, radiological treatment of carcinoma of the breast, stomach cancer, medical legislative problems, biological warfare, peptic ulcer, blood alcohol content, space age medicine, trauma systems, anesthesia, medical malpractice, Medicare participation, aging, and cost of surgery.

In the 1980s, annual meetings were held at various locations, such as North Lake Tahoe where the guest speaker was Covert Bailey, renowned exercise physiologist and nutritionist; Silverado Country Club in Napa Valley, again with Covert

Bailey; Furnace Creek in Death Valley; and Yosemite National Park featuring Reno pathologists who spoke about the tragic chartered airplane crash in Reno in 1983.

Unfortunately after about 1987, the keeping of scrapbooks and records regarding the activities of the organization, were discontinued, although some meetings did continue.

1998 was a landmark year for Reno Surgical Society. It celebrated 50 years in existence. Dr. H. Treat Cafferata, surgeon, and past president, spoke of the history of the organization and showed numerous slides dating back to the beginning of the group in 1948.

Treasured photos depicting enjoyable, enlightening, and humorous times brought back many memories. Dr. Cafferata says, "several talented individuals have presided over this organization which, I believe has provided a significant benefit to this community. It is unfortunate there are not more records of the events of the past decade."

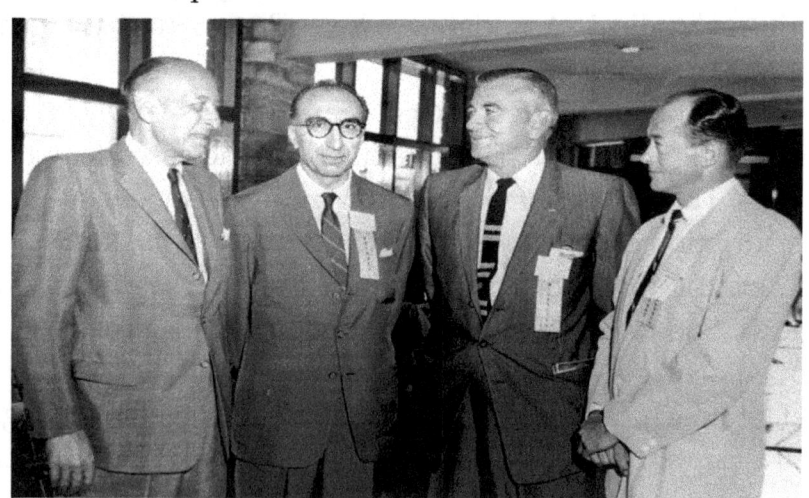

Reno Surgical Society, early 1960
Left: Dr. John Cline (President AMA, 1951-2),
Dr. Michael DeBakey (Renown cardiac surgeon),
Dr. Wesley Hall, Sr. (President AMA, 1971-2),
Dr. William O'Brien, Jr. (President RSS)

As of 2005, there were 65 members, one-third of whom were retired from practice. Thus organization would disband at the end of 2005 or in early 2006. (Records of RSS are in the History of Medicine Museum.)

## HISTORY OF DERMATOLOGY IN RENO, 1946-2005
### By Dr. Roderick Sage

Dermatology is a medica discipline that can be traced to antiquity and is thought by historians to be the oldest medical specialty.

The skin, being an external organ and visible to anyone interested, readily presents its afflictions for study and treatment. The fact that so many of those rashes look alike has led to great confusion, which in the course of time has been enhanced by the nomenclature of skin disease.

One practice has been to label a disease after some early observer, who gained immortality by attaching his name to a new mystery eruption. Further confusion results when a skin problem may be described with Greek or Latin whoppers. Here is a relative well-known example—pityriasis lichenoides et varioliformis acuta, also known by its eponym as Mucha-Habermann Disease.

Perhaps because skin diseases are rarely fatal, dermatology has been considered more of a minor specialty, but to those suffering with a skin problem it is a major issue. And more so if the problem is one of the viral poxes or blistering disease such as pemphigus—very serious indeed!

The American Board of Medical Specialties was conceived in the early 1920s and incorporated in 1932. Its initial organization was the American Board of Dermatology and Syphilology. Syphilis was a major cause of skin afflictions before the age of penicillin. The syphilis designation was dropped in the 1960s when penicillin had all but eliminated syphilis, but as it turned out only temporarily because syphilis made resurgence.

Dr. Charles McNitt was the first certified dermatologist to practice in northern Nevada. He was a medical graduate of Columbia University where he also trained in dermatology. He came to Reno in 1946 and practiced until 1957. Dr. Mortimer Falk came to town in 1952 and continued practicing until 2002. He graduated from the University of Michigan School of Medicine and trained in dermatology at the University of Pennsylvania. The third early skin specialist was your author, Dr. R.D. Sage, who came to Reno from Stanford University in 1958.

In earlier times, the first dermatologists served the northern half of Nevada and a wide swath into Northeastern California from Alturas to Bishop. With the retirement of Dr. McNitt in 1957, Dr. Falk had the sole responsibility for the dermatology problems of this large area until Dr. Sage arrived.

The situation was stable until the mid-1970s, at which time the population of Nevada and the numbers of new physicians, both specialists and generalists, began to surge. (The population of Reno, Sparks, Carson City, and contingent areas in the mid-1950s was close to 60,000; as of 2005 it has burgeoned to 1,000,000, while the state is 3,000,00.)

Until the last quarter of the twentieth century the number of certified American skin specialists was stable at 1,500, and they tended to cluster around larger cities, especially if a medical school was nearby. The most recent estimate of American dermatologists approaches 18,000.

Treatment modalities until the recent twenty years were rather stable. The most used and dependable was ultraviolet light for inflammatory ailments including acne, psoriasis pityriasis rosea, and many forms of eczema. We also treated acne and stubborn inflammatory dermatoses with x-ray therapy, but this method is now outmoded because of the fear of radiation side effects and the development of better treatment forms.

Topical management of skin problems was, and still is, the mainstay of the dermatologist, and more so fifty years ago. A fair amount of hocus pocus helped in the concoction of our various potions, lotions, and brews containing mixtures of tar, sulfur, salicylic acid, menthol, and phenol, to anchor our therapeutic arsenal in the control of itching and inflammations.

In recent years these "nasty-looking-stinky-messes" have given way to the more tolerable and effective steroid preparations for use both outside and inside the skin. To control itching, many older skin doctors used several sedatives, such as barbiturates, chloral hydrate, and even aspirin. Currently tranquillizers, antihistamines, and some of the recently developed immune modulating drugs are the mainstay of treatment. There was once a great reliance on dietary measures, the most memorable being the dictum against eating chocolate to control acne. We now know that is mostly nonsense.

The 1970s coincided with the establishment of the University of Nevada School of Medicine (UNSOM), which opened in 1970 as a two-year School of Medical Science with thirty-two students. It expanded to a four-year MD granting program in 1977.

The first four-year class of thirty-six graduated in with an MD degree 1980. With the growth of UNSOM, the facilities in Reno and Las Vegas have developed superb teaching programs.

Reno surgeon Dr. Fred Anderson was named the "Founding Father" of UNSOM, having been in the forefront of a lengthy struggle for funding from the Nevada Legislature. Ultimately, a multi-year donation from the Howard Hughes Foundation convinced the legislature to fund the school. Not to be forgotten are the numerous Nevadan physicians and generous lay persons, who helped make the new school possible. The class size has been steady at close to sixty in the last few years. At first males predominated, but in recent years the distribution by sexes is equal.

Initially, most of the medical classes were held on the UNR campus and at the Veterans Hospital. The early focus was on the preclinical sciences (anatomy, physiology, pharmacology, pathology, and biochemistry). Introductory clinical courses were offered in surgery, medicine, obstetrics and gynecology, and psychiatry, and believe it or not, in dermatology. Dr. Falk and I conducted a rather compact ten-day clinical review in conjunction with the student course in skin physiology.

Years later after the students had matriculated elsewhere, we learned in many cases our offerings were their only dermatological exposure in all their training.

With the advent of our medical program and its expansion to four years, parallel changes were evident with the growth of Reno, Nevada, and the whole country. Reno exploded from being a lively small city to a boomtown big city. In fact, Nevada showed the greatest percentage state population increase in the United States during the late twentieth-century. The new school helped to blunt the predicted shortage of medical practitioners.

For the two dermatologists who held the fort for so long, 1958-71, changes were underway. A half dozen new skin specialists came to town in the 1970s: Dr. Tom Standlee, Dr. McCarty, Dr. Steve Billstein, Dr. Larry Gardner, Dr. Victor Rueckl, and Dr. Charles Clemmensen. In the 1980s, we welcomed Dr. James Torok and Dr. Burdick. The 1990s saw more new faces, but in the current century the floodgates opened.

By 2010, twenty-eight dermatologists were available to serve the 300,000 area residents and an equal number of persons in contiguous and mainly rural Nevada and California counties. In keeping with the formation of group practice, Doctors Kevin Kiene and Bret Blackhart in Reno opened an office with seven partners and a modern new building. Dr. Clemmensen in Carson City has followed suit with a four-member group and a substantial building. In addition, smaller coalitions have formed.

In the last ten years, we have witnessed the coming and going of several itinerant skin doctors who rented space in rural communities such as Winnemucca, Fallon, Elko, and Yerington. For their monthly visits they would allegedly cram dozens of patients onto the schedule, charge what were said to be outrageous fees, then scurry back to their home base in southern California. Their commitment to the local community and patients was almost nil.

Fortunately, as more dermatologists have arrived, these services became provided on a permanent basis from Reno and the days of the medical nomads have ended.

The American Academy of Dermatology (AAD) is the heart of our specialty, boasting 16,000 members in 2010 compared to 1,500 in the 1960s. The AAD sponsors its annual convention each spring in various cities with a premier teaching program and a notable attendance from abroad. This is the one national meeting that members feel obliged to attend.

In recent years, all of medicine benefited from the tremendous surge of research leading to the development of innovative treatment techniques. A broadly expensive therapeutic arsenal abetted by pharmaceutical contributions and development of creative instrumentation is part of this modernization. There have been notable advancements in skin surgical methods such as Mohs Microsurgery to evaluate margins of skin tumors and laser surgery technology.

Corticosteroids also evolved to offer more effective treatment methods. With the advent of the topical and systemic retinoids (Accutane et al) we found a favorable treatment for severe acne.

New immune altering chemical agents related to Tumor Necrosis Factor (TNF) inhibitor type drugs nurture hope for eventual cure of some of the most difficult skin diseases. Antibacterial therapies are in a perpetual state of refinement, and we hope are keeping at least one jump ahead of the antibiotic resistant microorganisms. Also specific cosmetic modalities such as Botox became widely available.

At the latest count, the Reno area has twenty-eight specialists (board certified or board eligible dermatologists). The increased number of specialists has led to the increased availability of many procedures, many being cosmetic in nature such as liposuction, scar removal of all kinds often related to acne, hair transplants, wrinkle ablation, and laser treatment of tattoos and birthmarks. This phenomenon is related to the increased competition amongst dermatologists and the marked demand for more cosmetic procedures, aided by an expansion of residency training programs. Of major significance is the fact that cosmetic surgery is usually payment in advance of service. Insurance coverage for these procedures is minimal, thus the frequent hassles with carriers are eliminated.

An inspection of the practice of dermatology in Reno in the past fifty years reflects changes in American medicine in general. We have seen the numbers of dermatologists expanded 5-to-10-fold. We daily witness a broad range of advances in our ability to diagnose and treat skin problems. We note the availability of well-trained skin specialists now serving full time in areas previously without such care.

All in all, the outlook is excellent for dermatology and all of medicine to come to terms with the many significant problems mankind faces in a changing world.

## "The Mollie Folly," 1908
### By Ryan Davis

In 1910, *Carson City News* reported historic surgery by four prominent physicians, but current medical knowledge raises a doubt on their diagnosis. Like the men in the *Carson City News* lead article, these doctors contributed to the advancement of Nevada medicine during the early twentieth century.

On December 12, 1910, Drs. George McKenzie, Reine Hartzell, Ernest Krebs, and Donald Maclean took part in the removal of sixty to seventy pounds of tissue from a prison inmate named Mollie Marrison (Harrison). What was her diagnosis? Elephantiasis.

At first glance this event may not sound odd to the reader, but there are two glaring discrepancies in the medical report. "Well, for one, it is highly unlikely a patient in 1910 could have over sixty pounds of tissue removed and survive" says Dr. John Iliescu, a retired Reno plastic surgeon, who is one of the doctors featured in our book *The Cutting Edge*. "The amount of fluid that would be lost by the patient alone would be enough to result in massive complications."

The other anomaly present is the diagnosis of elephantiasis. What makes the diagnosis odd is the area in which it was diagnosed. According to Dr. Donald Maclean, who was the resident doctor at Humboldt State Prison and the man responsible for the diagnosis, the disease was present in the woman's breasts.

Elephantiasis is a disease caused by filarial roundworms that inhabit lymph nodes, causing infection, inflammation, and swelling. This inflammatory swelling occurs mostly in the limbs of infected patients or in the scrotum of some male patients.

"Since a female's lymph nodes that supply the breast are located primarily in the axillary region, it is highly unlikely that elephantiasis could ever occur in her breasts. In elephantiasis the patient's arms would become inflamed instead of her breasts" states Dr. Anton Sohn, pathologist at the University of Nevada School of Medicine.

Considering these revelations, one must wonder what, indeed, was Molly Marrison's (Harrison) diagnosis. Was she the recipient of a radical- record-breaking new procedure, or a doctor's misdiagnosis?

It isn't as if the doctors who led the procedure were a group of mad scientists. Dr. George McKenzie, the lead surgeon, was, in fact, one of the leading physicians not only in Nevada but the entire Far West. Along with being one of the founders of St. Mary's Hospital and its training school for nurses, he founded Mt. Rose Hospital.

Dr. George McKenzie was president of the Nevada Medical

Society at the time the surgery took place and a member of the American Medical Association and the American College of Surgeons. He graduated from Rush Medical College in Chicago and after taking graduate courses at Bellevue Hospital in New York, he studied medicine at universities in London, Edinburgh, Glasgow, and Dublin. According to Sister Eulalia Cramsie, who assisted Dr. McKenzie as a nurse at St. Mary's: "McKenzie was an exceptional performer in those small, white-tiled surgical rooms. He was a fast worker at a time when total sterilization of the operating room was impossible. He was a wonderful surgeon."

Further research reveals no case of elephantiasis was diagnosed in a woman's breasts. Furthermore, no case of sixty to seventy pounds of tissue being successfully removed in any type of surgery was found in a review of 1910 medical journals.

What exactly was Mollie's folly? Did she just have abnormally huge breasts?

**NOTE:**

Following is an email we received from Guy L. Rocha, Asst. Administrator for Nevada Archives & Records: "I read with great interest the article entitled *The Mollie Folly* by

Ryan Davis. I wanted to know more about this woman, so I looked for her prison inmate case file. Mollie was a black woman, age 23 in 1908, sentenced to 10 years in prison in Carson City for 2nd degree murder in Winnemucca, Nevada.

Dr. Donald McClean [Maclean] was the resident doctor at the State Prison in Carson City and not the Humboldt State Prison. For many years, the only state prison facility in Nevada was in Carson City.

Dr. Donald McClean [Maclean] mentions the operation in his report in 1910, which is part of the Prison Warden's biennial report in the Appendix to Journals of Senate and Assembly for 1911: "In Harrison's prison record when she was seeking release from prison in 1911, she mentions the medical procedure and that she still has health problems despite the surgery. There is nothing more about the operation. It appears she was released from prison in 1913 as there are no records in her file after 1913."

The surgeon was Dr. Donald McClean [Maclean] (1872-1938), the father of longtime Reno surgeon, Dr. Ken McClean [Maclean]. The prison record indicates "Mollie Killed a negro in her tent in Winnemucca with a knife." The record further states under marks, scars, moles, deformities, et cetera, "breasts abnormally large." She was paroled in July 1911 from her second-degree murder conviction.

## HISTORY OF MEDICAL MALPRACTICE IN NEVADA
### By Dr. Thomas Brady

Dr. Brady was a past president of Washoe County Medical Society, Nevada State Medical Association, and the Western Section of the American Urological Association.

Practicing medicine in Nevada, over the last forty years, has been complicated by medical professional liability issues. Perhaps one of the most serious adverse effects of malpractice from a doctor's point of view, is its impact on the physician-patient relationship. It is essential that an open, trusting, caring, and aggressive doctor-patient relationship exist for the best medical care. If physicians see patients as potential adversaries, medical care clearly will suffer. We have always been patient advocates, not their adversaries.

During the period 1935 to 1975, 80% of all malpractice lawsuits were filed in the last 5 years of that period. Amounts awarded to plaintiffs were going up because of the influence of inflation, increasingly liberal judges and juries, and aggressive trial lawyers.

From 1974 to 1976, under-prepared and under-funded professional liability carriers or insurance companies left the market and a crisis of availability of insurance developed. Some physicians went bare and had no insurance.

To help solve the problem, Nevada created a physician-owned, non-profit insurance company, Nevada Medical Liability Insurance Company (NMLIC). About the same time, Doctors Company was created in California. This relieved the availability of insurance problem. Nevada had ventured into voluntary medical-legal screening panels in the 1960s.

The idea was to keep frivolous lawsuits from going to court and provide quicker settlements when malpractice and injury occurred. Hopefully, this would also lower costs. In 1975, the Nevada Legislature made these voluntary panels mandatory for all claims. The panels were less than satisfactory because 30% of claims rejected by the panels went to court anyway.

There were so many claims that the panels were terribly backlogged, and the plaintiffs' attorneys used the panel as a means of discovery using the accumulated information in subsequent litigation. As frustration with the panels rose, trial lawyers, insurance companies, and doctors all joined in lobbying the legislature to again make this medical-legal screening panel voluntary, and this passed in 1981.

Costs for liability insurance continued to soar. Malpractice insurance premiums increased on average of 22% per year from 1980-1985. Multi-million-dollar judgments became more common in areas such as neonatal pediatrics, neurosurgery, and especially obstetrics. The coverage available was $1 million per case and $3 million total. Since almost all the babies delivered in rural Nevada were delivered by family practitioners, they simply could not afford the $36,000 per year cost of insurance and stopped delivering pregnant women. Obstetrics in rural Nevada was gone, and a new crisis developed.

In 1985, the Nevada State Medical Association (NSMA) began a long and ultimately successful lobbying effort for TORT Reform. This effort was opposed by the Nevada Trial Lawyers Association (NTLA). The four basic TORT Reforms proposed were:

1. Limits on liability (cap on awards for non-economic loss)
2. Periodic payments of court awards (in lieu of lump sum payments)
3. Limitation of attorney contingency fees (sliding-scale increments)
4. Collateral source payments (prevention of double payments in court awards)

I was involved in the lobbying effort and there were many intense discussions with the trial lawyers and legislators. Finally, a deadlocked legislature and the Judiciary Committee led by Bob Sader directed us to meet and make a compromise proposal.

Bill Bradley, David Gamble, Dr. Anton Sohn, and I met, and the outcome was a new medical/legal screening panel. The new panel was much more effective. The five basic parts were:

1. It was mandatory
2. It was based on records only (the plaintiff and defendant did not face each other)
3. The results were admissible in court
4. If the panel found for the defendant and the claimant lost in court, the defendant must be awarded costs and attorney fees
5. If the panel found for the plaintiff, a settlement conference must be held

The new medical-legal screening panel proved to be successful, but the battle for real TORT Reform was just started. The issue of medical malpractice would not go away despite the success of the screening panel. Medical liability created tension between legal and medical professions.

Physicians believe reform of the TORT system is needed because the present system is too slow, too expensive, unfair, and doesn't consider the life and death decisions that doctors face and make and confront daily. They believe a system which gives an average of 30 to 40 cents per dollar awarded to the injured patient is not effective.

Lawyers, on the other hand, see the TORT system as a fundamental part of our social system which rights civil wrongs and holds doctors accountable.

They see themselves as instruments of rectification and justice. As such, the face-off has stood. It would not end until 2005 when true TORT reform was passed through the initiative process on the public ballot and then enacted by the legislature. At that time, the medical-legal screening panel was abolished, and in retrospect, many wish it was still in effect.

## HISTORY OF GRAVE ROBBING
### By Todd Savitt PhD

The Great Basin History of Medicine Society held its annual fall meeting at the Airport Plaza Hotel in Reno on November 14, 1994. The meeting was well attended with about fifty medical students and other society members appearing for a nice dinner of Salisbury Steak, and the Airport Plaza's world-famous mashed potatoes, together with a splendid dessert.

The featured speaker for the evening was Dr. Todd L. Savitt, medical historian from East Carolina University School of Medicine. Dr. Savitt is currently a guest lecturer at the University of Montana School of Medicine in Missoula, Montana and is well-known as a medica historian.

Dr. Savitt's topic was *Resurrection and Dissection: Aspects of the History of Grave Robbing*. In his talk, Dr. Savitt traced the study of human anatomy from the days of Plato in the fourth century BC through the days of Galen, continuing through the Arabic spread of the Greek philosophy.

In the early days of medicine, anatomists had great difficulty obtaining suitable material for their study and dissection, and too often were forced to rely upon grave robbers (also called resurrectionists) to obtain specimens for dissection. During one period in England, body snatchers were accused of murdering the homeless to obtain bodies. It was a fascinating talk, well-illustrated with sometimes gruesome pictures made from old journals, and it served to demonstrate the problems encountered in the development of science.

**NOTE:**

Several early Nevada MDs mentioned grave robbing to study anatomy.

## PROF. WALTER MILLER MD, PHD, UNIV. NEV. 1ST PROF. OF SCIENCE, 1887

Dr. Walter McNab Miller was the first professor of science at the University of Nevada. He was born in Osborn, Ohio on July 10, 1859, and graduated from Columbus High School in 1875. After teaching school for years, he entered Ohio State University, graduating with a BS degree in 1885. While attending the University Walter McNab Miller taught natural science at Portsmouth High School and served as principal for two years.

In October 1887, Professor Miller began his duties at the University of Nevada as a chemist, bacteriologist, botanist, meteorologist, geologist, and curator of the museum. He was granted a "life diploma" in teaching from the University of Nevada soon after he arrived in 1887.

He made a fieldtrip to the valleys of the Humboldt and other rivers to gain first-hand knowledge of botany in Nevada. He published *Interdependence of Plant Life and Climatic Conditions in Nevada* from information gathered on the fieldtrip.

From 1889 to 1899, he was professor of anatomy, physiology, and geology at the University of Nevada. From 1896 to 1899, he served as bacteriologist and pathologist with the experiment station. He was frequently consulted about diseases of animals. During the time that he was at the University of Nevada he was registered as a student at Cooper Medical College (now Stanford SOM) in San Francisco and received his degree in medicine in 1895. Dr. Miller also attended Johns Hopkins University, Harvard University, and studied at the Universities of Leipzig.

He became professor of pathology and bacteriology at the University of Missouri in 1902 and became widely known for his role in formulating health programs and health legislation, both in Missouri and nationally. He was recognized as a pioneer in the field of public health. He lived in Columbia, Missouri until his death in 1942.

## Robert Koch & Arthur C. Doyle, "Quest to Cure Tuberculosis" *The Remedy* (Thomas Goetz) 1890

### By Louis "Gene" Toole

In *The Remedy*, Thomas Goetz provides us with a well-written and easily readable narrative on the history of medical progress in mid to late nineteenth-century Europe as the leading minds sought to understand cause, cure, and transmission of infectious disease. Great debates raged in the medical and scientific community for years and even decades.

Competing theories abounded and Goetz skillfully elaborates on the substance of the issues and the personalities involved with sufficient detail to inform, but not so much as to bore the reader with minutiae.

Today, the idea of "germs" as the cause of many diseases is regarded as common sense and obvious; but that was anything but the case at that time.

General acceptance of the "germ" theory was slow in coming even as professional and well-documented research offered ever more proof. Enter Dr. Robert Koch, a German physician trained at Göttingen University who became a central figure in the story. Early in his career he took a position as a local health officer in Wollstein, an agricultural town, where he enjoyed a thriving practice but, in the evenings, he conducted research in his kitchen. He established a protocol for his research which he followed meticulously as he begun to identify specific bacteria as the cause for various diseases. Rigid adherence to his well-developed protocol enabled him to convincingly defend the conclusions of his work and he rose rapidly to become one of the most prominent scientists in Europe.

He was promoted and given significant additional resources by the Kaiser so that he might continue his research on a grander scale and thus enhance the reputation of German science in the eyes of the world. In his new position, Koch decided to attack the problem of tuberculosis. It was a formidable challenge. Tuberculosis (or consumption as it was commonly known at the time) is a dreaded worldwide killer. In England fully one quarter of all deaths were due to tuberculosis.

In 1900, it was listed as the number one cause of death in the United States. There was a powerful incentive to find a cure. Whoever did so would provide not only an immeasurable benefit to mankind but to their own fame and fortune.

Meanwhile, the renowned French scientist, Louis Pasteur, became aware of Koch's work and is impressed with his methodology and results but Koch after all is; "gasp"—a German. Pasteur checked Koch's work by successfully replicating some of his research, which created animosity and a hostile exchange between the giants for a considerable time.

This eventually subsided, but an ongoing can-you-top-this competition between them took place to identify evermore causes and cures.

In 1882, Koch finally isolated the bacilli that causes tuberculosis and presented his findings to the medical community.

Those present were thoroughly convinced by his demonstration. The next obvious step was to determine a cure. Then, in 1890 Koch finally thought he had it. The very idea created worldwide euphoria at the prospect of a cure for this killer. Clinical trials began immediately to further quantify results.

Arthur Conan Doyle was a little-known English physician

trained at the University of Edinburgh in Scotland. He conducted a modest medical practice in Southsea, England, but his true passion was writing (he will later become the renowned author of Sherlock Holmes). He had followed the work of Koch for a decade and at the announcement of a cure he hastened to Berlin to observe demonstrations and to tour the clinic where patients were being treated. While touring the wards of treated patients he was taken aback. Koch's process appears uncontrolled and chaotic, and his documentation does not meet his historically rigid standards. Doyle cannot personally observe any difference between treated and untreated patients.

In addition, Koch was secretive about his cure, and he was reluctant to give samples to others so they can conduct independent trials. Doyle was suspicious the purported cure was not a cure at all. It seems Koch may have been premature in his announcement. Doyle summarized his observations in a letter to a British periodical. It was a bold decision because he, a relative nobody in the field of medicine, is challenging the great Dr. Koch. Others also express the same feelings as Doyle, but Koch's reputation protected him for a time.

Eventually additional samples of "the cure" were made available to others so they could conduct independent trials. As these additional clinical results began to come in from various sources, they were not favorable to Koch and his reputation suffers. The world would have to wait for the promised cure. The cure for tuberculosis was not found until World War II when antibiotics were discovered and found to kill the mycobacterium that causes tuberculosis. Goetz was an award-winning science writer and had a master's degree in public health from UC Berkeley and a master's degree in literature from the University of Virginia.

**NOTE:**

Every medical student/medical doctor knows <u>Koch's three Postulates</u> for infectious disease. ONE: The microorganism must be found in abundance in all individuals suffering from the disease, but not in healthy organisms, TWO: The microorganism must be isolated from a diseased individual and grown in pure culture, and THREE: The microorganism causes disease when introduced into an experimental host.

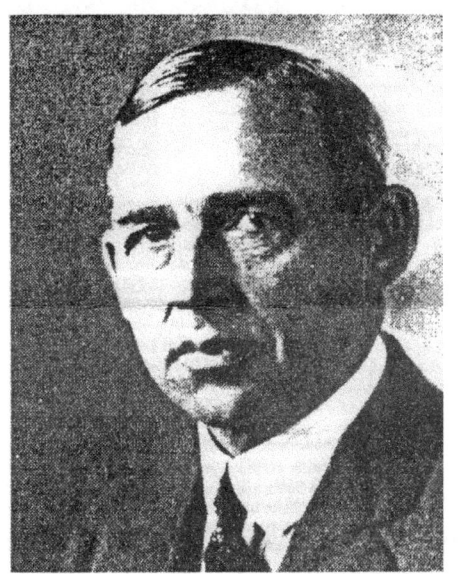

Professor Walter McNab Miller     Dr. Reine Hartzell

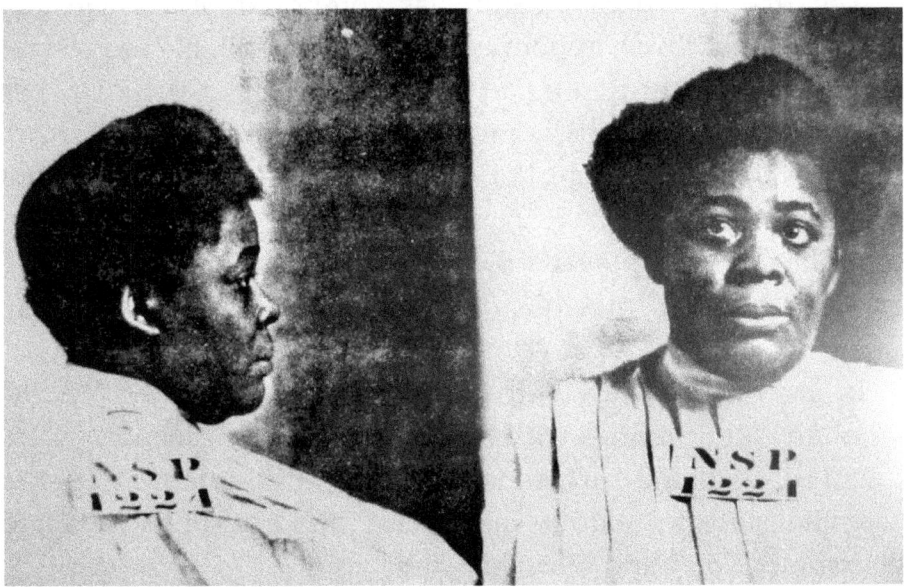

Mollie Harrison (From her Prison Record) 1908

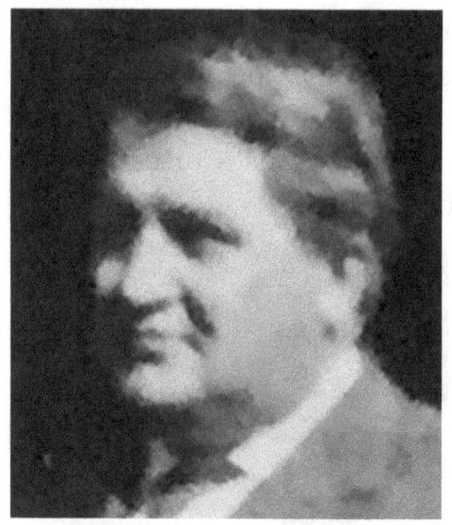
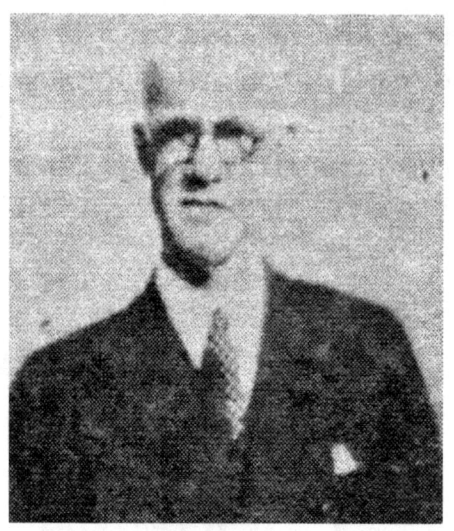

Dr. George McKenzie    Dr. Donald Maclean, Jr.

## PUBLIC HEALTH IN NEVADA, THE FIRST FIFTY YEARS
### By Dr. Donald S. Kwalick

In March 1992, Nevada began its centennial year of "organized" public health in the state. This report concerns the first fifty years in the rich history of our state.

The first Board of Health was composed of the Nevada governor and three appointed physicians—J.J. Henderson of Elko, J.A. Lewis of Reno, and S.L. Lee of Carson City. Dr. Lee remained an active participant for thirty-three years (until 1926). Over this time, a great deal of energy was spent in development of vital statistics.

As late as 1900, Nevada did not require physicians to report: ".... all cases of contagious disease... and all deaths from any cause."

In 1910, there were still no mandatory morbidity reports, although all counties (except Lander and Lincoln) were voluntarily making such reports. Finally, on March 27, 1911, a state vital statistics statute was enacted, and in 1912 Nevada had its first morbidity and mortality statistics:

| Disease | Cases | Deaths |
|---|---|---|
| Pneumonia | 330 | 102 |
| Pulmonary TB | 190 | 52 |
| Smallpox | 215 | 3 |
| Typhoid Fever | 228 | 24 |

In 1913, Nevada state law required the Boards of County Commissioners to appoint local health officials at not less than $25 per month. All physicians were required to report all cases of smallpox, diphtheria, and scarlet fever within 24 hours, and all "contagion" by the fifth of each month for the previous month. Willful neglect or refusal was subject to a fine of not less than $5 and no more than $25.

In 1920, Nevada was the only state without a full-time health officer. In 1929 Nevada finally adopted the U.S. model vital statistics law and therefore for the first time, became part of the Federal registration system for births and deaths. We were the last state in the Union to adopt this model law.

In 1934, forty years after establishing our Board of Health, Dr. John E. Worden became the first full-time State Health Officer. During the period from 1935-40, the State Board of Health, with 26 full-time employees, was the state's fourth largest department.

In the early 1940s, the Board was reorganized into the Nevada State Department of Health and was composed of eight divisions:
1. Administration and Training.
2. Vital Statistics.
3. Maternal and Child Health and Crippled Children's Services.
4. Dental Hygiene.
5. Public Health Engineering.
6. Local Health Administration, Epidemiology.
7. General Disease Control.
8. Laboratories.

During the first fifty years, the Health Department struggled to find qualified full-time staff. Development of an efficient system of reporting birth, death, and disease statistics was one of the major problems.

Only after the passage of state regulations for the reporting of communicable disease, enacted on January 24, 1992, did Nevada finally join the rest of the nation with an effective Public Health law.

**NOTE:**

Dr. Donald S. Kwalick was the State Health Officer for Nevada until January 1997 when he moved to Clark County Health Department.

## Public Health in Nevada, The Second Fifty Years
### By Dr. Donald S. Kwalik

During the first fifty years there were only four individuals who held the office of State Health Officer. The second fifty years of public health in Nevada, from 1942 until 1992, were times of enormous change in public health throughout the country. During the second half of the century there were twelve different State Health Officers, with two of them serving for more than 10 years. The position of State Health Officer was abolished by the State Legislature in 1983 and re-established in 1987. During this period Dr. George Reynolds served as acting State Health Officer.

In the early forties and fifties, the State Board of Health was composed of two physicians, one dentist, one lay person, and the Governor. This board selected its chairman and the State Health Officer, who served as Secretary to the Board but was not a member. The State Health Officer also served as executive head of the State Department of Health. It was a turbulent mixture of both public health and politics that formed the background for the current organization. These are some of the outstanding events that occurred during the second 50 years:

1. 1947—A branch State Health Laboratory was established in LV.
2. 1948—Dr. Daniel J. Hurley, was appointed State Health Officer and provided stable leadership for 16 years. Physicians were appointed as County Health Officer in all Nevada Counties.
3. 1949—The Clark County Health Department was formed, and a full time Health Officer appointed. Enabling legislation passed to receive Hill-Burton funding. Seven Hill-Burton projects were initiated.
4. 1950—Seven counties had public health nursing services, weekly news releases, and radio programs regarding public health activities.
5. 1952—There was an unusual outbreak of Rocky Mountain Spotted Fever. Nevada suffered the worst polio epidemic in its history with 108 cases and 8 deaths. Hospital surveys and inspections began.
6. 1953—Reportable disease list was revised. New confidential reporting form adopted.
7. 1954—Salk polio vaccinations began in Washoe County. Three fatal cases of botulism were reported.
8. 1957—Special Children's Clinics established in Reno and Las Vegas. The Nevada Dental Society purchased a mobile unit for rural dental services.
9. 1958—The Reno/Washoe County Health Department was organized.
10. 1959—Food and Drug lab activities transferred from University of Nevada to DOH.
11. 1960—Legislation enacted to provide care for indigent tuberculosis patients. DOH reorganized into six bureaus: Environmental Health, Preventive Medical Services, Mental Health, Public Health Nursing, Hospital Services and Vital Statistics. Nevada Public Health Association established.

12. 1962—Nevada had the highest birth rate in the U.S. Dr. John F. Carr resigned as Clark Co. Health Officer. District Health Departments established, with County assuming financial responsibility.
13. 1963—Dr. Otto Ravenholt appointed Clark Co. Health Officer. State Health Department became the Division of Health in the Department of Health and Welfare.
14. 1964—Bureau of Maternal and Child Health and Crippled Children's Program began. Dr. Hurley replaced by Dr. W.T. Weathington beginning an era of rapid turn-overs as Health Officer.
15. 1966—Nevada was the first state in HEW Region IX to have all participating hospitals certified for Medicare.
16. 1967—Dr. William Bentley appointed to the Board of Health, serving for 25 years. A rabies emergency discovered in Ely and White Pine Counties.
17. 1968—Deaths due to heart disease dropped to below 30% for the first time in Nevada. State was first in Southwest US to comply with Federal Clean Water Act.
18. 1969—Division of Health bureaus centralized in Carson City except for Laboratories and Preventive Medicine services. Infant death rate in Nevada was 3-5 points higher than U.S. average.
19. 1970— "Stop Rubella" campaign in Washoe Co. Rubella becomes a reportable disease.
20. 1972—Nevada became 24th state with Atomic Energy Department (AEC) agreement regulating radioactive material.
21. 1973—Department of Health and Welfare became Department of Human Resources. Air and water pollution programs transferred to new Division of Environmental Protection under the Department of Conservation and Natural Resources. Bureau of Mental Health became Division of Mental Hygiene and Mental Retardation within

Department of Human Resources. The Office of Emergency Medical Services was established.

22. 1980—Improved pregnancy outcomes program started with federal funds; infant mortality rate fell markedly.
23. 1981—State Laboratory Director, Biostatistician, and Medical Director of Community Health Services positions were eliminated.
24. 1983—State Health Officer, Consumer Health Bureau Chief positions were eliminated.
25. 1984—Federal Improved Pregnancy Outcome funds vanish. Infant Mortality Rate increases.
26. 1988—State Health Officer position reinstated. New positions created in Communicable Disease Control, AIDS prevention, Radiological Health, long term care facility regulation, and medical laboratory regulation. Two pediatricians were hired for Special Children's Clinics.
27. 1989—Health Educator, Laboratory Director, Biostatistician positions reinstated. State legislature strengthened communicable disease statutes.
28. 1990—State Health Officer, Laboratory Director, and Biostatistician positions were filled.
29. 1991-1992—Health Planning transferred to Division of Health. Budget shortfalls necessitated 20% cuts.
30. 1992—Cumulative AIDS cases exceeded one thousand. The 1980s began with budgetary problems. Despite a decade of shuffling positions, eliminating and reinstitution of positions and turnover in leadership, the budgetary problems persisted. Nevada continued to lead the nation in rates of lung cancer, deaths from trauma, liver cancer, low birth weight, and suicide. More planning for disease prevention, health promotion and wellness was needed to make Nevada a healthy environment.

**NOTE**

The photograph of Dr. Don Kwalik is from Bernhard & Williams' book.

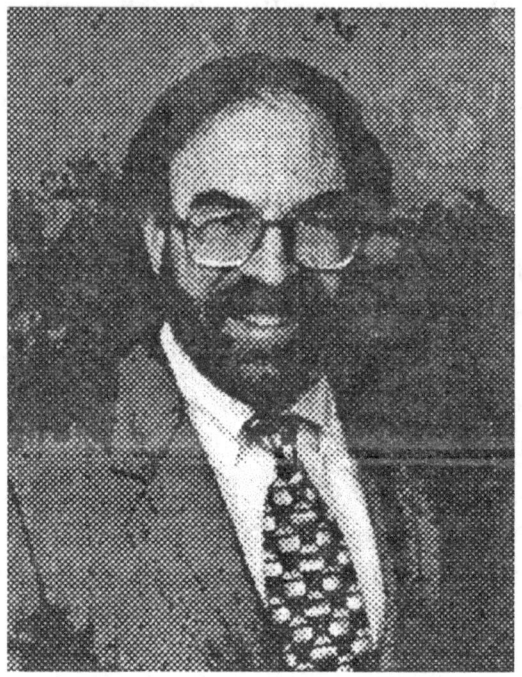

Dr. Donald Kwalik

### GALAXY 203 CRASH IN RENO ON JANUARY 21, 1985 (30TH ANNIVERSARY) RENO LED THE WAY IN AIRCRAFT ACCIDENT INVESTIGATIONS USA TODAY 10/28/14 HEADLINE "PLANE CRASH DIDN'T KILL THEM—FIRE DID"

### By Drs. Roger S. Ritzlin and Anton P. Sohn

In 1985, fatalities from commercial aircraft accidents surpassed all previous years, and Reno led the way with the first crash of the year on January 21. Of interest is the fact that in the ten years preceding 1985, thirty commercial aircrafts crashed, resulting in 2,500 deaths and only two investigators reported autopsy findings and injury patterns.

In all of Nevada's tragic accidents, the seventy deaths in the Galaxy crash is third to eighty-five deaths from Las Vegas' 1980 MGM Grand Hotel fire and eighty-five deaths in the Paradise Airline crash March 1, 1964, on Genoa Peak near Carson City.

Eric Moody and Phil Earl from Nevada in the West magazine provided information on the Genoa crash. Smoke inhalation and fire played a major part in the Las Vegas tragedy, and it also was a major cause (60%) of the deaths in the Galaxy crash. The following historical account will show the importance of studying all aircraft accident deaths to determine the cause of death. We also plotted and published where individuals were located at the crash site as related to cause of death, however this information is not included in this essay.

A Lockheed L-188 turboprop aircraft, shortly after take-off at 1:04 AM from Reno-Cannon Airport, crashed two miles south of the airport (See page 365) On board were six crew and sixty-five passengers, some of whom had attended the Superbowl at Stanford University and stopped in Reno to get other passengers before returning to Minnesota.

Immediately after takeoff the pilot radioed that he was experiencing an unusual vibration. He was instructed to return to the airport. The plane banked right, lost altitude, and crashed in a field east of South Virginia Street. It skidded across a field, impacted a drainage ditch, broke apart, caught fire, and smashed through an RV sales lot.

Debris from the plane ended in Virginia Street. The sound, smoke, and the light from the fire were witnessed by Drs. Anton Sohn and Roger Ritzlin in their homes in south Reno; both were several miles from the accident site. Within five minutes after the accident, fire and rescue personnel arrived at the scene.

There were three survivors. Two later died in the hospital and one survived with nonlethal injuries. The lone survivor, 17-year-old George Lamson, Jr., was sitting next to his father where the plane broke apart. They were ejected from the plane belted to their seats. George, Jr. landed on top of his father. (His father saved his life.) The father died on the eighth day of his hospitalization, and George Jr. walked away from the crash. In 1990, he moved back to Reno and lived anonymously, a testimony to Renoites who showed him kindness. In 2013, he was featured in a CNN documentary film called *Soul Survivor.* In 2021, he still lives in Reno.

Dr. Ritzlin: "Little did I know the noise we heard would result in sixty-eight autopsies waiting for us. David Melarkey, an autopsy assistant, showed up with his autopsy gear to assist us without our contacting him. I believe he was the weekend on-call-tech at the time. We were impressed with his initiative and support, which helped considerably."

During the next three days forensic pathologists Drs. R.S. Ritzlin, J.H. Gauthier, and A.P. Sohn did autopsies on the sixty-eight victims who died.

Dr. V.A. Salvadorini and Washoe County Coroner Vernon McCarty assisted with organizing the temporary morgue. Autopsies were necessary for five reasons:
1. To settle the estate when several members of a family with different heirs die in the same crash
2. To deny life insurance when the policy contains a clause that excludes payment to beneficiaries when the victim is intoxicated regardless of whether alcohol contributed to the death
3. To pay for pain and suffering prior to death which is permitted by Nevada law when negligence or wrongful death is proven
4. To make positive identification of victims
5. To gain knowledge to improve airline safety

Pathologists made the final determination of cause of death of those killed at the scene after reviewing autopsy and toxicology results. Three categories emerged. The first category, blunt trauma, included twenty-seven (40%) individuals who died immediately with lethal injuries and no evidence of smoke or carbon monoxide (CO) inhalation. The second group of eight (12%) individuals died from a flash fire, exemplified by rapid incineration and no lethal traumatic injuries or inhalation of smoke. The third and final category included thirty-three (48%) people who lacked lethal injuries, but who had marked elevation of blood CO, soot in the lungs, and toxic products from smoke inhalation. This finding indicated individuals who were not killed immediately on impact.

Dr. Ritzlin: "An attorney told me our categories of death were extremely helpful in determining the pain and suffering payout. He mentioned that the estate of someone who died instantly of traumatic head injuries would receive less than the estate of someone who suffered from smoke inhalation. This attorney said our categories of death were a reason that cases were settled without long court battles and pathologist's testimony."

Dr. Sohn: "Autopsy identification was necessary for one man because a dental examination at autopsy revealed no evidence of previous dental work, however, autopsy body X-rays revealed an old injury sustained when he played football at the University of Minnesota. I was also notified to be prepared to testify in a 1987 trial in Minnesota, but the case was settled based on the autopsy findings."

## Important:

An FAA investigation revealed the cause of vibration after takeoff was due to an unsecured cargo door. Furthermore, the pilot made the crucial mistake of reducing power to return to the airport when he should have maintained or increased power.

## Liability By Monique Laxalt, ESQ.

The liability insurer of Galaxy Airlines flight 203 was notified almost immediately after the 1:04 AM January 21 crash. It promptly utilized its resources to assist in the subsequent investigation and eventual settlement of claims. Per protocol, investigators and attorneys were involved.

Primary legal responsibility was given to Reno attorney Bruce Laxalt who, organized and directed investigators and attorneys on the early morning of the 21st. Priority one was to ensure the three surviving passengers were receiving the best available medical care.

The next priority was to secure and preserve the crash site, which encompassed over a square mile with debris strewn across U.S. Highway #395. Once bodies of the deceased were removed and their locations catalogued, investigators began the search of what remained of the aircraft.

An effort was made to locate every part and piece of the Lockheed Electra. Mr. Laxalt contacted the anthropology department at the University of Nevada, whose department head agreed to provide students to mark out grids, which were then searched for aircraft debris as well as personal effects of the passengers. There were many "finds" which had been previously missed prior to the implementation of the grid approach.

Mr. Laxalt, a former chief homicide prosecutor with the Washoe County District Attorney's office, coordinated with Doctors Anton Sohn, Roger Ritzlin, and Jay Gauthier to ensure autopsies performed on the deceased included a determination whether the deaths were due solely to blunt force trauma, post-crash fire/smoke inhalation or a combination of both. These findings were important for damages assessment in the evaluation and settlement of the prospective wrongful death claims. One aspect of the investigation that Mr. Laxalt handled with great sensitivity was ascertaining the identity of each individual passenger on board Galaxy 203.

The group had been at a Super Bowl party hosted by Caesar's Palace in South Lake Tahoe where Dallas Cowboy running back Tony Dorsett was the lead celebrity at the request of Caesar's.

The flight manifest did not contain all correct names and

relationships. To sort this out a meeting took place in the suite at Caesar's Palace with the host where the Super Bowl party had taken place. Verification and confirmation of the true names of the deceased passengers took days.

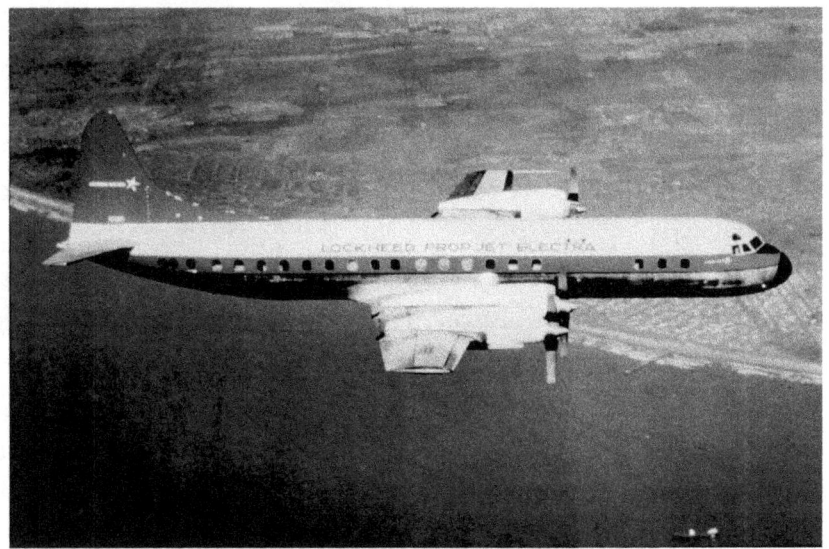

Reno Galaxy 203, 1985

## HOME REMEDIES IN NINETEENTH CENTURY NEVADA
### By Dr. Anton Sohn

Many cultural groups rely on the use of home remedies rather than treatment by a doctor. Consultation with family or friends for advice on medical problems is a natural process. Since acquaintances might have had similar problems that yielded to practical and accessible remedies; their advice was usually sought and followed. In the Great Basin, travelers, ranchers, miners, and settlers followed this simple natural process. In fact, today, we would consider much of what the educated civilian doctor practiced in the 19th century to be little more than application of home remedies. In Austin, Nevada, Dr. Riddle in 1868, treated typhoid fever with mustard baths and brandy rubs, an acknowledged Basque home remedy. It is reasonable to assume if someone else in the family showed symptoms like those of typhoid fever, they were treated in the same manner without contacting Dr. Riddle.

Furthermore, in a setting such as the Great Basin, professional medical care was frequently days away, in one of five or six populated areas. Due to the sparse population in the 19th Century West, the philosophy of self-help was prevalent to a much greater extent than in modern times.

Even today in remote areas of the Great Basin it is still necessary to rely on home remedies before professional help can be obtained.

When doctors were not available, the first white travelers in the Great Basin had to rely on their own medicine chest or get various drugs from other members of the party. A variety of medicines were available and were carried by the emigrants. One important group of drugs was narcotic—morphine, laudanum, opium, or Dover's powders—used for sedation, analgesia, and to treat diarrhea. A second group included purging agents. To achieve this effect, calomel (mercurous chloride) was administered for several ailments. Similarly, cream of tartar with antimony, Epsom salts, and castor oil were used as emetics. A third important group comprised the alcohol solutions which were stimulants. Alcohol was an important ingredient of patent medicines. Brandy, whiskey, and other spirits were used internally and externally. Also carried with the wagon trains were camphor, flaxseed oil, ginger, horehound, ammonia, carbolic acid, hartshorn, quinine, sulfur, turpentine, and many other herbs and chemical compounds. If the concoctions were not palatable, molasses, honey, and sugar were used as sweeteners.

When Raymond Doetsch crossed the Great Basin in a wagon, he described the medicine chest as containing "Elixirs, tonics, salves, balms, unctions, and ointments, together with physiking pills, laudanum, calomel (mercurous chloride), essence of peppermint, castor oil, and a few patent medicines."

Just as important as available medicine were the various

health care guidebooks that promulgated the various treatments and philosophies of medicine in the 19th century. In 1769, William Buchan wrote and published the first self-help book, *Domestic Medicine*, in Edinburgh, Scotland. Written to educate and inform the public on the prevention of disease, it appeared in America approximately 100 years later, and became popular. Written for the "rural elite" to treat their neighbors, the book contained description of the diseases and their symptoms, followed by their treatment.

Many other books were published in America, but probably the most important was John C. Gunn's *Domestic Medicine, or Poor Man's Friend*, first published in 1830. Gunn, an educated physician, thought every aspect of medicine could be practiced by the common man if the practice of medicine was reduced to principles of common sense. He directed his treatise "for families of Western and Southern States."

Many sects and ethnic groups relied on remedies indigenous to their culture. Latter Day Saints (LDS, Mormons) settled in wide areas of the Great Basin before and during the mining explorations, while the Basques came later with the growing sheep industry. Both groups had home remedies passed down by their elders.

A typical old-world Basque remedy consisted of a mixture of dried mustard and wood ashes added to hot water for soaking feet to ward off a cold. Whiskey rubs were also utilized by applying them to the chest, as were kerosene and lard plasters. Sore throats were treated by drinking hot water with ashes and crushed mustard.

A Basque remedy for earache involved plugging the ear with a cotton pledge after blowing smoke into the ear canal. Warm cooking oil was sometimes used in the ear instead of smoke. Garlic and vegetable oil were applied to boils, and the patient drank the purulent material extracted from the boil to effect a cure.

Garlic had wide use in Basque medicinal culture. Internally, it was used in soup to cure the common cold and externally, garlic cloves were bound to wounds to promote healing. Poultices were also made of bread dough, wrapped in a towel or sock, and applied to the sore neck or afflicted area.

Many Basques used superstition and magic to cure conditions such as warts. To effect a cure a potato was cut into four pieces to simulate a cross, rubbed on the wart and buried in a manner reminiscent of Native American practices. Cow manure was used on burns, as were some local plants. Urine had wide usage in Mormon folklore. It was used to treat chapped skin, sore eyes, earache, and was given internally to babies with the croup. Baby urine was also applied to normal skin to improve the complexion.

In addition to the use of excreta, pioneer Mormon home remedies included the use of animals and animal parts. Brains were rubbed on the gums of a child perceived to be suffering from teething. Chicken liver was rubbed on a wart, and the liver was then buried in a manner like Basque treatment. Live animals were also used to treat serious and life-threatening illness. Live chickens or pigeons were split open and applied to the chest as a poultice to treat pneumonia or applied to the neck to treat diphtheria.

More important to Mormon tradition was the use of herbs, sagebrush, and the divinely inspired Brigham tea. Widely used throughout the Great Basin, Brigham teas are made from several plants, but the most important ingredient was a septate reed-like grass known as *ephedra viderens* that contains a mild stimulant, ephedrine. Teas made from this plant and the common sagebrush were not only ingested, but they were also used topically on sores, sprains and in poultices. They were used as stimulants and tonics in the spring to purify the blood. Women used sagebrush tea to wash, invigorate and rejuvenate their hair.

**NOTE:**

This article was abstracted from Dr. Anton Sohn's book, *The Healers of 19th Century Nevada*.

## Ethan and Hosea Grosh, "Sad Story, 1857"

... A drama with tragic consequence was being played out in Gold Canyon where Gold Hill, Nevada, would be built. In mid-August 1857, the Grosh brothers (Hosea Ballou and Ethan Allen) were prospecting when Hosea accidentally struck his foot with his pick. An infection ensued, and despite improvement after poultices of rosin, then bread and soda, a friend was consulted who recommended a poultice of cow dung. Dr. Benjamin L. King agreed cow dung was the right therapy. The infection progressed and Ethan wrote his father, Rev. A.B. Grosh, requesting money to buy the services of Dr. Charles D. Daggett, the "best doctor" in the area. Unfortunately, the services of the "best doctor" never came, but Hosea's immortality was established.

His treatment, although ill-advised by today's standards, is the first recorded home remedy and medical treatment by a doctor in Nevada. The following is an abstract of that letter.

Ethan Grosh, Gold Canõn, Sept. 7th, 1857: "Dear Father, I take up my pen with a heavy heart, for I have sad news to send you. God has seen fit in his perfect wisdom & goodness to call Hosea, the patient, the good, the gentle to join his Mother in another & a better world than this....

"At the time of his death I had gone to see a physician in Eagle Valley, some 14 or 15 miles from here. It was very sudden-unexpected but very peaceful. Not a shudder, not a gasp, not a change of feature marked the parting of soul and body. He simply fell asleep. It was such a death as God blesses the good with.

"The immediate cause of his death was the wound in the foot I mentioned in my last. It occurred about the middle of the forenoon of Wednesday, Aug. 19, [by first letter] or Thursday the 20th. He died Wednesday, Sept. 2d. We were packing dirt from a small ravine to the right fork of the main Canon. I dug and Hosea drove the jack (mule).

"We had brought no water with us for drinking and becoming thirsty (it was very hot.) I started down to the main ravine for a drink. I met Hosea as he was coming back for another load and told him what I was going for and that I had not quite a load dug for him. On my return he was setting on the ground beside the dirt holding his left foot in his hand.

"I have done it now, he shouted as. I came within hearing, and on my asking what he had done, he said he had struck the pick into his foot. "Why how in the world did you do it," I asked as I first saw the wound. It was a frightful gash. The dirt we were digging was only 16 or 18 inches deep, and, though it dug hard, there were but few stones in it. He smiled and said he hardly knew how he did it. He then pointed to a large quartz rock laying loose on top of the ground just on the edge of the hole. "Somehow" he said "I hit that." He would not let me carry him to the house but rode the jack. The ground was rough, and the jolting caused him considerable pain.

"For about a week it got on finely, despite the hot weather here. But the evening of the eighth day, his foot was swolen [sic], and the wound was closed. The next morning, I lanced the foot in two places and got out considerable matter, which relieved the pain, and checked the swelling. I also changed the poultice from rosin soap to bread and soda. The bread & soda worked very well, and I think if we had continued it everything would have come out right.

".. Monday afternoon I went down to the store—four or five miles—to see if I could get either opium or laudanum, so he might get his necessary rest. I could find neither, But I saw Mr. Rose, and he told me he had some at his house in Eagle Valley. He also recommended me to try fresh cow dung as a poultice. I took some cows dung up with me and applied it immediately. I should have mentioned the leg had commenced swelling, and we could not check it. The poultice at once checked the swelling, and ...ed the pain, and next morning everything was looking well again. I found a man who was going up to Eagle Valley and sent by him for the opium, and for a little quinine, cayenne & several other things if they could be got. I could get nothing here & Hosea was quite billious [sic] besides touched with the dyspepsia—the result of his confinement to bed.

"I understood the man would be back that evening, but that evening found I was mistaken. This evening also occurred the misshap [sic] which I think sent Hosea out of this world. The cat jumped on the bed, and in doing so lit with all his weight on poor Hosea's sore foot. It caused him intense pain. That night he suffered great pain, and next morning he had a high nervous fever. He complained that during the night he had been slightly flighty. He was very cool & calm, and before I went to see Dr. B. King (formerly of Dearfield, N.Y.) & with whom we had some slight aquaintance [sic] we had considerable conversation, He [Hosea] said, that through God's mercy we had passed through as great trials as this—and to that mercy we must trust—without God's mercy what would we be?

"Dear Brother! he spoke as though the trial was as much on me as on him. He was so uncomplaining & made so little of his sufferings that it took close watching to see how sick he really was. After some little thought he consented to a proposition I made to send to you for $50. or $100 so we could, on the strength of it secure the services of Dr. Daggett (Dr. Charles Daggett), the only good DOCTOR in Carson Valley, should it be necessary. Little did either of us dream of the danger being so near at hand.

"I dressed his foot. It was rather cold. He quieted my apprehentions [sic] by saying it was the effect of the warm poultices. The poultice was warmer, a little, than blood heat. He felt it very sensible, and we both congratulated ourselves on the favorable symptom, as the poultice before that had been warmer and he had hardly felt it. He complained of being ... sick, just before I left, but felt no other pain.

"About 9:00 AM, I started for Eagle Valley to see Dr. King and get what medicine I could, leaving him in charge of Mr. Galphins, who came to the house a few minutes after I had left. I had not gone far before a feeling of uneasiness took hold of me. Twice I threw myself down behind a cedar bush, completely overcome with a great dread that it would terminate fatally. I prayed—Oh with what agony I prayed that he be spared—that the loss of the limb might be the worst. Finally, to get rid of this dreadful apprehension I struck across the mountains, which though it shortened the distance a few miles, was very rough, and I was almost barefooted. Dr. King was very kind to me. He recommended the continunance [sic] of the cow dung poultice, as being the best to be had here. He did not regard the swelling of the foot & leg—neither the coldness—as anything serious. He spoke-spoke [sic] as if a wound got along very slow in this country but did not seem to think that the danger was increased thusly. Hosea complained of pain in the back, and one particular-spot, near the shoulders on the left side, he said produced nausea if it touched the bed. The doctor regarded it only as the result of the pain & loss of sleep together with slight billiousness [sic] He gave me four pills of Blue Mass—which I took for fear of hurting his feelings.

"Though I could get no physic but aloes or Ep. Salts, both of which we had and would not use. I regretted very much that I could get no hops, as I had more hope of allaying the nausea with that than anything I could think of. From Mrs. Rose I got some Opium & a few ounces of garden peppers. I started back with a lightened heart. It was just dark as I got back. Mr. Galphins met me a few steps from the house. "You must prepare yourself for bad news, Allen," he said. I heard strange voices in the cabin, and I thought that either Dr. Daggert [Daggett], or some physician travelling across the plains had come on to the Canõn & had been sent up by the miners below, (as Hosea was thought a great deal of) and that it might have been pronounced necessary to amputate the foot. I was quite unprepared for the answer to my

'What is it?' 'Hosea is dead! Oh, the terrible force of that blow! Oh! the utter desolation of that hour....

Truly and Affectionately your son, E.A. Grosh."

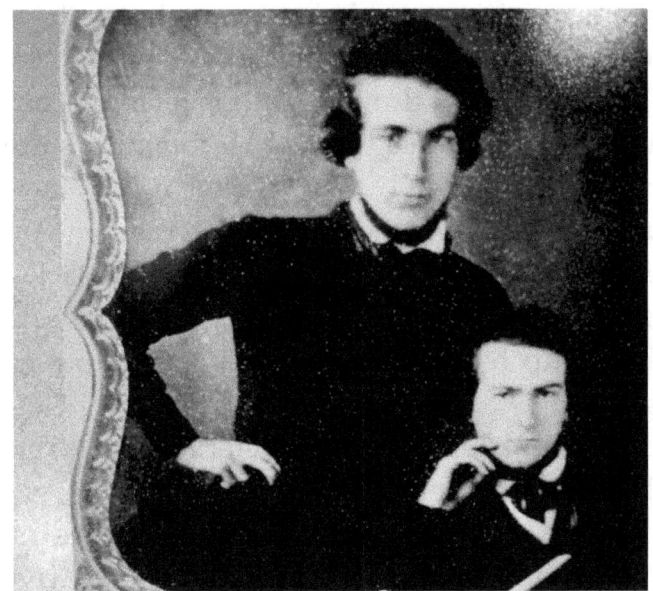

Grosh Brothers, 1857

**NOTE:**

The original letter is in the possession of Charles T. Wegman of Bloomfield, NJ. His great-grandfather was Warren Rhinehart Grosh, a brother of Hosea and Ethan Grosh. A typed copy sent to Eric Moody of the Nevada Historical Society is used with Mr. Wegman's approval. The complete letter is printed in Dr. Anton Sohn's book, *19th Century Medical Practitioners in Nevada*.

## "SMALL-TOWN" VETERINARIAN A.A. CUTHBERTSON

Perhaps no branch of medicine is more dangerous and physically demanding than the practice of veterinary medicine— at least in the experience of Elko Veterinarian Arlynn Alexander Cuthbertson. During the 45 years he has been practicing in Northeastern Nevada, he has been kicked by horses, rolled his pickup, squeezed by cattle, run over by his own truck, suffered at least six airplane accidents, been infected with Brucellosis, and he still loves the practice of veterinary medicine!

Born in Sterling, I, in 1922, he was the son of small-town Veterinarian Arthur Alexander Cuthbertson. Early in his life he was exposed to medicine as he helped his father with his practice. During the "Great Depression years" following the stock market crash of 1929 and years of drought and crop failures on the farms of the mid-west, his father suffered economic hardship and foreclosure.

He was forced to join the federal government program of farm relief. In those hard years of depression and lack of feed for cattle, beef prices dropped to new lows and the government tried to prop things up by buying up cattle for $5 per head, then destroying them.

The government hired hungry veterinarians to inspect the cattle and supervise their destruction. Later the government hired veterinarians to participate in tuberculosis eradication programs, which involved testing every animal in every herd for tuberculin reactivity. During this time, the Cuthbertson family moved quite a bit, first to Mississippi, then to I.

When World War II came, Arlynn first tried to enlist in the U.S. Marine Corps but was rejected because of his eyesight. He was accepted by the U.S. Army. Probably because of his already considerable knowledge of horses, he was sent to Fort Riley, I, where he joined a horse cavalry. After a period as an instructor at Fort Riley, he was transferred to a cavalry reconnaissance troop attached to the 96th Infantry Division. The division was sent to the Philippine Islands where the troop was detailed to carry supplies across the mountains with a pack train, but in short order the trail became too muddy for the horses.

It was necessary for them to use native carabao (water buffalo) to transport the guns and ammunition. Eventually the terrain became so rough that they were forced to abandon both the animals and equipment and continue on-foot. The mission was aborted, and the Americans were forced to retreat in the face of

Japanese sea-borne invasion. Arlynn Cuthbertson emerged from the conflict unscathed, holding the rank of 1st Lieutenant. He married Carol F. Main, completed a course at California State, then graduated from University of California, Davis in 1953 with a DVM.

He went into practice with a friend of his father, Dr. C.H. Kennedy, in Elko, Nevada, soon after graduation and learned to fly. Since his arrival he has logged 9,000 hours flying time and covered a 40,000 square mile area in his practice.

His flying has not been without incident. When taking off from a ranch in Ruby Valley in the 1960s one ski of his ski-equipped Piper "Super Cub" hit a cow's back and flipped the aircraft over. Doc emerged unhurt, but the airplane was totaled. On another occasion his ski-equipped plane hit a rock while landing near Mountain City and flipped over, damaging the propeller, and tearing the wing fabric. While the rancher took the prop back to his shop to hammer it out, Dr. Cuthbertson sewed up the fabric on the wing using a curved surgical needle and suture, then flew the jerry-rigged plane back to town for repair.

Once, a ski hit a rock as he tried to set down in a sudden snowstorm north of Ely and flipped again, but neither plane nor pilot suffered any serious damage. Another time, while flying a Helio Courier near Diamond Valley the rudder jammed. Unable to turn left after take-off, he turned to the right, made a circle, and landed safely. After removing a piece of metal jammed in the rudder, he took off again and flew home.

His most serious aircraft accident occurred in May of 1986. Flying from Battle Mountain to North Las Vegas to attend a meeting of the Nevada Health Department, he encountered a sudden severe windstorm. While attempting to land on a dirt road in Dixie Valley turbulence caused a wing to hit the ground. The plane cartwheeled, destroying the aircraft, and pinning Cuthbertson in the wreckage with both legs broken.

As he hung by his harness, listening to the fuel dripping out of the tank he said, "I kept waiting for it to blow up." He was found by a passing motorist and flown to Washoe Medical Center, where he underwent multiple surgical procedures before he recovered. He states, "I would still be flying if I could pass the physical exam."

During his long career, Dr. Cuthbertson has earned numerous accolades. He belongs to the American Veterinary Medical Association, the U.S. Animal Health Association, and the Nevada Cattleman's Association.

He is a member of the Nevada Veterinary Association and has twice been named as Nevada State Outstanding Veterinarian, first in 1966 and again in 1987. He was listed in *Who's Who in Veterinary Science and Medicine.*

He has received a special award from the Nevada Cattleman's Association, served on the Nevada Board of Health, taught at the Northern Nevada Community College, and served on the board of trustees for the Elko General Hospital. Dr. Cuthbertson has donated his time to the Elko County and Livestock Show for over 30 years. He is a Rotarian, an elder in the Presbyterian Church, and has been awarded a special Nevada Mental Health Award. He served as a County Commissioner for two terms.

Although his practice has included all manner of animal care (he has taken care of everything from boa constrictors to elephants) he enjoys caring for large animals—cattle and horses—more than small animals. He refers to them as "companion animals." For a pet, Dr. Cuthbertson enjoys cats more than canines: "Cause they don't hold a grudge."

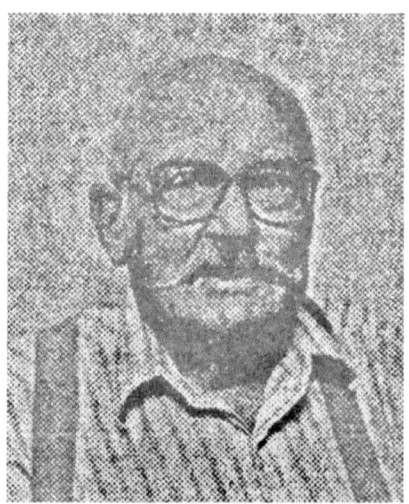

Arlynn Cuthbertson DVM

Prior to his near-fatal accident in 1986, he was an accomplished horseman, winning a jumping contest in 1974. Sadly, his injuries have made it too uncomfortable to continue riding.

The Cuthbertsons have been married for 50 years and have five children—four daughters and a son, Alan, who is a third-generation veterinarian practicing with his father in Elko. They also have nine grandchildren.

**NOTE:**

This story is from a history by Marcia Barker-Browning, Nevada Museum and *Elko Daily Free Press* and *Elko Independent*.

## SILICOSIS IN DELMAR, NEVADA, 1894
### By Lauran Evans, Second Year Pathology Student

With the boom of gold mining in the West came an insidious, deadly disease that continues to plague the mining industry today. Little did nineteenth century pioneers know that inhalation of dust would cause an incurable century lung disease years later. Their westward migration to strike gold ended in death and the creation of ghost towns. The U.S. government was reluctant to protect or compensate these workers, enacting policies decades too late. However, these deaths could have been prevented by simple measures adopted in modern times. This slice of history serves as an opportunity to examine the past, especially in Nevada, to help improve patient care.

Dust clouds did not seem particularly dangerous to the pioneers of the West, as they lived in an environment constantly surrounded by dust. Unbeknownst to them, one specific particle in the dust called silica, or crystalline quartz, was being released into the air in and around the mines. Once inhaled, silica particles deposit in the lungs and cause mass destruction, leading to a disease known as silicosis. Exposure is cumulative and may cause disease in as little as seven months of exposure.

Most silica dust inhalation in the late 1800s, and in the modern-day world, occurs in an occupational setting. Sand blasting, quarrying, and especially mining all create deadly dust clouds that precipitate silicosis.

Families of exposed workers described their loved ones as suffocating, with their lives slowly being drained away. Affected individuals presented with a gradual onset shortness of breath and radiologically exhibit fibrosis and nodules in the lung. Over time, the disease might accelerate, especially if chronically exposed, and could lead to pneumonia, chronic obstructive pulmonary disease (COPD), respiratory failure, and death. If silicosis itself does not kill the patient, there is an increased risk for tuberculosis and lung cancer. Of the estimated 17,000 deaths from silicosis between 1968-2006, 14% ultimately died from tuberculosis.

Recent advances in tuberculosis and cancer treatments have provided better outcomes for those affected by silicosis. However, there are no curative treatment for silicosis, so prevention is key. This disease has been known for some time, even dating back to the Roman Empire, but we have been slow in progress for research.

During the Roman times, it was first realized that dust from rock drilling had detrimental effects on workers' lungs. Because of this, silicosis is believed to be one of the earliest occupational diseases in history. The disease remained elusive to scientists until the late nineteenth century, when mining boomed in the U.S. Silica was finally identified as the mysterious deadly particle, but it would take years until its detrimental sequelae would be fully recognized. Before silicosis could be definitively linked to mining, the gold rush attracted countless pioneers to the West. Nevada was deemed fit for mining, and towns were quickly built throughout the state. Delamar, once a thriving town, was a place where acute successes were met with chronic pain.

In 1894, a gold mine in Delamar, Nevada, was established, with special promise for the state's depressed economy. For the next five years, the mine was one of the most productive in the state— turning over 300 tons of gold ore per day. For the residents of Delamar, work was fruitful, and gold was plentiful, but not for long.

Over time, workers developed illnesses ranging from malaise to intractable cough. Disease progression led to many deaths, and nearby physicians took notice and collaborated. In 1900, Dr. Winthrop Betts published a study in Journal American Medical Association (JAMA) detailing the morbidity and mortality at the mine in Delamar. Overall, 166 worker deaths were attributed to dust inhalation. The natural history and autopsies of thirty of those workers were examined, all of whom had been previously healthy 20 to 40-year-old men. The longer a worker was exposed, the less time he survived afterwards. The average exposure time was 14 months, with an average survival time of 10 years after exposure.

Dr. Betts' autopsy reports showed widespread lung damage with silica deposits, which provided pathological evidence. Unfortunately, after Dr. Betts' publication, silicosis deaths continued, transforming the once prosperous Delamar into a ghost town. Delamar is only one of many towns in the U.S. where this tragedy has occurred.

Western U.S. is not the only area that has been affected by silicosis. However, it was the deadliest area due to several factors. The West had a higher prevalence of quartz deposits in the land than Eastern U.S., thus creating dust clouds with higher concentrations of silica. Mines out west also implemented air-cooled drilling and end-of-shift blasting, which reduced silica to smaller, more dangerous particles that could lodge deeper in the lung. In addition, the gold strike brought an unstoppable boom of pioneers to the West who were hoping to make large financial gains.

It is estimated over 25% of western miners developed some form of silicosis in the early 1900s. Around the same time, the rest of the country also began noticing that miners contracted a tuberculosis-like disease, termed "minor's TB" or "miner's puff." In 1910, John Haldane published a study entitled *Effects of Mine Dust Inhalation*. He demonstrated a causal correlation between silica dust inhalation and silicosis, which greatly contributed to public and government awareness of the issue. Great Britain proceeded to pass the Workmen's Compensation (Silicosis) Act of 1918, and shortly after, Canada implemented similar policies.

Employers were subsequently forced to compensate workers who developed silicosis, which in turn incentivized greater prevention efforts. The U.S. would then trail Great Britain and Canada in compensation policies by over 20 years.

Unfortunately, the U.S. was one of the last developed nations to implement laws to protect workers from silicosis. Instead, the U.S. government placed responsibility on mining companies to control hazards; companies then carelessly deferred responsibility to their employees. Individuals could purchase their own army gas masks or respirators to wear during work, but due to the uncomfortable nature of these devices, they were rarely used.

As a result, western states were confronted with lawsuits filed by workers, union protests, and public upset before they took the initiative to create their own policies.

After much back and forth between corporations, unions, and lawyers, the U.S. ratified the 1943 Occupational Disease Act. This act mimicked the compensation policies from other countries and states but was long overdue. The U.S. government and mining companies were largely to blame for this political battle and delay in policy creation. Earlier action by the government would have provided sick patients with relief from medical and funeral costs. In addition, the policies that were eventually enacted only provided compensation after workers contracted disease; they did not create a framework for prevention. It would take almost 30 more years for the U.S. government to pass rules to protect the workers from future exposure.

In 1971, the same year OSHA (Occupational Safety and Health Administration) was created, specific protection rules were imposed on construction and mining employers. These rules provided strict dust control guidelines and required health screenings for employees. OSHA updated these standards in 2015, giving companies more flexibility in the type of dust control used, while providing workers with more protections.

The new provisions require companies do the following: control dust with water or ventilation, comply with the permissible exposure limit of airborne silica (50 micrograms/cubic meter of air), limit worker exposure, inform all employees regarding the risks of exposure and protections available, and provide medical screenings and support to highly exposed workers. The government has come a long way in the past century regarding occupational protections, and we must ensure these rules continue to be strictly enforced to prevent history from repeating.

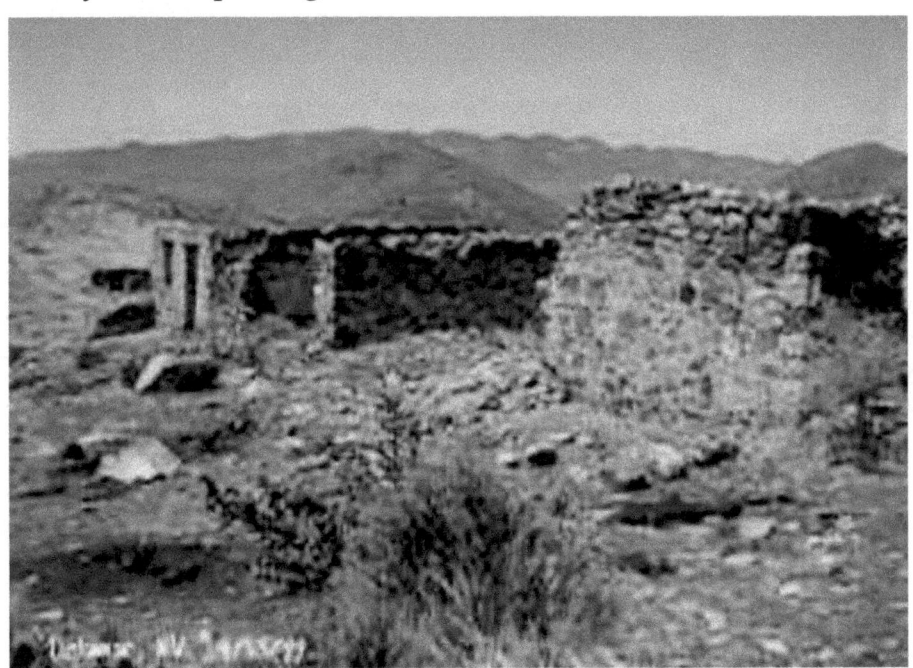

Delmar Building Ruins, 1990s

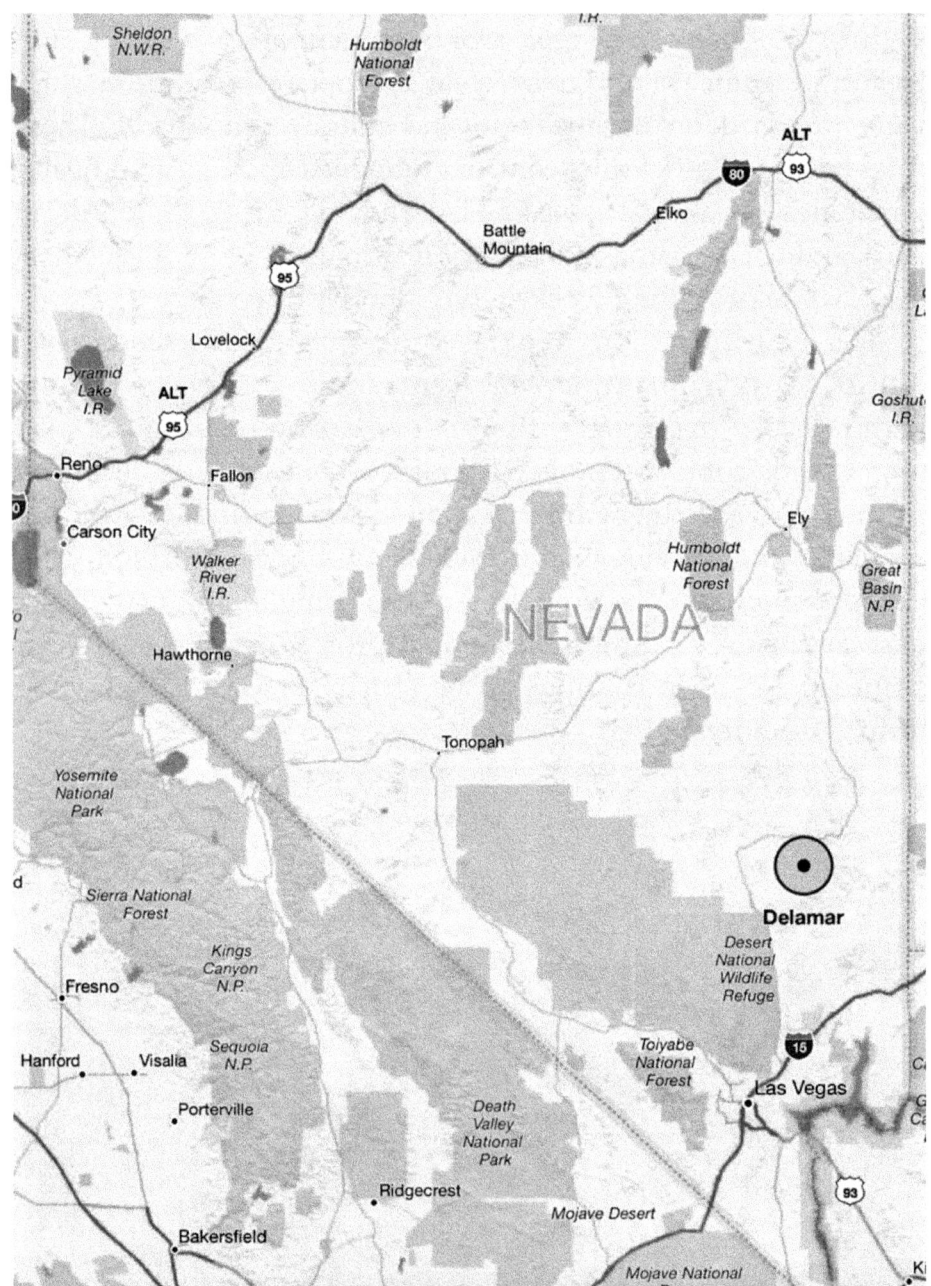

Delamar, Located 111 Miles North of Las Vegas

In our own backyard of the western U.S., great suffering and loss of life took place. The danger of silicosis started by affecting ancient Romans, extended to pioneers in the western U.S. and continues today. Nevada is currently the leading gold producer in the U.S., and it is estimated two-million U.S. workers are currently exposed to silica per year.

As citizens, we must continue to improve and enforce life-saving prevention techniques by encouraging fair policies. Physicians must inquire about occupational exposures and discuss strategies with patients to reduce such exposures. Finally, we must be aware of emerging disease and not be afraid to speak out when governments or corporations ignore its signs. It is our duty to insist on further examination and studies, as did Dr. Winthrop Betts. The story of silicosis provides a glimpse of both the evolution and stasis of medicine throughout history, and we must apply what it has taught us to improve future healthcare.

## PHARMACIES IN EARLY NEVADA, 1862-1939

History Student Intern Peter Aylworth and Dr. Anton Sohn were inventorying the museum's extensive medicine bottle collection when they decided to highlight Nevada's pharmacies. As a result approximately 100 medicine bottles and pillboxes that were either engraved or labeled from early Nevada were placed in a separate showcase with pill making equipment, balance scales, and prescription books, dating from the 1860s.

Pharmacies' showcase shown on page 383 are from the following:
1. Biter & Lernhart Drug Store, Virginia City, 1897
2. Cannan Drug Store, Reno, 1935
3. Cole Drug Store, Virginia City, 1862
4. Dupont Pharmacy, Elko, 1919
5. Hale's Drug Store, Reno, 1939
6. Hilp's Drug Store, Reno, 1915
7. Johnson's Drug Store, Carson City, 1897
8. Jones' Drug Store, Gold Hill, 1864
9. McCullough's Drug Store, Reno, 1891
10. Morris-Loring, Fallon, 1912

11. Nevada Drug Store, Carson City, 1897
12. Pioneer Drug Store, Virginia City, 1897
13. Red Cross Drug Store, Reno, 1908
14. Shaw's Drug Store, Virginia City, 1897
15. Steptoe Drug Store, Ely, 1908
16. Twiaba Medicine Bottle, Elko, 1871
17. Whitley Drug Store, Truckee, CA, 1910

A large book in the History of Medicine Museum contains original signed prescriptions by doctors from 1867, including several signed by Dr. Anton Tjader, hero of the 1860 Pyramid Indian War. The museum also has Carson City pharmacists Stephen C. Haydon's and Charles S. Hammer's 1860s prescriptions. Our exhibit includes large bottles with bulk ingredients that were weighed or measured to fill prescriptions. Of interest is a twelve-inch mortar and pestle that was used to crush and plants for "herbal" prescriptions.

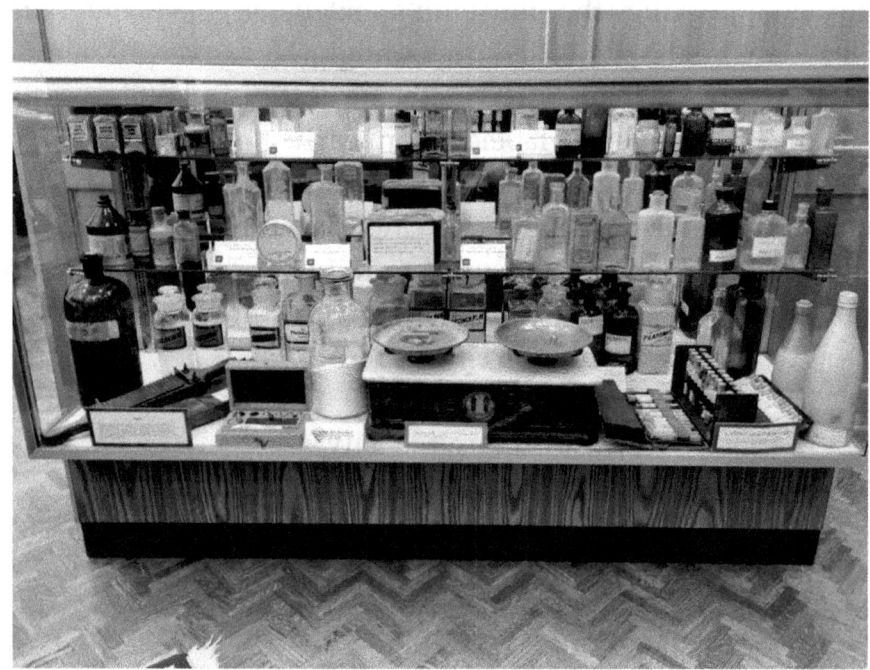

Pharmacy Exhibit
(History of Medicine Museum)

## More on Nevada Pharmacies
## By Peter Aylworth and Linda Valle

William E. Pettis, born in 1901, graduated from the University of Mississippi School of Pharmacy and came west to Winnemucca. He moved to Reno in 1927 where he was a pharmacist for over fifty years. William Pettis began his career with Hale's Drug.

Mr. Pettis owned the following pharmacies:
1. Lake Street (Mizpah Hotel)
2. Riverside (Riverside Hotel)
3. B Street (Sparks)
4. Sterling (Near UNR)
5. Town and Country (Reno)
6. Empire (Empire, NV)
7. Carson (Carson City)
8. Greenbrae Drug Company (Sparks)

Pettis' son-in-law, F. Ted Lemons, born in 1925, graduated from George Washington School of Pharmacy in Washington, D.C. He served in Hawthorne, Nevada, during WW II while in the U.S. Navy.

While in Hawthorne, he met his future wife, Alice, who is Linda Valle's mother. F. Ted Lemons worked for Pettis, and both had outstanding careers and were presidents of the Nevada Pharmaceutical Association. William Pettis died in 1982, and F. Ted Lemons died in 2012.

**NOTE:**

Linda Valle read our article on Nevada Pharmacies and met with Peter Aylworth to provide information on Nevada Pharmacies.

## Prison Doctor Karen Gedney, "*30 Years Behind Bars*"

This fascinating book recounts episodes revealing the mindset of criminals and how Dr. Gedney dealt with their demands and executions.

Dr. Karen Gedney: "When I retired as a prison doctor after three decades, I knew I had to decide my next act in life. It had to be different, something that would test me, have a positive impact, and which would allow me to use my background in corrections and medicine.

"One of the things that came to mind was writing my memoir, *30 Years Behind Bars*. As an internist I was trained to look at the whole person, understand problems and treat them. I found the prison and medical system to suffer from the same problem. They spend their time, energy, and money on taking care of the symptoms vs. the problems that caused them in the first place.

"I experienced many complex issues in the prison. I share the true stories from the perspective of a healer and problem solver, not a person oriented to punish and shame. It is my hope the reader will remember the true stories and characters that bring to life, the conflicting interests and views of custody, the inmates, and the young physician caught between them. It is my goal to emotionally make people aware and cause them to ask themselves how they can be part of the solution to end mass incarceration in the United States.

"There has never been a book written by a female prison doctor about the correctional system, let alone one who chose to turn it into her calling, even after being taken hostage. If you love underdog stories that leave you with hope, check out my memoir, *30 Years Behind Bars*."

Caroline Ford, Former Director of Rural Health at UNRSOM: Dr. Gedney was one of the first Nevada trained physicians in 1987 to receive an assignment in the National Health Service Corps program to repay her medical school debt through service to a medically underserved community. The Nevada State Office of Rural Health forged a relationship with the Nevada State Prison System to focus on incarcerated populations of medically underserved. Dr. Gedney embodied the core values of the program that was national at the time but was developing a state component finalized legislatively in 1989. Those values compelled practitioners with roots in the community to commit to medically underserved areas within the state. Dr. Gedney's prison medical practice and experiences will help to improve patient care for the future.

**NOTE:**

Dr. Gedney graduated from University of Cincinnati SOM in 1984, did a residency in internal medicine at University of Nevada Reno School of Medicine, and in 1987, became physician at Carson City's State Prison.

## NEONATAL INTENSIVE CARE UNITS IN NORTHERN NEVADA
### By Drs. Kristin Sohn Fermoile and Anton Sohn

Drs. Louis Gluck at Yale and Mildred Stahlman at Vanderbilt are foremost among U.S. pioneers in premature infant care (1950-60s). Their many contributions include the first modified neonatal respirator by Dr. Stahlman, and Dr. Gluck's organization of an ICU for preemies and sick infants. Neonatology became a certified sub-specialty of the American Academy of Pediatrics in 1975.

In 1973, Reno's pioneering neonatologist, Dr. Donald Pickering established the first Neonatal ICU (NICU) in northern Nevada at Washoe Medical Center (now Renown Regional Medical Center) to transport and care for infants. Dr. Steven Missall was also involved in the unit. By 1978, it was growing, and the Fleishmann Foundation donated $372,000 for expansion.

A tragic incident occurred in 1980 when Pediatric Cardiologist Ali Monibi was transporting an infant to San Francisco for surgery.

The plane crashed on Mt. Rose; the infant died, but 4 passengers survived.

In 1982, Dr. Pickering moved to Alaska, leaving Dr. Missall as Reno's only neonatologist. Saint Mary's Hospital opened a NICU, and he moved to their unit. To maintain accreditation,

WMC Chief of Staff Dr. Anton Sohn, recruited Neonatologist Bonnie Lees from UCLA. Senator Paul Laxalt got approval from the U.S. Department of Labor for her, a Canadian, to practice in the u.s. After she arrived in 1982, WMC's NICU was certified as the Regional Unit; SMH was not approved to transport infants. They ignored this mandate and the "Baby War" continued.

St. Mary's hired a San Francisco attorney in 1984 and sued for restraint of trade. Two years later the hospitals agreed to join efforts and signed an agreement with Pediatrix Medical Group to share neonatologists. In 2020, Pediatrix formed a separate team for each hospital due to hospital demand and increased patients and acuity level. Today, WMC (Renown) has 39 NICU beds with an average census of 36 infants. SMH's NICU has an average census of 10 infants.

**NOTE:**
The term "Baby War" originated 4 June 1976 by *Nevada State Journal* to describe competition between WMC and SMH.

## Southern Nevada's First Neonatal Intensive Care Unit

### By Founding NICU Director Dr. Bernard Feldman

"The development of neonatal intensive care in Las Vegas is a great story of starting a local NICU by a distant perinatal program. In 1974, there were about 5,000 deliveries/year in Las Vegas' six hospitals. Newborns requiring intensive care were flown to Salt Lake City or Los Angeles.

"Dr. Harrison Sheld, a local obstetrician contacted Dr. Louis Gluck at the Univ. of Calif. San Diego for help. A two-year grant from the Las Vegas March of Dimes (MOD) was obtained which paid for on-site UCSD neonatal fellows to provide training in resuscitation, fetal stabilization and monitoring, nurse education, and staffing in the NICU.

"Sunrise Hospital was chosen because it had more respiratory, laboratory, imaging, and back-up services than

Women's Hospital and So. Nev. Memorial Hospital (UMC) although they had more deliveries.

"Sunrise CEO Nathan Adelson gave assurances that all patients, insured or not, would be accepted. A space adjacent to labor and delivery, with six incubators and an overhead warmer, was provided.

"I was in the first group of four San Diego fellows at Sunrise. We ate, slept, and spent a month on-call, 24 hours-a-day in the hospital, attended high risk deliveries, rounded with nurses and physicians, and provided training. Local non-pediatric specialists in supporting disciplines willingly consulted whether an infant was insured or not. Dr. Don Christiansen performed most of the abdominal surgeries. Pediatric specialists from UCSD held follow-up clinics and teaching conferences in Las Vegas.

"Dr. Charles Vinnik, president of the MOD chapter was very supportive of the UCSD fellows. Board members entertained us in their homes. The Italian/American Club provided a furnished apartment with a rarely used kitchen. They provided a hatchback shift car for transport, not realizing infants needed care during transport. As the oldest, I was the only one who knew how to drive a shift car! Later, an ambulance company volunteered personnel and an ambulance.

"Jet-Avia donated a Lear jet to transport infants who needed more extensive surgical care. Initially, they had three jets, but one crashed in 1977 with Frank Sinatra's mother and another was impounded in South America allegedly for transporting drugs. Jets were preferred as reports showed a higher accident rate for helicopters. Also, helicopters are noisy, making it difficult for monitoring. Whenever possible, ground transport was used to not risk lives.

"After six months Sunrise's unit became overcrowded with babies doubled in incubators. I described this to Nate Adelson. Within a week, workers put up sheets for protection, knocked out concrete walls, and doubled the unit's size. New incubators, overhead warmers and ventilators arrived within two weeks. I asked Nate how he accomplished this in so short a time. He replied, 'I have juice!' Later I found out how much 'juice' Adelson's name had in Las Vegas.

"All did not run smoothly. Disagreements developed when morbidity-mortality conferences revealed OB care could have been better.

"We encouraged maternal transport to Sunrise for a high-risk delivery. Physicians at Women's Hospital were hesitant to support this. They disagreed that a problem could have been ameliorated by a different intra-partum approach. These differences stemmed from Women's Hospital desire to have the NICU and difficulty in accepting advice from a 'fellow.'

"I later learned dissension stemmed from the origins of the hospitals. Women's was started by Obstetrician Sol DeLee whose uncle, Dr. Joseph DeLee was considered the father of modern obstetrics and the founder of Chicago Lying-In Hospital where he introduced portable incubators. Sol, who founded the Las Vegas Obstetric and Gynecologic Society had similar ambitions for Women's. Sunrise, on the other hand, was built by Merv Adelson (Nate's son), Irwin Molasky, Allard Roen, a casino developer and Moe Dalitz, a gangster and casino owner. At one medical society meeting, an obstetrician from Women intimated 'fellows' were brought to Sunrise to care for the babies of Mafia prostitutes! Women's Hospital eventually hired a pediatrician to care for infants in their Level I nursery.

"I had an advantage of being the oldest fellow, having served as a medical officer in the United States Navy for five years and in private pediatric practice of for eight years. This afforded me stature to better handle inter-personal problems.

"The experiment in regionalization was successful. When I became director, the neonatal mortality was about 14/1,000 births, one of the worst in the nation. Ten years later, in 1985, it dropped to 8.5/1,000, ranking Nevada first in the nation.

Medicaid funding for newborn care was higher than any other state and such results helped encourage Senator Harry Reid's continued support for such funding. A curious twist to this story is that Harrison Sheld was a classmate of mine at SUNY, Downstate. We received MD degrees in 1959 but had not been in contact until I arrived in Las Vegas in 1974. What a pleasant surprise!

"In 1963, I was a pediatric resident at Bethesda Naval Hospital when our peds and OB departments were eagerly preparing to care for President Kennedy's baby, Patrick Bouvier, who unfortunately died after birth.

"I was a 'Fellow' in Neonatal/Perinatal Medicine from July 1974 through June 1976; at which time I became director of Sunrise's NICU and assistant professor of pediatrics at UCSD. Dr. Sheld was appointed chair of obstetrics at the School of Medicine (now UNRSOM), and in 1998, I was appointed its chair of pediatrics." (A "fellow" is a doctor-in-training to become a specialist after a residency.)

**NOTE:**

Dr. Feldman was responsible for bringing pediatric subspecialists to Las Vegas. UNRSOM Dean Dr. Robert Daugherty and Pediatrics Chair Dr. Trudy Larson hired Dr. Feldman to start a pediatric residency in 1996. The department expanded under Dr. Feldman's leadership. He recruited Drs. Beverly Neyland and Charles Snavely as the first clinical instructors. By 2003, the department had 36 residents, 22 full-time faculty, and a community faculty of 80.

## Neonatal Intensive Care Unit in Northern Nevada
## "Next Thing I Knew I was Hanging Upside Down"
### By Anne (Knox) Williams RN

"At the end of my Feb. 22, 1980, 3-11 PM shift I volunteered to fly Shane Swenson to San Francisco for open-heart surgery. We took off in a twin-engine Cessna around 10:30 PM. Pilot Leroy and Dr. Ali Monibi were in the front seats. I took care of baby Shane with Kim Stearns LPN.

"I saw clouds at my window and Lake Tahoe level with us in the distance. WE WERE TOO LOW!!! The stall signal was going off. The next thing I knew; I was hanging upside down with my seatbelt on and my swollen lip covering my nose. Kim crawled over and released my seatbelt.

"Shane was dead from injuries!!!

"I fell on Kim's broken leg. We disengaged ourselves to locate where the roof and sidewall meet. I noticed Ali's bloody face with a large head wound. We placed him on the wall of the plane so he could breathe easier. He had no shoes, so I tucked his feet in my coat. Snow was inside the plane. Leroy was laying on my legs. He wouldn't get out of the plane to see where we were, so I hit him. After he got back in, he said we were 10 miles from the nearest light, and the snow was super deep.

"It was a long night. Ali and I passed out for about 45 minutes each hour. When awake I'd check on him. He had so much blood on him, I was worried. My shoe was gone. My right foot was frozen.

"At daylight search and rescue found us. Due to my head trauma, things were blurry. Because Ali and Leroy could walk, they removed them first.

"They told us the plane rolled three times between two rock outcrops. We were in a 70-degree avalanche area. They tied the plane to trees and put us in baskets to lift us out around 12:30 PM.

"Kim and I were hospitalized for two weeks. I had a lumbar-sacral compression fracture, severe frost-bitten feet, and frostbite of the right leg. Kim had rods placed in her spine and her ankle fused. The FAA said our injuries were due to Leroy not tying down the transport. When the plane rolled, the transport hit us on our heads and legs.

"We found out from our lawyer that the control tower told Leroy three times to turn on the lights. He also falsified his logbook and had not flown enough hours for transport qualification. Even though he was not certified for Instrument Flight Rules (IFR), he was flying by instruments. We sued him; his transport license was permanently revoked, and his private license was revoked for two years.

"I was out of work for two years and on workmen's compensation. I relearned to walk and regain feeling in my feet. I am afraid of helicopters, turbo-planes, and small aircraft. I will fly in jets. I figure if they go down, there will be no recovery. Ha-Ha."

## RENO'S FIRST ACCIDENTAL NICU DEATH, FEBRUARY 1980
## By Dr. Ali Monibi

"I regained consciousness with excruciating pain in my side and blood on my head and face. I was upside down with the pilot on me, making the pain intolerable. When I gained full awareness, I saw the lit instruments and heard a buzzing. Panic overtook me with impending death, thinking an explosion imminent!! It was a miracle there was no explosion.

"We crashed!!! I heard moaning in the back seat. I yelled to make sure they responded. Nurse Anne Williams said baby Shane had died. We were transporting him to California for heart surgery.

"He was born in Winnemucca and transported by ground to WMC's ER and admitted when I was on call. Transport was arranged with Pilot Leroy, Nurses Anne, and Kim, and me in the co-pilot seat.

"The procedure was to go to an altitude to clear the mountains, but the pilot was unfamiliar with the downdraft on the east side of the mountains.

The last memory I had was flying by the top of the trees and the altimeter reading 9,000 feet. We were not gaining altitude, going down in a draft, unable to gain altitude.

"Yes, we had crashed!!! Everyone was alive except the baby,

who had a scarce chance of survival because of his heart condition. We took extreme measures to give him a chance, but his destiny was in this catastrophe.

"All night we wondered where we were. The pilot did not seem to have his faculties and could not tell me if we were discoverable.

"The next morning, we noted National Guard helicopters landing on the meadows about 1000 feet below us. We had crashed on Mount Rose. They were unable to land at night for fear of causing an avalanche.

"Divine intervention saved us. The right-wing detached when hitting a tree. The fuselage glided forward, on a bed of snow. After about 150 feet, the plane hit a granite wall. We sat there till 11:00 AM when we finally got covered with blankets brought by a Nevada National Guard helicopter. The warm bouillon they brought was the most delicious I had ever tasted.

"I held pressure on the gash on my head all night and tamped the bleeding wound. I was found to have a very low red blood count after transport to the ER. I was surprised I did not go into shock.

"Yes, I survived for my little daughter, Farrah, who was still in her mother's womb."

## NEONATAL INTENSIVE CARE UNITS IN LAS VEGAS
## By Founding NICU Director Dr. Bernard Feldman

"Without Drs. Don Christiansen and Bill Stephan (photo page 283), the Sunrise NICU would not have achieved the success it did. I also recall our first ligation of a Patent Ductus Arteriosus (PDA) on a premature infant was performed by Dr. Harold Feikes with Dr. William Stephan as anesthesiologist.

"I don't recall the size of the infant, but it was a preemie who would not come off the ventilator. I diagnosed the PDA, but the baby was too sick to fly to UCLA where my cardiac surgeries were being done under the direction of Dr. William Friedman, chair of pediatrics. I had worked under Dr. Friedman at UCSD during my fellowship and he was the pediatric cardiologist consulting on the infants in Las Vegas. When he moved on to UCLA, he continued his consultation visits to Las Vegas and gave Grand Rounds which I arranged monthly at Sunrise Hospital.

"Anyway, being the infant was too sick for transport, I called Don Christensen who recommended Dr. Harold Feikes. I put in a call to Harold who was in the surgical dressing room. He did not know who I was, so I went through a lengthy explanation of the infant's condition.

"I was quite sure of the diagnosis trying to convince him to operate. He was completely silent during the entire phone conversation and when I was finished, he said, "bring the baby down to the OR at lunchtime, I'll do him between cases." I was dumbfounded but relieved. I took the baby down to the OR, and Dr. Bill Stephan gave some whiffs of anesthesia. I helped Harold identify the PDA which at this point was as large in diameter as the aorta and all went well.

"I'll never forget that first encounter with Harold and I told the story at the ceremony when, in 1991, I was given the Harold Lee Feikes Memorial Physician of the Year award by the Clark County Medical Society."

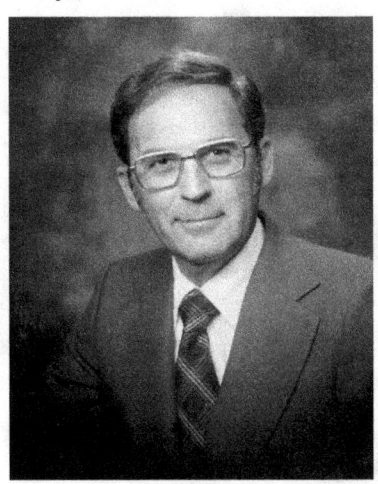

Dr. Bill Stephan, 1974

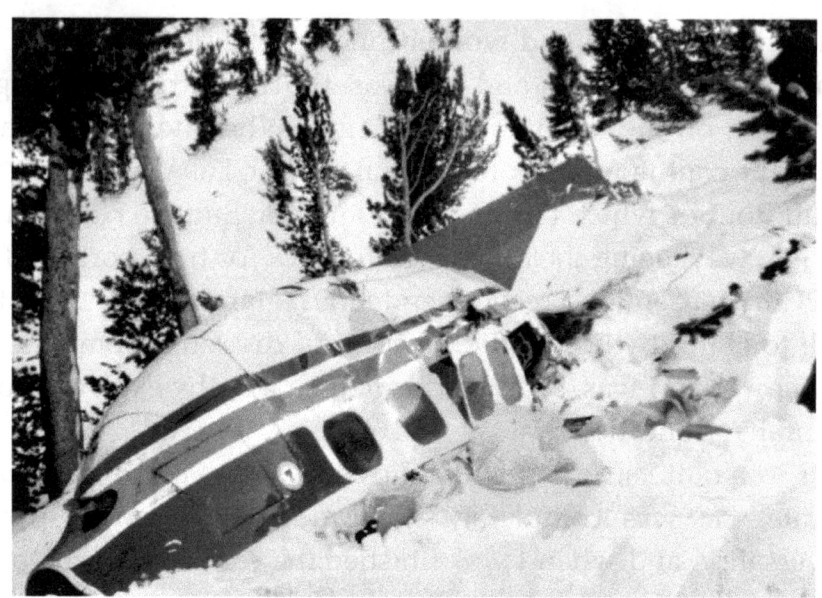

NICU Transport Crash, Mt. Rose

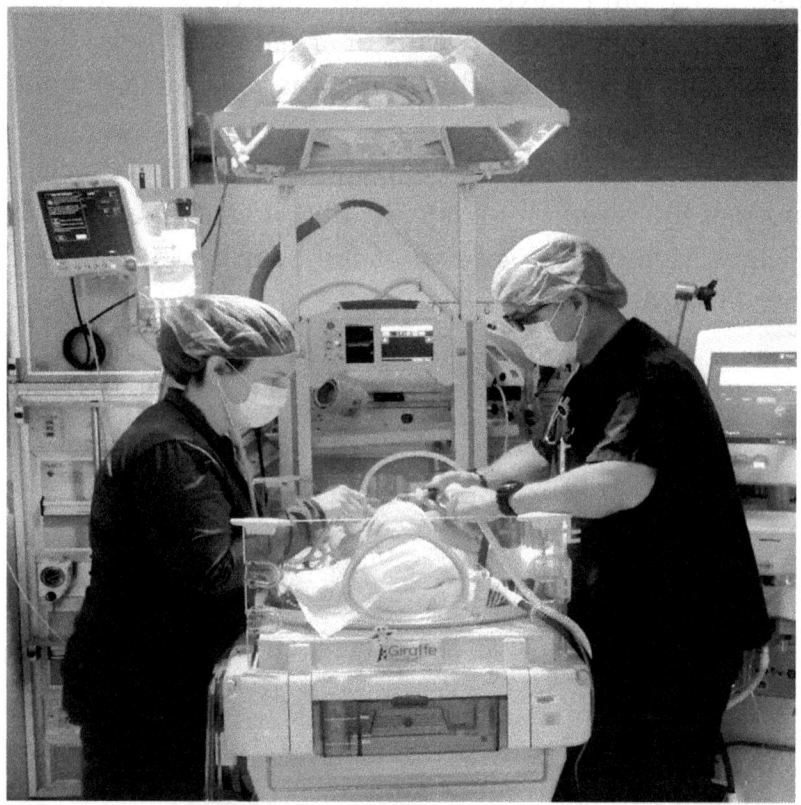

Erin Madsen RN, Brian Walsh RT, Renown NICU, 2020

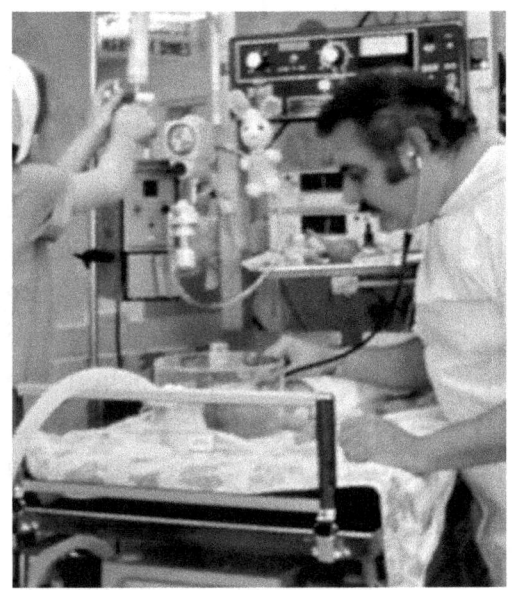
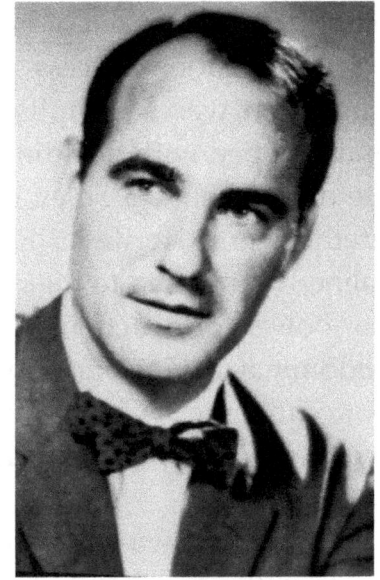

Dr. Feldman, Sunrise NICU, 1976   Dr. Pickering, 1973

## Another Dr. Christensen, "To the Rescue"

Dr. Bill Stephan commented on Dr. Don Christensen's repair of a newborn with gastroschisis (defect in abdominal wall with the GI tract outside of the abdomen) at Las Vegas' Sunrise Hospital. Following is an account by Dr. G. Norman Christensen of a repair he did of gastroschisis at Ely's Hospital in 1990s: "My wife and office nurse and I had been cross-country skiing on Ward mountain. It was snowing so hard that we quit and returned to town. As was my custom, I stopped at the hospital before going home. As I was walking down the hall to go out the back door, the delivery nurse excitedly stopped me in the hallway and said, Dr. Christensen you need to see this baby.

"I opened the delivery room door to see a large group of family members around a lady who had just delivered a male infant with gastroschisis. The infant was in a Kreiselman (infant warmer). I got all the family members out of the delivery room and summoned my surgery group. It was apparent we could not move to the OR because we needed to keep the infant warm. Therefore, I did the operation with the infant in the Kreiselman without changing out of my ski clothes.

"Intravenous access was obtained, and endotracheal intubation was accomplished. The operative field was draped and prepped with Betadine. A urethral catheter was needed, but we did not have a Foley catheter small enough to insert in the urethra, so a sterile #5 French feeding tube was used. Warm saline was applied to the intestines, and I determined there were no bowel obstructions. The intestines were placed in the abdominal cavity and closure begun. As we approached the bottom of the incision there was a clear structure protruding, which obviously was the urinary bladder. The tube in the urethra had come out.

"This area was re-prepped, and the sterile tube replaced. Faced with a recurrence, I asked the tech for a cutting needle with 4-0 silk.

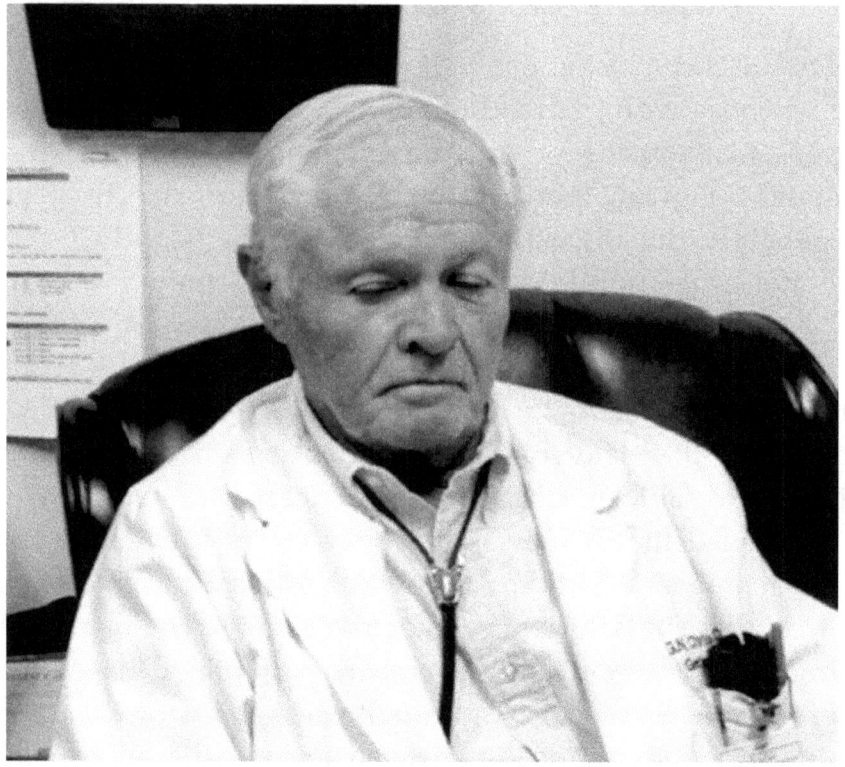

Dr. G. Norman Christensen, 1990s

"The needle was used to impale a portion of the plastic tube and sutured it to the foreskin. "The closure was finished, and dressing was applied. Due to the need for warming, the patient remained in the Kreiselman with covers. The family practitioner who had delivered the child, the anesthetist, nursing personnel, and I monitored the child, who was on ventilation until a neonatal crew from Sunrise Hospital arrived the following day. The next day I received a call from Sunrise giving a report on the newborn and expounding on the technique for maintaining bladder drainage.

"Due to medical records outdating, I do not have records from those days (approximately thirty-years-ago). In fact, I do not have the exact date this happened. The family moved to Winnemucca, so I lost follow-up information on the baby."

## Nevada's Medical Heritage
## Great Basin History of Medicine Museum and Library

The HOM Library (HOML) is named after the six Doctors Hood who practiced in our state. Dr. William Henry Hood came to Battle Mountain in 1886 and in 1899 received Nevada medical license #1 for the grand sum of $2. Five Doctors Hood followed. The three HOM Museum rooms are the Dr. Donald Mousel Lounge, the Dr. Robert Daugherty Study Room, and Dr. Owen Bolstad Conference Room. The late Dr. Mousel was on ophthalmologist and dedicated humanitarian who treated patients in poor countries and communities where eye care was difficult or impossible to obtain. The Daugherty Study Room recognizes former Dean Bob Daugherty, who made the area available to the Great Basin History of Medicine Program (GBHMP). The Dr. Owen Bolstad Conference Room is in honor of Dr. Bolstad, who created the GBHMP with Dr. Anton Sohn.

Satellite HOML exhibits are located at the entrance to the Savitt Library, the entrance to the Nevada State Public Health

Laboratory on the SOM campus, and the entrance to the Savitt Medical Education building.

The HOM Collection displays historical medical artifacts, books, and photographs. The collection contains 121 oral histories; written documents; and over 7,000 photographs related to the school of medicine, the Nevada State Medical Association, frontier military medicine in the Great Basin, Nevada hospitals, and doctors in Nevada, dating as early as 1851 when Dr. Charles Daggett arrived in Genoa. The collection includes all the published issues of *Greasewood Tablettes* (quarterly history of medicine bulletin) since its inception in 1989, and 120 oral histories related to public health, hospitals, and the practice of human medicine, veterinarian medicine and dentistry dating from 1939. Also included in the museum archives are 15 file cabinets with documents of historical importance.

The medical instrument collection includes over 900 medical artifacts, including Dr. Donald Mousel's collection of over 100 eyeglasses dating from the 18th century when Benjamin Franklin created the bifocal lens.

Dr. Fred Anderson's collection of early Nevada Indian medical artifacts and medical instruments, nineteenth century surgical instruments, and early twentieth-century medical furniture and instruments are in the exhibit. The Savitt entrance showcase at one time contained a collection of early obstetrical instruments and artifacts donated by Dr. George Furman, who was the founding member of the obstetrical department at the SOM.

Two objects of importance to Nevada are Dr. Simeon L. Lee's microscope (Nevada's first Microscope) and a 7-inch wooden stethoscope used by an unknown doctor in Austin, Nevada in 1863.

Dr. Rene Laennec in Paris invented the stethoscope in 1816. Before that time a doctor put his ear on the patient's chest to hear heart and lung sounds. Laennec observed young students on a street in Paris listening to tapping sound hear over a long wooden pole. He quickly deduced that heart sounds would transmit over a similar device and rolled a notebook and placed one end on the patient's chest and the other at his ear. Thus, he invented and named the stethoscope (*Stethos* [breast] *skopein* [look at]). Years later, a 7-inch wooden stethoscope was made. Later came the stethoscope as we know it today.

Dr. Simeon Lemuel Lee came to Pioche in 1872 and became one of Nevada's most prominent nineteenth century doctors, but it is unknown when he brought his brass microscope to Nevada. The microscope was invented in the 1600s, but illumination crucial to seeing details of microscopic objects was developed in 1893. Therefore it is reasonable to assume Dr. Lee obtained his microscope sometime around 1900. It is the first known microscope in Nevada. Dr. Lee died in Carson City in 1927.

The book collection includes over 750 medical books, 16 books published by the Greasewood Press, books on Nevada history with reference to medicine, approximately 73 nineteenth-century medical books, and 17 eighteenth century books including a 1702 rare edition of Mead's *Mechanic Account of Poisons* donated by Dr. Ken Maclean, who was a longtime secretary of the Nevada Board of Medical Examiners.

The museum/library contains over 120 oral histories.

A recent addition is a gift by Dr. Tom Hall, retired St. Mary's Hospital pathologist, of a 1787 book. The HOML book collection includes 110 current monographs on the history of medicine; 50 books on military medicine; early issues of the *Bulletin of the Nevada State Medical Association*; the complete New York Academy of Medicine Library Catalog and the *Index-Catalogue of the Library of the Surgeon General's Office*, U.S. Army, 1880-1955. We also list more than 700 doctors who practiced in Nevada between 1857 and 1900. The complete collection of the *Classics of Medicine* is housed in the medical library.

The beginning of western medicine Is chronicled in the

museum. The oldest and maybe the most important relic in the museum is a Greek Marble column with a carved snake, the emblem of medicine. It relates to the beginning of western medicine in ancient Greece. Hippocrates, who was born around 460 B.C. on the Island of Cos taught disease was a natural process and not from supernatural sources as was formerly taught. Before Hippocrates prayer to Aesculapius and interpretation by the temple priest was essential to healing. The Aesculapians believed in the healing power of snakes, which dwelt in the unknown beneath the ground. Their symbol was a single serpent wound around a staff. From this we get the modern symbol of medicine, the *caduceus*.

The U.S. military added a second snake and wings to the staff as part of a military doctor's uniform. The serpent symbol is displayed in the museum on an ancient 12-inch marble pillar from the city of Byblos (now Jubayl), a 5,000-year-old Phoenician city. In Biblical times the city was known for its papyrus used for written records. Bible derives its name from Byblos. U.S. Ambassador Robert Borden Reams, who was appointed by President Eisenhower, gave the marble column with the serpent to Dr. Fred Anderson, who gave it to the museum.

Hippocrates and associates refuted the Aesculapian supernatural cause of disease and taught that sickness arises in the patient or from the environment. Writings of Hippocrates known as the *Hippocratic Corpus* were recorded over approximately 200 years.

The *Hippocratic Corpus* contains 70 different texts, which are characterized by clarity of thought, scientific method, and moral teaching. The most famous declaration is: *"Life is short. The art is long. Opportunity is fleeting. Experience is delusive. Judgment is difficult."*

Hippocrates' teachings have guided medicine for thousands of years. Its disciples emphasized that maintain equilibrium between the four humors (Blood, Yellow Bile, Black Bile, and

Phlegm) was necessary for good health. This theory resulted in bloodletting and purging to maintain equilibrium, a practice that existed into the nineteenth century.

Great Basin History of Medicine Museum's Earliest Artifacts

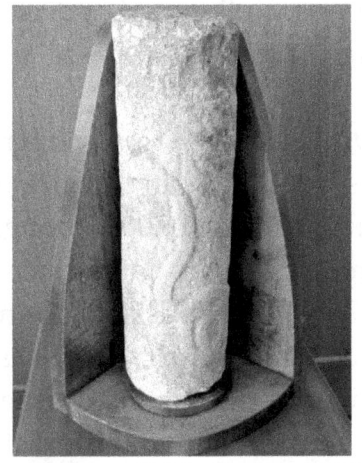

Byblos Column With Snake, 500 B.C.      Wooden Stethoscope, 1863

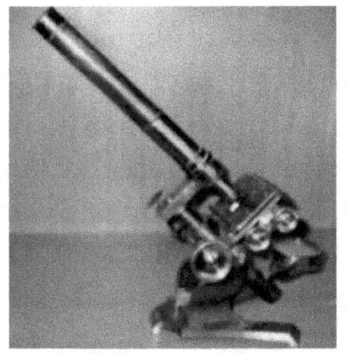 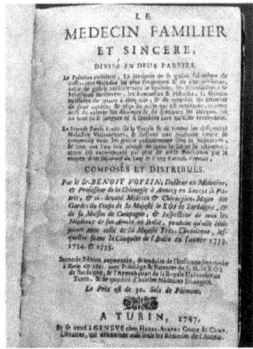 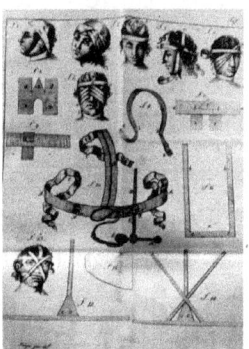

Dr. Lee's Microscope, 1900      1747 Book on Medicine

## DR. CHRISTIAN B. ZABRISKE, "1868 DISINFECTANT"
### By Dr. Anton Sohn

Dr. Christian Bevoort Zabriske was no ordinary Polish descendent. He had a dream to explore the unknown and help others overcome illness. He was born in Haversack, New Jersey, on June 29, 1801, into a family that had emigrated from Poland in the 1660s.

He received a medical degree from Columbia University in 1832. However, a vision led him west. He and son, Elias, moved to Jacksonville, Illinois, where he joined as a volunteer for the Mexican War in 1846. After the war he was back in New York as a surgeon for the California Union Association that had plans to go to California's goldfields through the Panama Canal and up the coast to California.

Initially, landing in Panama with his fellow passengers, he found over 2,000 other travelers stranded and waiting for passage to California. The group raised $6,000, bought a dilapidated schooner, and sailed up the coast to San Francisco.

The 1862 Silver City directory lists Dr. Zabriske as living on Second Street between High and Main with son, Elias, an attorney. Various directories and advertisements during the 1860s and 1870s list seven additional doctors living or practicing in Silver City.

His patient ledgers start October 12, 1862. They show appointments through October 4, 1868. Many of the notations were after midnight. Irene Brennan's article on august 12, 1975, in *The Nevadan* notes Zabriske's fees ranged from $2 to $10, but his collections were about thirty percent. For example, during September 1863, his charges were $1,013.50, and payments were $368. Brennan further notes, "By Cash (Greenbacks) $70.00." To further add to his collection deficit woes, Greenbacks sold at the local banks for between 68¢ and 72¢ on the dollar.

Zabriske's ledgers give some insight into this practice. He used the lancet, as was the practice at the time, to bleed patients. In addition, he used blistering, scarification, and cupping.

Blistering was a procedure when blisters were produced by applying intense heat and lancing the blisters to drain fluid.

Scarification resulted when a flat surfaced gadget with six or eight spring-loaded lancets pierced the skin or mucus membrane to produce oozing of blood or serum. To increase oozing a heated glass cup placed over the wounds for suction.

Dr. Zabriske charged $50 for a delivery and on one occasion, he charged $15 for delivering a placenta. Smallpox was a threat to nineteenth century citizens of Nevada, and the doctor charged Lyon County for treating the illness. He also vaccinated patients to prevent the dreaded disease. The following was in the *Gold Hill Daily News* 12.11.1868.

<u>Zabriske's Disinfectant</u>—speaking of chloride of lime, carbolic acid and other popular disinfectants, Dr. Zabriske said, "The best way to fortify against the smallpox is to eat plenty of good grub, keep your bowels in order, use a reasonable amount of choice whiskey, gin, brandy—whichever you prefer—and keep out of the way of the disease as much as possible." It was said, "The doctor's head is pretty level, but what's a poor fellow to do who hasn't got any mouth for whiskey?"

There was professional courtesy among doctors in Silver City. Zabriske and Dr. Seldon McMeans amputated a badly broken leg after teamster Ezekiel W. Culliver splintered his leg in two places. On another occasion Dr. Zabriske set Joseph Todman's broken femur and charged $50. He consulted with Dr. Minneer regarding Todman and after seven visits found it necessary to perform a bleeding. He sometimes used a starch bandage to immobilize a fracture. His ledger showed he charged $50 for syphilis treatment. He treated fourteen cases of syphilis (three were secondary syphilis) and eight cases of gonorrhea.

Dr. Christian Zabriske died at the Reno Asylum, November 1886, and Candelaria's True Fissure noted in an obituary: "Dr. Zabriske… represented Lyon County in Republican conventions many times. An able physician, possessed of a gigantic brain, one of the handsomest men the writer ever saw."

# X

## NURSING
## "CONTENT TO HELP PEOPLE"

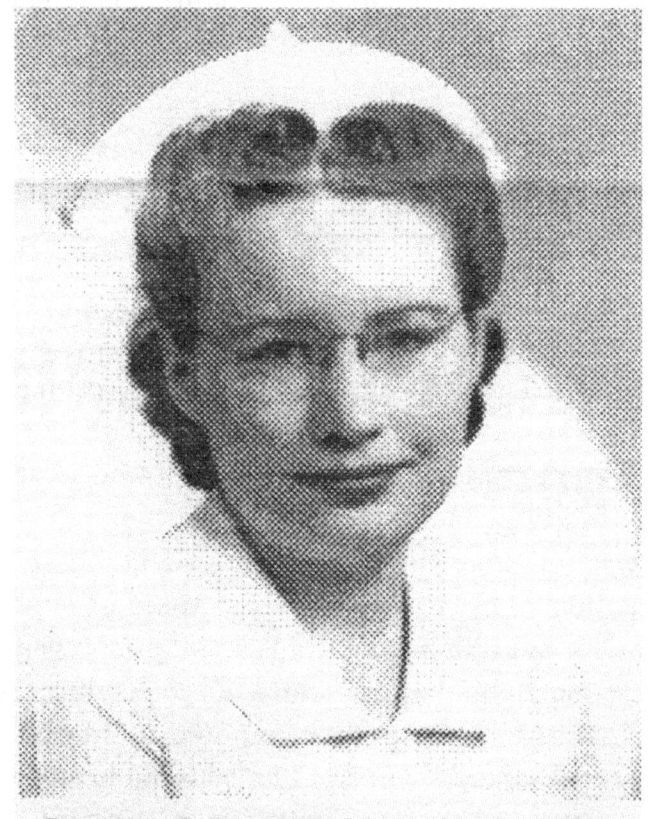

*DOROTHY GEORGE RN 1943*

# MIDWIVES IN NEVADA, 1878-1908
## By Phyllis Cudek

The wagon trains bearing pioneers included pregnant women and midwives who could attend to them during childbirth. Isolated communities through which the wagon trains passed also had a need for the knowledge and experience brought by midwives. Outbreaks of smallpox, influenza, and other such illnesses required as much medical assistance as could be found in the area, and midwives were often the only persons available with any medical experience. Their knowledge of home remedies and use of herbal ingredients was often invaluable to the settlers' health. So scarce were medical supplies that cactus fiber was occasionally used to suture wounds.

Although the importance of midwives was undeniable, they rarely listed themselves as "professionals" in county census reports or city directories.

For example, in *Bishop's Directory of Virginia City, Gold Hill, Silver City, Carson City, and Reno, 1878-79*, professions such as dressmakers, milliners, domestics, teachers, and ladies' nurses were listed; however, only two midwives, Mrs. Julia Bellmerre of Virginia City and Mrs. S.M. Drannan of Reno were acknowledged in addition to Mrs. Helen Anderson of Reno, who was listed as midwife and physician. Midwives were crucial to the sustained population growth of rural communities. They enabled the West to grow and prosper because of their maternal and childbirth attention and skills.

The Church of Latter-Day Saints (LDS or Mormons) contributed widely to the presence and importance of midwifery in Nevada in the 19th and early 20th centuries. Settlements established under the direction of the Mormon Church in Salt Lake City took families to remote areas of the state. The proliferation of children demonstrated the need for childbirth assistance; therefore, women were often chosen from their communities to travel to Salt Lake City to be trained in the techniques of midwifery and who then would return to their communities to practice.

In 1891, Panaca in southeastern Nevada was such a community. One of its midwives was Mariah Berdilla Rich (nee Atchison).

This woman delivered W. Driggs, who later wrote an article for *Nevada Historical Quarterly* describing childbirth in a small western town. Two other women from the Mormon Church, well known in their community of White Pine Country were Mrs. Mary Leicht Oxborrow and Mrs. Margaret Christina Arnoldus Windous.

Author Effie Oxborrow Read writes about midwives, Mary Leicht Oxborrow (her grandmother), and Margaret Christina Arnoldus Windous, in *White Pine Lang Syne, A True History of White Pine County, Nevada.*

"In 1900, Mrs. Mary Leicht Oxborrow came from St. George, Utah. She had been set aside by the Church authorities as a midwife and doctor for the community of Lund. She already had sons and daughters there. Her excellence as a doctor cannot be over-commended. She made her own medicines, salves, face cream, and had keen knowledge of herbs. She accomplished tremendous medical feats in care of broken bones. She delivered 235 babies, two of whom were her own great grandchildren. She was an excellent musician and was a beloved character."

Read continues later in her book with information on another much-admired midwife and doctor, Margaret Christine Arnoldus Windous.

"In 1908, the Latter-Day Saints Church requested each ward of the Church send at least one Relief Society member to Salt Lake City to train under the direction of Dr. Ramona B. Pratt. Mrs. Windous had eight children and limited education, but she accomplished this mission and received certification for practicing obstetrics and nursing. She was the country doctor, and it was necessary for her to make many lonely trips across the desert in the dead of night with her little black buggy and faithful horse, Dolly."

Mrs. Windous lived in Nevada since 1899, had a maternity home in Lund, and delivered more than 1,000 babies. "Her patients were of all nationalities and religions," writes Read. Most communities had their own midwife who could be summoned for an expected birth. Midwives, unlike physicians, gave family assistance in ways other than delivering a child.

A midwife would leave her own family while she gave physical and emotional support to the expectant woman, often cooking meals, doing laundry, housecleaning, and caring for other family members after the birth of a new baby. This service would often last several days before and/or after the childbirth. On the frontier women helped women in any way.

In Nevada's early days, it was not unusual for a mother to be a midwife to her daughter, daughter-in-law, her granddaughter, or for a sister to be a midwife to her own sister. Although a midwife was usually a woman who had given birth to children herself, it was not uncommon for a young girl to assist a family member in the birthing process, thereby providing her with experience to assist others as she grew older.

A few illustrations of midwifery activities follow. Anna Mueller Engel Neddenriep was a German immigrant and qualified midwife who wore a long black cape as a symbol of her profession. She was referred to as an "Angel of Mercy" by Carson Valley neighbors.

Around 1900, Mrs. Mary "Granny" Dakin offered hospital services in Elko after having been a midwife for many years. She also having taught midwifery to her daughter, Mrs. Tillie Roach.

Mrs. Bill Bradley, a midwife for the White Pine County area was untutored but would often... "tie her own small baby to her back Indian-style, saddle a pony, and ride twenty miles or more to be on hand for the blessed event."

Mrs. Scott from Osceola was midwife for Anna Day Swallow in the Shoshone area around the 1880s. Despite her lack of formal medical training "Little Mrs. Dr. Swallow" treated burns, pneumonia, and delivered babies in her community. She would often travel in the dead of night by horse and sleigh in two feet of snow to reach a patient. There are certainly hundreds of untold similar incidences of the unselfishness and devotion displayed by 19th century women in the vast state of Nevada.

The treatment given by midwives was usually non-interventionist. Although forceps had been used for hundreds of years and were sometimes present in the medical bag of a midwife, they were often reserved for use by a physician for a difficult delivery.

Administration of ergot, a commercially prepared medicine formulated from a rye grain fungus, was used by midwives and physicians to produce contractions of the uterus to curtail postpartum bleeding. Other home remedies known by midwives were no doubt used to provide comfort, but generally, childbirth was on the frontier without aid or medication.

Puerperal fever, commonly known as childbed fever, was a constant threat to the life of a delivering mother. However, once the importance of cleanliness and sterilization became known, this condition became less prevalent. As Nevada's population grew, some of the larger communities, such as Elko, Ely, and Reno, had maternity homes or hospitals, which were usually operated by nurses or midwives. Some women would come for the birth of a child and then remain for several days to heal and regain strength.

Anonymity was common of many midwives in Nevada's wide-open spaces. Finding and documenting names of women who aided and performed medical services for their communities was difficult.

Terminology in reference to midwives adds frustration to research efforts; midwives may also be referred to as "ladies nurses" or "Doctresses" which could also refer to female physicians, or merely those who treat sick or injured people. Also present were a few men who signed birth certificates as *accoucheur*, which can be interpreted as male midwife or an obstetrician, but not necessarily a physician. The moral atmosphere of the 1800s and early 1900s contributed to the obscurity of midwife identification in that "genteel women" did not discuss birthing nor intimate personal life in general. By 1900, births in the United States were assisted approximately equally by both midwives and physicians. This was not true in the sparsely populated state of Nevada.

**NOTE:**

This article was abstracted from the chapter entitled "*Early Midwives*" in the book, *Healers of 19th Century Nevada* by Dr. Anton P. Sohn and published by Greasewood Press. The chapter was researched and written by Phyllis Cudek.

Dr. Bethenia Owens, born in Oregon, was one of nine children. She married at 14 but divorced after two children.

Fiercely independent, she supported her family by taking in laundry and doing nursing. After her children graduated from college, Bethenia attended the University of Michigan School of Medicine and earned an MD.

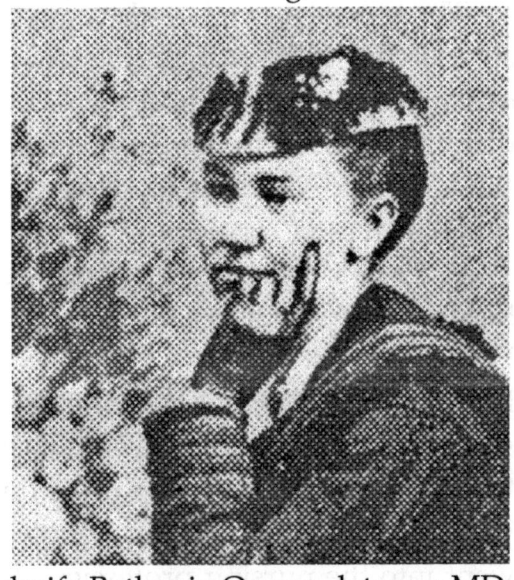

Midwife Bethenia Owens, later an MD

# Dorothy George RN, "Content to Help People"
## By Lisa Puleo and Annie Blachley

Dorothy O'Donnell (George) RN, always wanted to be a nurse. As she says, "I wanted to take care of people and be a bedside nurse, and that's what I was." During her nurses training at St. Mary's Hospital in Rochester, Minnesota, before World War II, nurses were taught to do everything. In the morning they bathed patients, gave them backrubs, and changed linens. Before the patients napped or were prepared for sleep at night, nurses gave the backrubs, turned them, and made them comfortable. Nurses changed linens twice a day—more often if necessary—and were responsible for treatments and medications as well as bedside care. Dorothy recalls that because of the severe shortage of registered nurses (RNs), they worked 12 hours a day, six days a week, and earned $125 ($2,482 in 2022) a month.

During and after WW II, while serving with the U.S. Army Nurse Corps in Okinawa, she oversaw a makeshift orthopedic ward, a tent much like MASH unit. When a typhoon hit the island, everything was washed into the China Sea.

The nurses moved all the patients on litters into caves in the side of the hill until the storm abated, when patients were evacuated to stateside hospitals. "It was very hard work, but you couldn't leave them there in the beds, nor do any nursing care of the wounded, because the tents and everything washed out to sea," she recalls.

After her 1946 discharge, she went home to Wisconsin, then headed west. At Las Vegas' Clark County General Hospital (now University Medical Center), she worked in obstetrics from 11:00 PM to 7:00 AM. She recalls nurses typically worked eight-hour shifts, six days a week, earning around $250 a month. Dorothy: "Nurses didn't complain a great deal in those days. They were very content to be helping people because that was why they went into the nursing profession. There were no such things as unions for nurses or strikes to interfere with nursing care."

While working obstetrics, Dorothy had many conversations with the doctor on call, Dr. Joseph M. George, Jr., who delivered many babies. They were married in 1950 and became partners in a calling that is fast disappearing—solo general practice. Dorothy George assisted her husband throughout most of his 42 years in practice in Las Vegas, as secretary, receptionist, nurse, and she adds with a smile, occasional janitor.

When Medicare became a reality, Dr. George's bills were routinely rejected because Medicare clerks didn't understand the coding. Dorothy would constantly have to explain procedures. Justifying services for Medicaid-insured patients sometimes required sending letters seven or eight times to collect 54 cents on the dollar of the authorized fee. Dr. George: "Before Medicare and Medicaid we didn't have many regulations. Doctors of my vintage universally felt we practiced in the 'golden era' of medicine." "Many nurses feel that way also," added Dorothy.

By the early sixties, something else in medicine had changed. When Dorothy asked if bedside nursing was being taught at a local hospital, a nursing professor replied, "We don't teach our nurses to be slaves." Dorothy: "That really shocked me—and it hurt—because to me, nurses are supposed be there to take care of patients, to be compassionate and caring."

Nurses don't do bedside nursing anymore—mostly the RNs do the bookwork, the paperwork, except in specialty units such as intensive care or recovery. Just recently I had a friend who was in the hospital for six days following major surgery and didn't have a change of bed linen the whole time. To me, hospitals will profit more if the patients have a good rapport with the hospital- and the patients would recuperate faster.

Looking back, Dorothy says she enjoyed her nursing career during the years she worked and was proud to say she was an RN. Dorothy: "But unfortunately, that is no longer true. Florence

Nightingale would turn over in her grave if she knew what was happening in her chosen profession today!"

**NOTE:**

The article about Dorothy George RN, is from an oral history by Lisa Puleo, which was edited by Annie Blachley.

## ELLEN HOUSE DNSc
### HISTORY OF NURSING IN NEVADA

The following History of Nursing information was extracted from Dr. (Fries) House's doctorate dissertation.

For hundreds of years, approximately twenty-seven tribes of Indians occupied the Great Basin. Their sole ownership expired when trappers and gold-silver seekers invaded the area in mid-nineteenth century. Most of these new arrivals were young and healthy. However, smallpox and other epidemics were common, and immunization was a new form of prevention. As mentioned earlier, Saint Mary Louise in Virginia City, staffed by the Catholic Daughters of Charity was the first hospital in the territory.

The medical profession was largely unregulated until Dr. Henry Bergstein ran for the legislature in 1874 with the intent of passing legislation to license doctors. Dr. Henry Bergstein was alarmed a local druggist treated miners with quicksilver (mercury) when they presented with constipation due to lead poisoning. The druggist succeeded in giving them a [quick] passage to the grave.

Dr. Bergstein sponsored legislation entitled, "An Act to Prevent the Practice of Medicine or Surgery by Unqualified Persons" in the 1875 legislature. The act required physicians to register with the county register. Unfortunately, they had no way to verify the doctor's word that he was a trained physician.

During the nineteenth century there were only two or three graduate nurses in Nevada. Most nursing care was provided by neighbors, midwives, and family. Later, according to a report filed by the American Medical Association (AMA) on March 27,

1943, there were 169 graduate nurses in Nevada. The first attempt to regulate nursing was years earlier on September 11, 1907, when an article appeared in the *Nevada State Journal* announcing local nurses attempting to form a labor union. The union was formed the following year in 1908, and the Nurses' Association (RNA) was formed.

Dr. George McKenzie was one of the first doctors at Saint Mary's Hospital when it opened in 1908 and is acknowledged as the first supporter of nursing education. Fifteen years later, Assemblywoman Marguerite Gosse, who had worked with the Red Cross during WW I, introduced the first Nurse Practice Act in the Nevada Legislature. Approved March 20, 1923, it directed the governor to appoint a Board of Nurse Examiners (BONE). The board consisted of three registered graduates. Nurses who applied for registration prior to July 1, 1923, were registered by endorsement.

On March 23, 1931, an Articles of Incorporation for the Nevada Nurses' Association (NNA) were filed with the Secretary of State John Koontz. The primary purpose of NNA was to establish a code of ethics.

Saint Mary's training school for nurses closed in 1922, and Nevada had no program for training nurses until 1957 when UNR established a Bachelor of Science (BS) program in nursing. It was named Orvis School of Nursing (UNR) after Arthur E. Orvis, who donated $100,000 in gratitude for previously receiving excellent nursing care. The first Dean of UNR Nursing was Doris Yingling. In 1961, NNA bought nursing pins for the 109 members of the first graduating class.

In 1965, an Associate Degree (AD) program in nursing was established at UNLV. Western Nevada Community College (later Truckee Meadows Community College) in Reno established an Associate Degree in 1971. UNLV added a Bachelor of Science in Nursing degree to its curriculum in 1972. By 1960, education and certification for nursing was well established in Nevada.

# Books By
# Nevada History of Medicine Foundation, Inc.

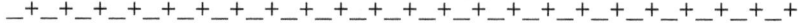

1. This Won't Hurt a Bit: The Life and Practice of Reno Dentist Harry Massoth, Eileen Barker, Editor A.P. Sohn, 1995
2. The Healers of 19th Century Nevada: 19th Century Chinese, Indian, Midwives, and Physician Healers, A.P. Sohn, 1997
3. People Make the Hospital: The History of Washoe Medical Center, A.P. Sohn & Carroll Ogren, 1998
4. Good Medicine: Four Las Vegas Doctors and the Golden Age of Medicine, Annie Blachley, Editor A.P. Sohn, 2000
5. Serving Medicine: Nevada State Medical Association and The Politics of Medicine, R.G. Pugh, Editor A.P. Sohn, 2002
6. Pestilence, Politics, and Pizzazz: Public Health in Las Vegas—Dr. Otto Ravenholt, Annie Blachley, Editor A.P. Sohn, 2002
7. Cutting Edge: Reflections and Memories of Doctors on Medical Advances in Reno, R.G. Pugh, Editor A.P. Sohn, 2002
8. Better Medicine: The History of the University of Nevada School of Medicine (Now UNRSOM), Phyllis Cudek and A.P. Sohn, 2003
9. Nevada Veterinarians: Profiles of Doctors in a Caring Profession, R.G. Pugh, Editor A.P. Sohn, 2007
10. Frontier Surgeon and Georgetown Medical School Dean: Reminiscences of George Martin Kober, Editor A.P. Sohn, 2008
11. The Birthplace of Nevada Medicine: Carson City, R.G. Pugh & A.P. Sohn, 2009
12. Doctoring in Nevada: Inspiration, Dedication, and History, Editors A.P. Sohn & R.M. Daugherty, 2013

13. 150 Years 0f Nevada Medicine (and more), A.P. Sohn & R.M. Daugherty, 2014
14. Medicine is History: Nevada's Great Basin History of Medicine, A.P. Sohn, 2017
15. Idaho Wildflowers in the River of No Return Wilderness at Pistol Creek, R. Montgomery, W. Payne, A.P. Sohn, W.J. Thompson, and L.E. Toole; 5th edition, 2018
16. With These Hands: A lifetime of Art and Crafts, A.P. Sohn, 2020
17. Growing up in Irvington, A.P. Sohn, 2020
18. Traveling the Globe, A.P. Sohn, 2020
19. Addendum to Traveling the Globe, A.P. Sohn, 2020
20. My Honor to Serve Mankind, A.P. Sohn, 2020
21. Call of the Mountain, A.P. Sohn, 2020
22. Vietnam War (Sohn, Myers, Brady, and Ganchan), A.P. Sohn, 2022
23. 1,000 Years of Medicine in Nevada's Great Basin, J.M. Grove and A.P. Sohn, 2022

# Abbreviations

_+_+_+_+_+_+_+_+_+_+_+_+_+_+_+_+_+_+_+_+_+

| | |
|---|---|
| AB | Bachelor of Arts Degree |
| | Assembly Bill |
| AD | Associate Degree |
| AFB | Air Force Base |
| AFIP | Armed Forces Institute of Pathology |
| AIDS | Acquired Immune Deficiency Syndrome |
| AMA | American Medical Association |
| ARDS | Acute Resp. Distress Syndrome |
| CBC | Complete Blood Count |
| CDC | Center of Disease Control and Prevention |
| BONE | Board of Nursing Examiners |
| BSN | Bachelor of Science in Nursing |
| BUN | Blood Urea Nitrogen (kidney function test) |
| DIHS | Division of Indian Health Serv. |
| DMD | Doctor of Dental Medicine |
| DNA | Deoxyribonucleic Acid |
| DNSc | Doctor of Nurse Science |
| DO | Doctor of Osteopathy |
| DVM | Doctor Veterinarian Medicine |
| ENT | Ear, Nose, and Throat |
| HFRS | Hemorrhagic fever with renal symptoms |
| HIS | Indian Health Service |
| HOML | History of Medicine Library |
| HOMM | History of Medicine Museum |
| HPS | Hantavirus Pulmonary Syndrome |
| ICU | Intensive Care Unit |
| LV | Las Vegas |
| MASH | Mobile Army Surgical Hospital |
| MD | Licensed Medical Doctor |
| MOD | March of Dimes |

| | |
|---|---|
| mRNA | messenger Ribonucleic Acid |
| NICU | Neonatal Intensive Care Unit |
| NNA | Nevada Nurses' Association |
| NPS | National Park Service |
| NSMA | Nevada State Medical Association |
| OR | Operating Room |
| OSN | Orvis School of Nursing |
| PA | Physician's Assistant |
| PhD | Doctor of Philosophy |
| PHS | Public Health Service |
| RN | Registered Nurse |
| RNA | Reno RN As. Ribonucleic Acid |
| SNV | *Sin Nombre* (No Name) Virus |
| SOM | School of Medicine |
| STR | Short Tamden Repeat |
| TB | tuberculosis |
| UCLA | Univ. California, Los Angeles |
| UCSD | Univ. of Calif. San Diego |
| UMC | Univ. Medical Center (So. Nev. Memorial Hosp) |
| UNLV | University of Nevada, Las Vegas |
| UNLVSOM | University of Nevada LV SOM |
| USPHS | U.S. Public Health Service |
| UNR | University of Nevada, Reno |
| UNRSOM | University Nevada Reno SOM |
| UNSOM | University Nevada School of Medicine |
| VC | Virginia City |
| V&T | Virginia & Truckee Railroad |
| UV | ultraviolet light |
| WHO | World Health Organization |
| WMC | Washoe Medical Center |
| WW I | World War I |
| WW II | World War II |

# Chronology of Medical Events

_+_+_+_+_+_+_+_+_+_+_+_+_+_+_+_+_+_+_+_+_+_+_

1851   NV's 1st MD; Dr. Charles Daggett
1858   Dr. Benjamin King's Revival of the Dead
1859   Pyramid Lake War Hero; Dr. Anton Tjader
1859   Mexican War Hero; Dr. Seldon McMeans
1860   NV's 1st Autopsy by Dr. Anton Tjader
1860   Civil War Heroes; Drs. Elias Harris and George Thoma
1861   Dr. Gideon Weed, Washoe City
1861   NV's 1st Female MD; Dr. Ada Weed - Washoe City
1861   Dr. Charles Kirkpatrick, Fort Churchill
1862   Dr. Christian Zabriske's Disinfectant
1862   Dr. John Veatch, Virginia City
1863   NV's 1st Black MD; Dr. W.H.C. Stephenson
1864   Homeopath Dr. Frederick Hiller sets Fractured Leg
1865   NV's 2nd Female MD; Doctress Hoffman, Virginia City
1865   Dr. Zetus Spalding, Fort Scott
1867   Dr. George Thoma, Eureka
1869   NV's 3rd Female MD; Doctress H. Jones, Treasure City
1869   Dr. Harris Herrick, Hamilton
1870   Dr. George M. Kober; Blood Ingest to Treat Tuberculosis
1872   Dr. Henry Bergstein, Important Jewish MD
1872   Dr. William Patterson, Fort Bidwell
1874   Dr. H.H. Hogan, Washoe County
1874   Registration required for NV MDs
1875   "Irregular" Dr. Samuel L. Lee, Pioche
1876   NV's 1st Hospital; Saint Mary Louise, VC
1879   NV's 4th Female MD; Dr. C. Post-Van Orden
1884   Dr. Samuel Weaver, Paradise Valley
1884   Dr. Simeon Bishop, NV Hospital for Insane
1884   NV's 5th Female MD; Dr. Eliza Cook

| | |
|---|---|
| 1886 | Nevada's 1st Forensic Exam; Dr. William Kendall |
| 1888 | 1st Abd. Surg. in NV; Drs. Dawson, Bergstein, J. Lewis |
| 1890 | Dr. John D. Campbell's "Phantom Hand" |
| 1890s | 1st Dr. Hood; William H. Hood, Battle Mountain |
| 1894 | 2nd Dr. Hood; Charles J. Hood, Elko |
| 1896 | Dr. Raymond St. Clair's "Missing Leg" |
| 1896 | NV's 1st Pediatrician; Dr. Anthony Huffaker |
| 1899 | Licensing required for Nevada MDs |
| 1900 | Dr. James W. Gerow, Delivery in Indian Country |
| 1900 | 1st University of Nevada Hospital |
| 1900 | "Unverified" Dr. A.P. Lagoon |
| 1901 | "Romantic" Dr. Washington L. Kistler, Wadsworth |
| 1901 | "Sink-or-Swim" Dr. Morris R. Walker |
| 1903 | 3rd Dr. Hood; Arthur J. Hood I, Elko |
| 1905 | 1st Las Vegas MD; Dr. Royce W. Martin |
| 1905 | 1st Las Vegas Hospital; Dr. H.L. Hewetson |
| 1905 | "Colorful" Dr. F.H. Wichmann, Lovelock |
| 1905 | NV's 1st Female Dentist; Helen Shipley |
| 1905 | "Serious-over-Study" Dr. T.P. Tyson, Washoe County |
| 1905 | Dr. E.S. Grigsby, Bullfrog |
| 1907 | Dr. George "Spunky-Kid" Gardner |
| 1909 | NV's 1st Pathologist; Dr. Oscar Johnstone |
| 1910 | Dr. John Fuller, Las Vegas to Reno |
| 1917 | WW I Heroes; Drs. D. Turner, W. Samuels & Alice Thompson |
| 1917 | "Blue Blood" Dr. Alice Thompson |
| 1920 | NV's 1st Blood Transfusion; Dr. Vinton Muller |
| 1920 | Dr. Mary Fulstone, Smith, NV |
| 1920 | Dr. Royce W. Martin, Las Vegas Hospital |
| 1921 | 4th Dr. Hood; Arthur J. Hood II, Reno |
| 1923 | RN practice act passed |
| 1924 | "One-of-a-Kind" Dr. Jack C. Cherry |

|  |  |
|------|-------|
| 1929 | 5th Dr. Hood; Dwight L. Hood, Reno |
| 1930 | Dr. W.B. Ririe, Ely Hospital |
| 1931 | Clark County Indigent Hospital |
| 1932 | Dr. Clare Woodbury, Las Vegas Hospital |
| 1935 | Dr. Kurt Hartoch's "Dueling Scar" |
| 1935 | NV's First Anesthesiologist; Dr. Olga Kipanidze |
| 1935 | Dr. Leslie Moren, Elko, Nevada |
| 1936 | NV's 1st Health Officer Dr. John E. Worden |
| 1939 | Carlin Canyon Train Wreck |
| 1939 | "Revered" Pediatrician; Dr. Roland Stahr |
| 1943 | Dr. James Swank, "Gem of Discovery" |
| 1945 | WW II Heroes; Drs. Robert Locke & Leonard Miller |
| 1946 | Dr. Ken Maclean, "A Doctors' Doctor," Reno |
| 1948 | 6th Dr. Hood; Tom K. Hood, Elko |
| 1952 | Dr. Laurence Nelson, Snow-bound Train Rescue |
| 1954 | Korean War Hero; Dr. Laurence Nelson |
| 1954 | NV's 1st Licensed Black MD; Dr. Charles West |
| 1955 | Dr. Jack Gilbert, Cedarville, CA |
| 1956 | Sunrise Hospital established in Las Vegas |
| 1957 | UNR establishes BS RN Degree |
| 1960 | Dr. Kirk Cammack, "Frontier Justice" |
| 1960 | North Las Vegas Community Hospital |
| 1962 | NV's 1st Neonatal Intensive Care Unit, Reno |
| 1962 | NV's 1st Neonatologist; Dr. Donald Pickering |
| 1963 | Nellis Air Force Base Hospital established |
| 1964 | Dr. James Barger, President, College of American Pathologists |
| 1969 | VN War Heroes; Drs. Treat Cafferata, Tom Brady, Richard Ganchan, and Anton Sohn |
| 1971 | 1st Class; University of Nevada Reno School of Medicine |
| 1976 | 1st Neonatal Intensive Care Unit, Las Vegas |
| 2017 | 1st Class; Univ. of Nev Las Vegas School of Medicine |

# Postscript Photos

_+_+_+_+_+_+_+_+_+_+_+_+_+_+_+_+_+_+_+_+_+_+_

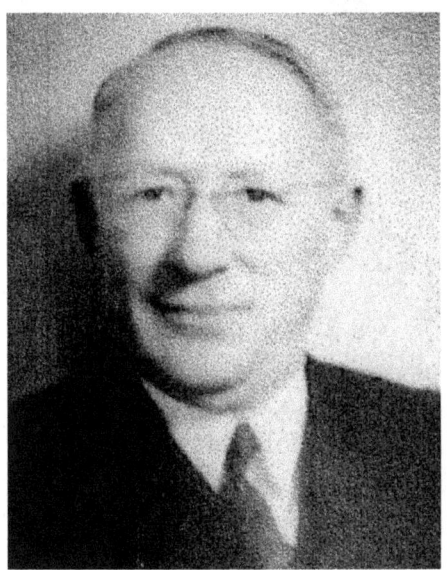

Dr. Ralph Bowdie, 1920

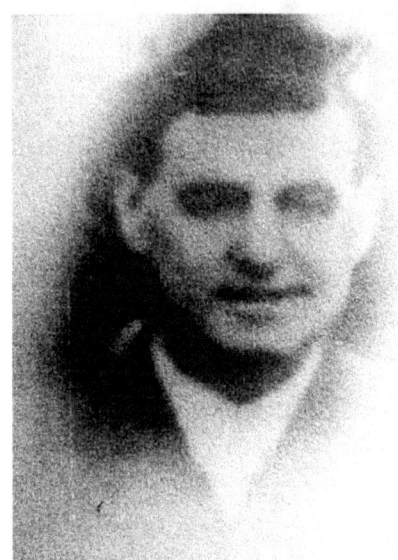

Dr. John L. Robinson, 1922

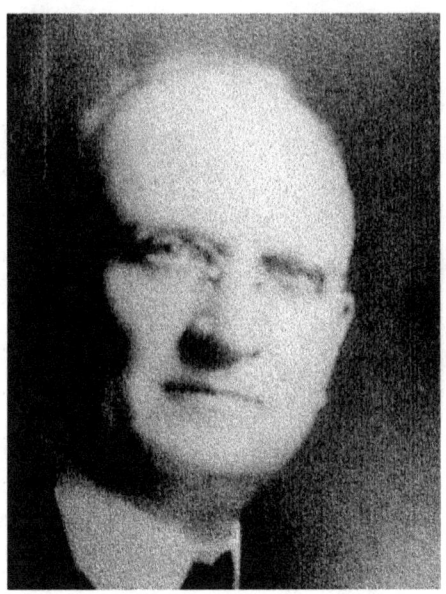

Dr. Horace Brown, 1923

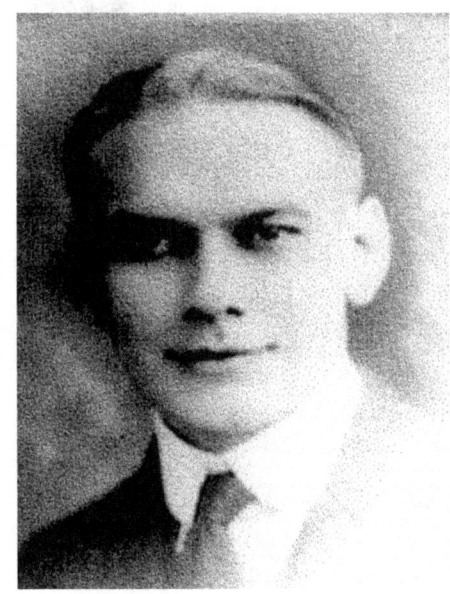

Dr. R.P. Roantree, 1930

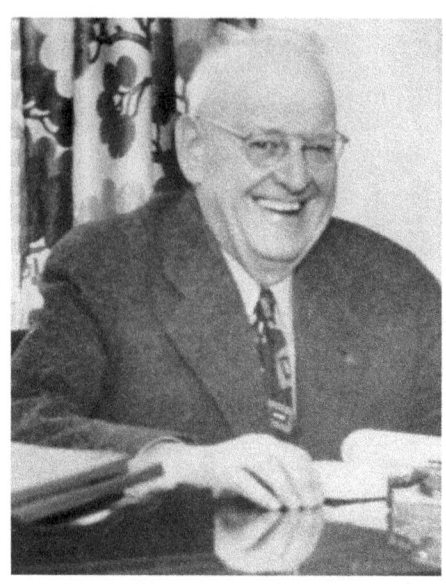
Dr. Charles E. Secor, 1936

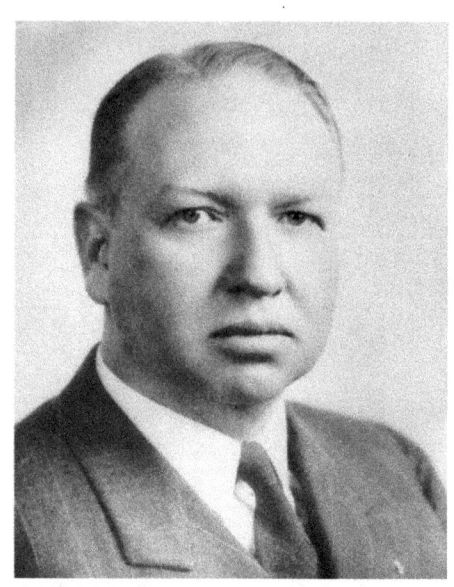
Dr. Daniel J. Hurley, 1942

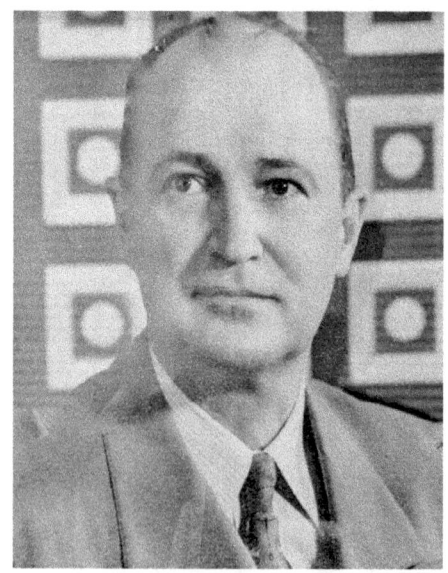
Dr. Edwin Cantlon, 1956

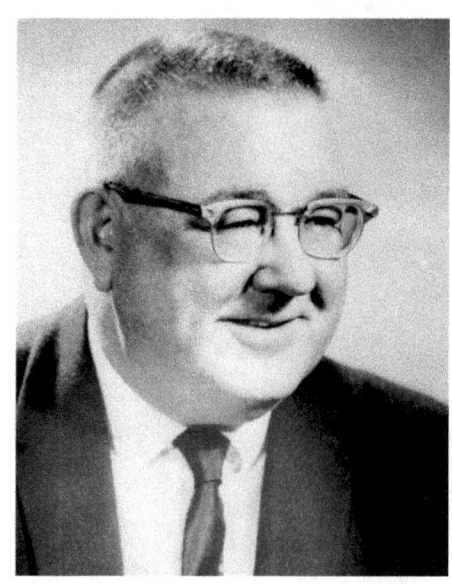
Dr. Stanley L. Hardy, 1957

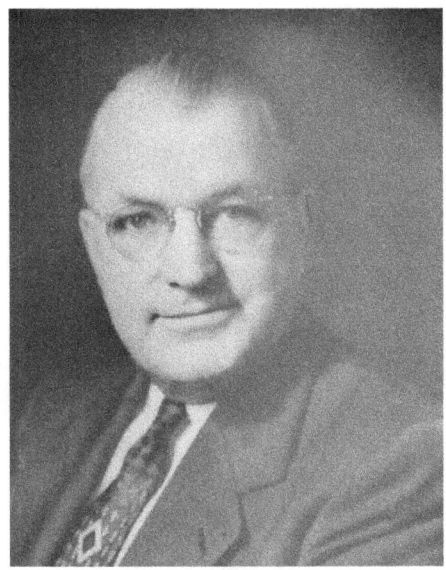
Dr. Roland Stahr, 1958

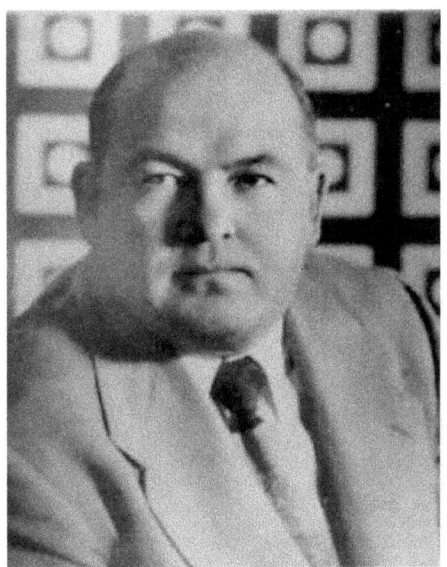
Dr. Ernest Mack, 1959

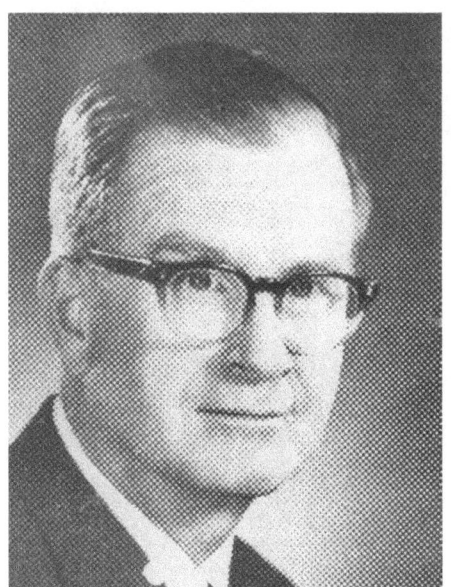
Dr. Joe George, 1965

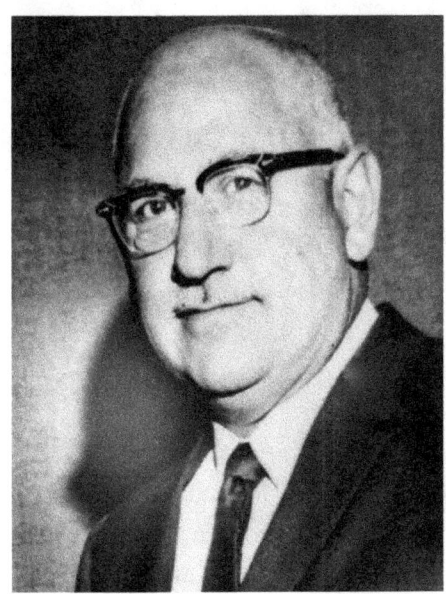
Dr. V.A. Salvadorini, 1969

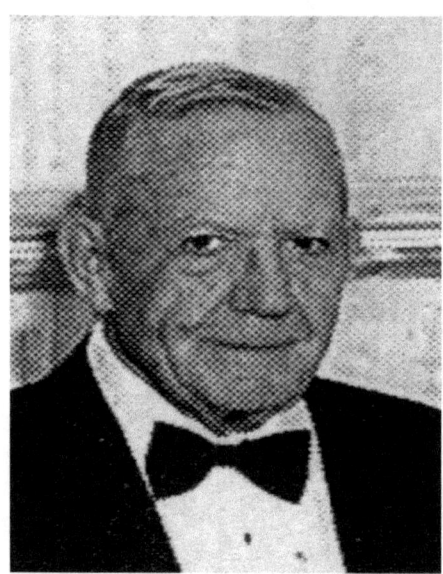 Capt. Treat Cafferata, 1987

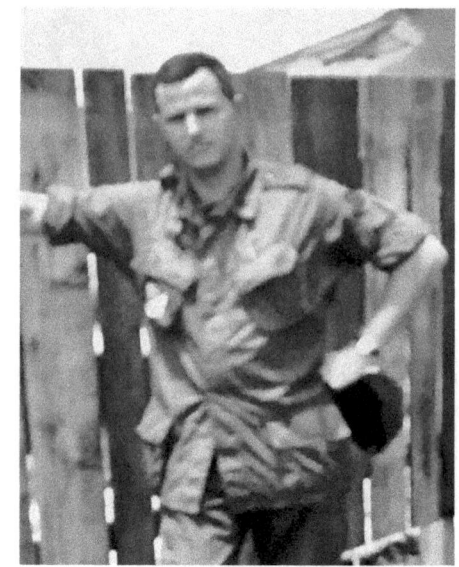 Capt. Tom Brady, VN 1968

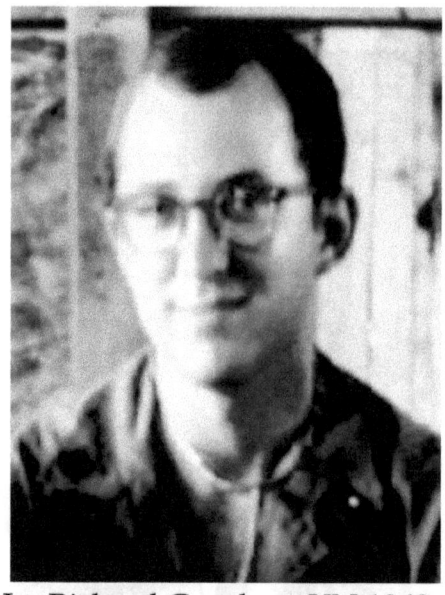 Lt. Richard Ganchan, VN 1969

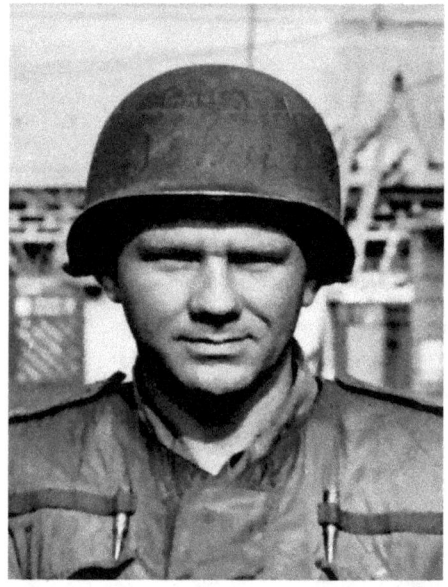 Capt. Anton Sohn, VN 1968

# Index

_+_+_+_+_+_+_+_+_+_+_+_+_+_+_+_+_+_+_+_+_+_

## A

Acuff, Star—281
Adelson, Merv—430
Adelson, Nate—429, 430
Ainsworth, Ronald—299
Allen, Mrs.—270
Allen, Richard—128
Allen, Sheri—261
Allen, T.C.—161
Allen, W.L.—273
Alvord, Lori—4
Ancker, Louise—95
Anderson, Frederick—XIII, 111, 292, 293, 308, 310, 332, 379, 440, 442
Anderson, Helen—447
Anderson, Mr.—271
Andrews, M.A.—372
Arbonies, William—111
Archer, W. Andrew—2
Arnold, Jim—107
Asclepius—36
Atcheson, Don—111
Aylworth, Peter—X, 232, 423, 425

## B

Bacon, Ted—299
Bailey, Covert—375
Baker, Mabel P.—216
Balcom, R.D.—108. 273, 277
Baldwin, Bud—302
Baldwin, E.J.—195
Banting and Best—368
Barengo, Bob—315
Barger, Janie—221
Barger, Jim—220, 309
Barger Jr, Jim—221
Barger, Josephine—221
Barger, Susie—221
Barger, Thomas—220

Barker, Eileen—X, 76, 161, 309, 323, 364, 456
Barker-Browning, Marcia—417
Barry, Patricia—99
Basie, Count—237
Bath, Dr.—83
Bazzini, Joe—92, 93
Beemer, Bill—158
Belliveau, Bob—222
Bellmerre, Julia—447
Bender, Bertha—369
Berger, Emmanuel—332
Bergman, William—366
Bergstein, Henry—X, 31, 49, 51, 94, 454
Bentley, William—398
Betts, Winthrop—419, 423
Bianchini, Joe—92
Bice, B.D.—359
Biddulph, Genette—309
Biddulph, Glen—309
Big Mouth Charlie—14
Bigley, Kim—309
Billstein, Steve—380
Bishop, Simeon—52, 53, 162, 164, 366
Blackhart, Bret—380
Blackwell, Eliz.—135
Blake, Dr.—209
Blachley, Annie—XI, 452, 456
Bolstad, Anne—141
Bolstad, Carol—141
Bolstad, Katie—140
Bolstad, Owen—X, 55, 58, 123, 136, 139, 239, 259, 308, 364, 439
Bolstad, Roger—141
Bolstad, Susan—141
Bonham, B.B.—161
Boniface, (Sister)—187
Bonner, Ernest C.—14, 16
Boyd, Mark—156, 157

Boyden, Fred—375
Boyer, Harold—309
Bowdie, Ralph—85
Bower, H.S.—366
Bowers, Lemuel S.—364, 365
Bowers, Persia—364
Bradley, Ann—104
Bradley, Mrs. Bill—449
Bradley, L.R.—52
Bradley, William—387
Brady, Tom—XI, 309, 385
Bradshaw, Jim—369
Bradshaw, Mark—209
Bremmer, Roger—314, 316
Brennan, Irene—444
Brisbee, Samantha—111
Broili, June—158
Brookhyser, Joan—300, 303
Brower, H.S.—366
Brown, Curtis—XI, 16, 309
Brown, D.D.—52
Brown, Horace—83, 84
Brown, John W.—16
Bryant, Edmund G.—104
Bryant, William Cullen—104
Bryarly, Wakeman—37
Buchan, William—407
Bulette, C.E.—277
Bulette, Julia—104
Burdick, Dr.—80
Burgan, J.F.—253
Burnside, Allan—296
Burgoyne, Gussie—X, 309
Burrow, Rodney—262
Bush, Asahel—114
Byfers, Bell—272

## C

Cafferata, Treat—309, 376
Caffaratti, Barbara—147
Caffaratti, Darius—143, 145
Caffaratti, John—143, 147
Caffaratti, Rose—147
Callister, T. Brian—337
Calvanese, Jerry—299
Cammack, Kirk—207

Campbell, Ainslie—218
Campbell, Edith—218
Campbell, Kimberly—219
Campbell, Floyd—218
Campbell, John D.—217
Campbell, Linwood W.—219
Campbell, Maggie—218
Campbell, Wilkes J.—218, 219
Cann, George—111, 167
Cann, William—75
Cantlon, Edwin—92, 93, 111, 287, 309, 332
Cantlon, Vernon—111, 332
Carlson, A.W.—309
Carlson, Kurt—148
Carr, John F.—398
Carter, J.W.—90, 91
Cashell, Bob—314
Chamberlain, Jay—299
Charleton, Elizabeth—181
Charleton, E.P. II—309
Charleton, Thelma—181
Charlie, Big Mouth—14, 15
Cherry, Bernard—1198
Cherry, Jack C,—208, 213, 278, 279
Cherry, Jack—213
Christensen, Mr.—21
Christensen, Norm—XI, 309, 437
Christiansen, Don—429, 434, 435, 437
Clark, W. Van Tilburg—37
Clemmensen, Charles—380
Clift, Bob—309, 315
Collett, George A.—137
Collett, Hugh—184
Colletti, Pat—299
Collins, Walt—309
Combs, William—173, 174
Console, David—309
Cook Eliza—65
Cooper, Eunice—372
Cooper, Thomas—372
Corkill, Bunny—148
Cowan, Alison-364
Cowgill, Dr.—380
Cramsie, (Sister)—384

Craven, Alice—271
Crittenden, Florence—270
Crook, George—15
Crosby, Robert—332
Crowley, Joe—313, 314
Cudek, Phyllis—XI, 276, 309, 374, 447, 451, 456
Cudek, Ronald—XI, 309
Cunningham, Ben F.— 359
Cunningham, Miss—271
Cunningham, Miss—271
Cuthbertson, Arthur A.—414
Cuthbertson, Arlynn A.—268, 269, 270, 413

## D

Daggett, Charles—98, 198, 409, 411, 440
Dagsen, Patricia—100
Dakin, Mary—449
Dales, Jerry—303
Dalitz, Moe—430
Daugherty, Bob—307
Daugherty, Christopher—307
Daugherty, Robert—X, XIV, 117, 185, 296, 297, 300, 307, 308, 309, 313, 317, 431, 439, 456
Daugherty, Karen—307
Daugherty, Kim—397
Daugherty, Sandra—305
Davis, Jefferson—104
Davis, John—111, 309
Davis, Ryan—94, 98, 382
Davis, Sam—33, 35, 107, 163
Dawson, Alson—94
DeCorte, Jarrett—230
DeLee, Joseph—430
DeLee, Sol—430
DeQuille, Dan—126
Desmond-Hellman, S.—299
Denton, Ralph—311
DeTar, Edward—186, 188
DeTar, John—186, 188
DeTar, Josephine—186, 187
DeTar, Michael—186, 188
DeTar, Tom—186

DiGrazia, Peter—323
Dilley, Thatcher—108
Dingacci, A.J.—144
Dingacci, Michael—149
Dingacci, Pat—149
Dini, Joe—299
Dinsmore, Dr.—368
DiSalvo, Art—309
Doetsch Raymond—406
Dodge, Frederick—132, 134
Dooley, John—XI, 79
Dorsett, Tony—404
Doten, Alfred—37, 125, 171
Doyle, Arthur—390
Drannan, S.M.—447
Driggs, W.—448
Drury, Wells—165
Duensing, Margaret—216
Dufurrena, Linda—170, 261

## E

Earl, Phillip—XI, 174, 204, 331, 401
Edmiston, Malcolm—303
Edwards, Charlotte S.—109, 110
Edwards, L.W.—273, 274
Edwards, Thomas G.—117
Eisenhower, Dwight D.—58, 441
Elgas—67
Elia, Joseph—79, 332
Elliott, Joan—144
Elliott, Russell—71, 73
Elliott, Verlyn—18, 144
Elliott, Fred—XI, 331, 332
Ellis, Joseph—366
Ellison, Bob—337
Ernaga, Stephanie—89
Ervin, Susan—369
Evans, Lauran—417
Evans, Mary E.—272
Exline, Angela Caffaratti—143
Ezell, Mike—XI, 2

## F

Falk, Mortimer—378, 380
Farwell, Frank—2214
Faust, C.B.—329

Fay, Alice—167
Fee, Dr.—272
Feikes, Harold—279, 434
Feldman, Bernard—XI, 428, 434
Fellows, (Sheriff)—254
Feltner, Barbara—309
Feltner, William—309
Ferguson, Ferdinand—108, 273, 277
Fermoile, Kristin Sohn—X, 112, 427
Flanary, Jack—148
Foch, Ferdinand—331
Follmer, Hugh—281
Ford, Caroline—426
Ford, Harrison—302
Fortier, Quincy—281, 309
Fothergill. LeRoy—362
Foxx, Clyde—332
Francis, C.H.—359
Frandsen, Peter—111, 112, 310, 360
Franklin, Benjamin—440
Freir, Evert C.—280
Friedman, William—434, 435
Friedriechs, C.W.—366
Frydenlund, Conrad—148, 149, 150
Fuller, Joe—196
Fuller, John—79, 83
Fulstone, Fred—44
Fulstone, Georgia—299
Funston, Frederick—73
Furman, George—299, 302, 440
Fulstone, Mary—41, 43, 188

## G

Galen—388
Galsgie, C.C.—271
Galphins, Mr.—412
Gamble, David—387
Gamboa, Rafael—323
Ganchen, Richard—457
Gardner, Larry—380
Gardner, George—83, 160, 195
Gardner, Matthew—195

Garrison, Teresa—XI, 309
Gates, C.R.—37
Gauthier, Jay H.—402
Gawande, Atul—299
Gedney, Karen—425
George, Chester—279
George, Dorothy—229, 230, 309, 452
George, Joseph—229, 230, 309, 453
Gerow, James—46, 83
Gerow, Lynn—46, 111
Gerow Jr, Lynn—49
Getto, Virgil—299
Gibson, Jay—309
Gibson, Mrs. Jay—309
Gilbert, Jack—99
Gillette, Denise—319
Gillette, Jim—299
Gillette, Philip—303, 316
Gillette, Rick—319
Glick, Milton—298
Gluck, Louis—427, 428
Goetz, Thomas—390
Gold, Jay—56, 58
Goodhue, Janice—299
Gordier, Henri—172, 173
Gosse, Marguerita—296, 455
Gossi, Pop—85
Grant, John—268
Grant, Ulysses S.—122
Grayson, Dr.—222
Green, C.C.—126
Greenspun, Hank—236
Gregory, Samuel—135
Grigsby, Edward—106
Grimsbo, Raymond—372
Grosh, A.B.—409
Grosh, Ethan—409
Grosh, Hosea—409
Grosh, Warren—413
Grove, Jennifer—X, 457
Gunn, John C.—407

## H

Hadfield, Dale—137
Hahnemann, Samuel—171

Haldane, John—420
Hall, Shawn—260
Hall, Tom—XI, 300, 441
Hall, Sr., Wes.—332, 375
Hammer, Charles—424
Hanson, Elmer—335
Hardy, Mrs. Roy—123
Hardy, Stanley—273
Harper, T.C.—83, 287
Harris, Elias B.—105
Harrison, Mollie—382
Hart, Thelma/Thomas—298
Hathaway, Pierre—90
Hartoch, Carole—170
Hartoch, Julia—169
Hartoch, Kurt—166, 261
Hartoch, Mark—169
Hartoch, Marlese—170
Hartoch, Wilma—170, 261, 309
Hartzell, Reine—382
Hay, Ing—239, 242, 244
Haydon, Stephan—424
Hayes, Hank—339
Heinrichs, James—2
Henderson, Joe—394
Heppner, Albert—75
Herrick, Harris S.—70
Hershey, Miss—19, 20
Herz, James—111
Hess, George—318
Hewetson, Halle—80, 83, 106, 276
Higgins, Sally—352
Hildreth, Martha—XI, XIV
Hiller, Frederick—37, 126, 171, 172
Hillhouse, J.D.—90
Hinkle, Bliss—174
Hinkle, George—174
Hippocrates—442
Hockenberry, Tim—148
Hoffman, Doctress—134, 135
Hogan, Henry H.—162, 163, 164, 366
Hogan, Roy—141, 259
Holmes, Janet—3
Hood I, A.J.—137, 175, 178
Hood II, A.J.—111, 175, 180

Hood III, A.J.—181
Hood, Charles J.—175, 176, 196
Hood, Dwight—111, 175, 287
Hood, Edith—179
Hood, Eunice—175
Hood, Florence—183
Hood, Henry—183
Hood, Irene Hunter—179
Hood, Jacqueline—184
Hood, Juliette—181
Hood, Keitha—183
Hood, Mary—175
Hood, Patricia—179
Hood, Tom—XI, 174, 175, 184, 259, 309
Hood, Mrs. Tom—309
Hood, Victoria—184
Hood, William H.—83, 175, 330, 359, 361, 362, 439
Hoover, Herbert—160
Hopkins, Alice—271
House, Ellen—XI, XII, 454
Huffaker, Anthony—106, 108
Hughes, Howard—207
Hull, Kevin/Frances—309
Hurley, Daniel J.—397, 398
Hughes, Howard—291, 292
Hussman, Ada—157
Hyde, Orson—98

## I

Iliescu, John—XI, 308, 309
Immenschuh, Dick—260
Ingle, Richard—296
Ingalls, W.D.—91
Isom, Chelsea—337

## J

Jack, Captain—215
Jenner, Edward—347
Johnson, A.M.—210
Johnson, Lyndon B.—237
Johnson, Red—332
Johnstone, Bertha—157
Johnstone, Eric—157
Johnstone, Oscar J.—75, 156, 362

Johnstone, Thorwald—157
Johnstone, William—157
Jolson, Al—167
Jones, Helena—134
Jones, Paul—211
Jones, W.W.—75
Joslin, S. Lees—91

## K

Kearns, Sam—90
Keeler, Ruby—167
Kendall, William P.—253
Kennedy, C.H.—415
Kennedy, Patrick Bouvier—431
Kern, Davey—261
Kern, Susan Miller—261
Kiene, Kevin—380
King, Benjamin L.—75, 172, 198, 411, 412
King, Tom—XI, XIV
King, William—309
Kinnegar, Andy—253
Kipanidze, Olga—157
Kipanidze, Vladimir—158
Kirkpatrick, Charles—248
Kirman, Richard—127
Kistler, Washington—77, 359
Klimek, Sandy—281, 282
Klubert, Barbara—143
Klubert, David—143
Kober, George M.—30, 127, 263, 346, 456
Koch, Robert—390
Koontz, John—455
Kords, L.—161, 163
Kozel, Tom—302, 303, 317
Krebs, Ernst—11, 12, 382
Kreisler, Leonard—309
Kreisler, Mrs. Leonard—309
Kwalick, Donald—XI, 127, 394, 396

## L

Laennec, Rene—440
Lagoon, A.P.—66
Lake, Myron—155

Lamb, Mary—172
Lamson, George Jr.—401, 402
Landis, S.N.—X
Landsteiner, Karl—38
Larson, Pansilee—261
Larson, Trudy—XI, 127, 431
Lawson, (Nurse)—327
Laxalt, Bruce—403
Laxalt, Monique—403
Laxalt, Paul—292, 300, 313, 428
Laxalt, Robert—348, 349
Lee, Simeon L.—68, 394, 440, 441
Lees, Bonnie—428
Lemons, F. Ted—425
Lenz, Gilbert—22, 283
Levine, Phillip—220
Lewis, John—94, 359, 394
Lewis, Parker—75, 83, 84
Littlefair, Ciligia—144
Lissak, M.A.—75
Lissak, Mrs.—271
Lister, Joseph—37, 118
Locke, Bob—XI, 111, 227, 332
Lockhart, Jacob—336
Lombardi, Louis—111, 234, 292
Loper, Mr.—187
Lovel, Joseph—255
Lund, Grant—274
Lyons, Colleen—XI, 309

## M

Mack, Ernest—111
Mack, W.B.—350
Mackay, Marie Louise—104, 268
Mackay, John—104, 268, 269
Maclean, Donald, Jr.—83, 118, 119, 382, 383, 384, 385
Maclean, Donald, Sr.—118, 119
Maclean, George—122
Maclean, Kenneth—111, 117, 190, 332, 385, 441
Magee, George R.—288
Magee, Catherine—288
Maher, Michael—161
Makley, Michael—161, 174
Malin, Jacob—188

Manning, George—299
Manogue, Patrick—268
Manville, Doris—309
Manville, H. Ed—291
Marden, J.P.—255, 261
Marschall, John—X, 51
Marsh, John—64
Martin, Nellie Cotton—205
Martin, Royce W.—80, 204, 272, 276
Maryanna, (Sister)—187
Masefield, John—142
Massoth, Louise—309
Massoth, Grainelle—309
Massoth, Patricia—309
Massoth, Harry—309, 323, 455
Matern, Dr.—184
Matthews, Washington—344
May, Jerry—318
Mayo, William—118
Mazzaferri, Ernie—313, 319
McCarran, Patrick—75, 212
McCarty, Dr.—380
McCarty, Vernon—402
McCloud, Percy—210
McConnell, Bill—262
McCormack, J.M.—54
McCubben, Dr.—270
McColley, H.H.—254
McDaniel, John—273
McDonnell, Patrick—107
McDowell, Ephraim—94, 116
McDowell, Samuel S.—196
McFarlane, Steve—299
McGirk, Blair—XI, XV, XVII
McKenzie, George—75, 83, 84, 271, 382, 383, 384, 455
McLellan, Lynda Mulvey—X, 229, 309
McLellan, S.A.—103
McMeans, Selden—103, 445
McMeans, Walter—103
McMillin, Anne—VI, 298
McNitt, Charles—378
Measom, Reuel J.—347
Melarkey, David—402

Mello, Don—299
Mercy, (Sister)—221
Metcalf, Gay—79
Michelson, Albert—54
Michelson, Pauline—52
Mienhimer, Carolyn—241
Mildren, Forest R.—277
Miles, Hoyt—309
Mill, Pearl—272
Miller, Blanche—197
Miller, Leonard—144
Miller, N. Edd—298
Miller, Nena—298
Miller, Walter McNab—389
Minarik, Melanie—127
Minor, W.H.—253
Missall, Steve—427
Mitchel, Millie—160
Mitchell, A.P.—161, 163
Molasky, Irwin—430
Montgomery, Robert—457
Monibi, Ali—XI, 427, 432, 433
Monibi, Farrah—434
Moody, Eric—401
Moore, A.B.—75
Mooser, Charles E.—75, 359
Moran, Bruce—XI, XIV
Father Moran, (Priest)—280
Moren, Jim—299, 304
Moren, Leslie—38, 136
Morrison, Sidney K.—83, 157, 359
Moseley, John O.—288
Moulton, Olin—332
Mousel, Carol—309
Mousel, Don—308, 439, 440
Mowbray, Jerry—X
Mozingo, Hugh—XVII
Mullen, John—173, 174
Muller, Vinton—37
Mullins Dr.—157
Munckton, George—198, 336
Myers, Warren—457
Myles, Robert—303

# N

Nannini, Leo—111

Neal, A.C.—88
Neddenriep, Anna—449
Neilson, Norm—174
Nelson, Alberta—58
Nelson, Erven J.—274
Nelson, Henry—299
Nelson, Laurence—55, 58
Nemec, Frank J.—309
Newbold, Richard—XI, 231
Newman, Fred—309
Newman, John—104
Nielson, Norm—174
Neyland, Beverly—431
Nichole, Stuart—341, 343
Nightingale, Florence—453
Noble, Jim—299
Noah, Doc—32
Norton, L.A.—99
Nylen, Bob—262

# O

O'Brien, J.P.—75
O'Brien III, William—269, 270, 332, 333
O'Callaghan, Mike—312
O'Donnel, Dr.—281
Ogren, Carroll—XI, 282, 456
O'Hara, Frances—271
Oliver, F.E.—373
O'Malley, Paul—211
On, Lung—239
O'Neal, R.McW.—359
Orvis, Arthur—291, 455
Overton, Nathan—270
Owens, Bethenia—451
Owens, Dr.—184
Oxborrow, Mary L.—448

# P

Paher—67
Palmer, Jack—332
Pardini, Ron—XV, 34, 299
Parks, Sam—309, 318
Parish, Barbara—367
Pasek, John—231
Pasteur, Louis—348

Patterson, Edna—260
Patterson, John—214
Patterson, William H.—213
Pauly, Ira—297
Paulson, Alberta R.—125
Paulson, Fred—39
Payne, William—457
Pearce, Bob—259, 260
Pearlman, Dr.—230
Pelter, Andrea—299
Pennington, William—298
Perrin, Sol—172
Pettis, William—425
Phalen, Steve—190
Phillips, Rodney—296
Pickard, John—83
Pickering, Donald—235, 427
Pierczynski, Ed—299
Pike, Pearl P.—78
Pinson, Wilkie—168
Pinto, Cynthia—XI, 268
Pittman, Vail—121
Platt, Virginia—270
Post-Van Orden, C,—65, 135
Poulson, Fred—39
Powning, C.C.—51
Powning, Clara Poor—54
Pratt, Ramona—448
Price, Jack—196
Prida, James—262
Priest, Richard—299
Pringle, Maida—332
Prosser, David—11
Prouty, Hugh—88
Prupas, Malin—299
Pugh, Rick—XI, 92, 125, 456
Puleo, Lisa—XI, 220, 223, 452

# Q

Quinn, Renee—332

# R

Rand, M.J.—187
Ravenholt, Otto—398, 456
Reams, Robert Borden—442
Record, Edward—351

Redd, Effie Oxborrow—448
Redfield, Neil—298
Reid, Harry—431
Reed, Mike—317
Reese, Enoch—172
Reese, John—172
Rey, Beatrice—216
Reynolds, George—396
Rhodes, Mark—299
Rice, R.L.—359
Rich, Maria—448
Richie, L.J.— 359
Riddle, Dr.—406
Ridenour, Gary—XI, 148, 150, 151, 152, 172
Rigelhuth, Mrs.—271
Ring, Orvis—455
Riordan, Mr.—187
Ririe, Evelyn—194
Ririe, William—183
Ritzlin, Roger—188, 309, 400
Roach, Tillie—449
Roantree, R.P.—39
Roberts, Dr.—359
Roberts, Frank—303, 309
Roberts, Jean—309
Robinson, Benjamin—52
Robinson, J. LaRue—83, 271, 359
Robinson, Martin A.—83
Robinson, Robert—314, 316
Rocha, Guy—X, 98, 112, 127, 198, 323, 384
Roctor, E.H.—75
Roen, Allard—430
Roff, N.J.—365
Romero, Lori—193, 194
Ronzone, Dick—311
Rose, Chuck—187
Rose, Perry—136, 208
Ross, Mrs.—75
Ross, Silas—67, 156, 269
Rowe, Peter—190, 332
Rueckl, Victor—380
Ruediger, Gustav—2
Ruggles, Charlie—167
Rulefson, Dr.—272

Rulison, Charles—322
Rulison, David—322
Rusco, Elmer—XI, 199, 203
Russell, Frank—332

## S

Sader, Bob—387
Sadler, Reinhold—216
Sage, Erwin—225
Sage, Rodney—XI, 144, 160, 161, 189, 223, 224, 285, 309, 377
Salk, Jonas—331
Salvadorini, V.A.—188, 402
Salvin, Hale—278
Samuels, Jr., Frank—64, 111
Samuels, W.L.—157
Sandahl, Dr.—277
Sanders, Moses—88
Satchell, Charles—201
Saunders, Rosalie—75
Savitt, Tod—309, 388
Savoy, Barbara—333
Sawyer, Grant—375
Sawyer, Paul—260
Sawyer, W.A.—350
Schablitsky, Julie—372
Schmidt, Elwood—XI, 17
Schwenk, Thomas—308
Scott, Arthur—332, 333
Scott, Evelyn—158
Scott Sr., John—332
Scott, Mrs.—490
Scott, Walter—210
Scully, Celia—312
Scully, Tom—293, 303, 312, 319
Secor, Charles—39, 137
Sedway, Marvin—297
Segelhorst, Irene—184
Servoss, George—83
Seyfarth, Hermann—324
Sheld, Harrison—428, 431
Shipley, Helen—322
Silvers, Albert—209
Simpson, William—332, 333, 334
Smith, Dorothy—49
Smith, Elizabeth—214

Smith, George T.—292, 293, 300, 303
Smith H.H.—66
Smith, Harold Sr.—49
Smithson, Allison—307
Smithson, Doug —307
Snavely, Charles—431
Snelling, Josiah—64
Snow, Asa—173
Sofie, Gene—87
Sohn, Anton—XIV, XVII, 23, 37, 43, 68, 87, 108, 122, 127, 134, 139, 143, 155, 156, 160, 170, 187, 188, 200, 229, 260, 308, 331, 343, 346, 353, 359, 360, 363, 372, 387, 408, 409, 413, 423, 427, 428, 439, 451, 456, 457
Sohn, Arlene—308, 309
Sontag, Ed—332
Spalding, Noah—89
Spalding, Zetus—87
Sparks, John—62
Sparks, Mrs. John—62
Sprangler, Nita—253
Springmeyer Sallie—158
St. Clair, Louise—197
St. Clair, Nancy—160
St. Clair, Raymond—83, 160, 359
St. Jeor, Steve—337
Stackpole, J.S.—161
Stahlman, Mildred—427
Stahr, Roland—223
Standerwick, Eunice—175
Standerwick, Harry—175
Standish, Miles—301
Standlee, Tom—380ed
Stearns, Kim—432
Stephan, Bill—XI, 434, 435, 437
Stephenson, Jane—202
Stephensen, W.H.C.—199. 237
Stock, Wilbourn—329
Stoetzel, James—18, 19
Stubbs, J.E.—286. 361
Sullivan, Dr.—83
Sumin, Richard—94
Summer, Hall—328

Swain, Clement C.—272
Swallow, Anna—490
Swank, James L.—229
Swank, Megan—229, 231
Swenson, Shane—431
Sylvain, Gerald—211, 274, 309

## T

Talbot, J.A.—75
Tappan, William—190, 303, 332
Taubenberger, Jeffery—330, 331
Taylor, N.G.—336
Terry, Wallace—38
Thom, Ruth—108
Thoma, George—94, 122, 123
Thompson, Alice—155
Thompson, David—189
Thompson, William—457
Thorrington, Bill—172
Tilton, James—255, 256
Tjader, Anton—128, 131, 198, 424
Tjader, Gary—131
Toll, David—160
Toole, Louis E.—XI, 390, 457
Torok, James—380
Toulouse-Lautrec, Henri—160, 197
Trall, Russell, T.—112, 114
Train, Percy—2
Treacher, Arthur—167
Turner, Ephram—232
Turner, D. Ashley—232
Turner, Ken—120
Twain, Mark—69, 82, 105
Tyson, Howard—91
Tyson, Jerry—89
Tyson, Thomas P.—89

## U

Uband, Myra—242

## V

Valle, Linda—XI, 425
VanSykle, Lloyd—55, 56
Van Zant, John—52
Veatch, John A.—109

Verglies, Jack—316
Vinnik, Charles—429
Vollum, Edward P.—344
Voorhees, Walter—18

## W

Wah, Bob—240
Wah, Eddie—159
Walker, Morris R.—60, 62, 359
Ward, Chris—339
Ward, Dr.—40
Warns, (Sister)—268
Watson, Anita—170, 171
Weathington, W.T.—398
Weaver, Samuel—93
Weed, Ada—112, 117, 134
Weed, Gideon—112, 117, 161, 163
Wegman, Charles T.—413
Wentworth, Cornelia J.—270, 272
West, Charles—236
West, William—83
West, W.W.—178
Whisman, Ray—329
White, Juanita—311
Whomes, Willi—148
Wichmann, Frederick—73
Williams, Lynne—XI, 293
Williams, Anne—431, 433
Willis, Park W.—116
Wilson, Frank—369
Wilson IV, Nathan—367
Wilson V, Nathan—369
Winder, Cheryl—296
Winder, James—296
Windous, Margaret C.A.—448, 449
Wines, Mr.—26
Wingfield Sr., Mrs. George—123
Winiham, W.P.L.—161
Winne, B.A.—18
Winnemucca, Chief—216
Ed.Wise, Mulchyor—75
Wixson, Margaret—365
Woodburn, William—75
Woodbury, Clare—273
Woods, C.H.—359
Worden, John—127, 395
Worden Jr., John—128
Worden., Shirley—128
Wullschleger, A.W.—75

## Y

Yingling, Doris—455

## Z

Zabriske, Christian—443
Zabriske, Elias—444
Zanjani, Sally—157
Zeigler, Mrs.—91
Zenan, Joan—XI, 229

This is the Story
of Medicine in the
Silver State from
the Beginning

www.ingramcontent.com/pod-product-compliance
Lightning Source LLC
Chambersburg PA
CBHW071359160426
42811CB00111B/2285/J